SIRTFOOD DIET

3 BOOKS IN 1

Complete Guide to Burn Fat Activating Your
"Skinny Gene" + 200 Tasty Recipes Cookbook
For Quick and Easy Meals + A Smart 4 Weeks
Meal Plan to Jump-start Your Weight Loss

KATE HAMILTON

First published in the United States of America in 2020

Copyright © 2020 Kate Hamilton

Typeset by Leah Jespersen.

Images from Unsplash.

ISBN 978-1-80109-984-4

CONTENTS

SIRTFOOD DIET

SIRTFOOD DIET MEAL PLAN

SIRTFOOD DIET COOKBOOK

SIRTFOOD DIET

A Quick Start Guide to Lose Weight and Burn Fat Fast Activating Your "Skinny Gene." Feel Great in Your Body. Learn to Stay Healthy and Fit, While Enjoying the Foods You Love!

KATE HAMILTON

First published in the United States of America in 2020

Copyright © 2020 Kate Hamilton

Typeset by Leah Jespersen

Images from Unsplash.

ISBN 979-8670554534

SIRTFOOD DIET

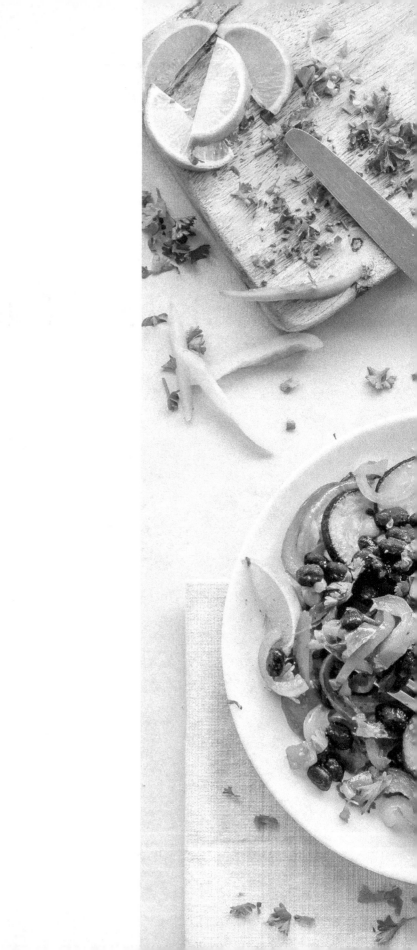

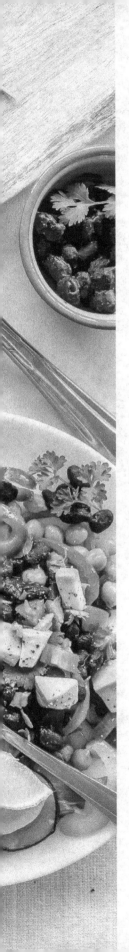

INTRODUCTION

The Sirtfood Diet was created by celebrity nutritionists Aidan Goggins and Glen Matten in 2016. Designed to include certain foods that will trigger the body's skinny gene, the diet is intended to help people rapidly shed excess weight without the consequences commonly seen in other diets.

Some diets require you to starve yourself, causing muscle loss along with fat loss. Others require you to give up foods that you enjoy, making them so restrictive that they are difficult for most people to keep up with.

On the other hand, the Sirtfood Diet encourages you to focus on sirtuin-rich foods combined into delicious and satisfying meals for both mind and body, making it very sustainable and effective.

With a mild calorie restriction for a short time and the increase in sirtuin-rich foods, your body will let go of excess fat even with low intensity or no exercise. From the tests completed before the diet's release, Matten and Goggins proved that the vast majority of people lost a significant amount of weight, 7 pounds on average.

However, it's not just a matter of weight loss. The Sirtfood Diet is proven to improve mental health and general wellbeing. Overall, there are some pretty compelling reasons to start considering the Sirtfood Diet— if you want to lose weight, gain muscle, and be healthier; this is a great way to do this. It will take diligence and dedication, but if you commit to this process, you, too, can reap these benefits. You can begin to be a healthier individual, inside and out.

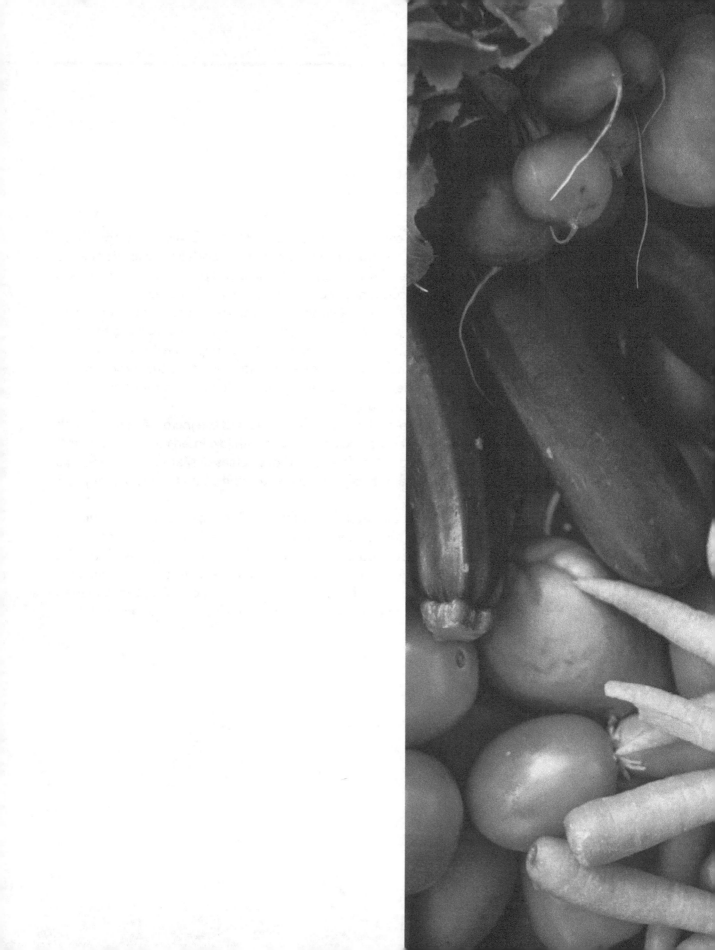

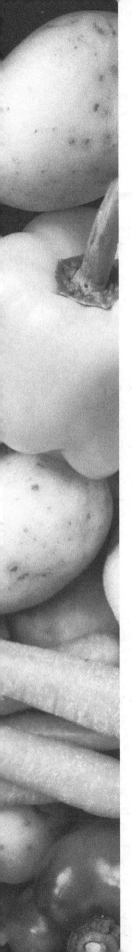

THE SIRTFOOD DIET EXPLAINED

The Sirtfood Diet is very famous due to its scientific benefits and amazing transformations of the body's metabolic capacities. Thousands of people have unlocked incredible and aesthetic physiques by following the Sirtfood Diet.

These results are not coming from myths attached to the basic philosophy of dieting; in fact, the Sirtfood Diet has a robust and growing scientific background. It is essential to understand how and why it works to fully appreciate the value of what you are doing to improve your health and well-being.

THE PROCESS OF FAT BURNING

The most significant benefit of the Sirtfood Diet is its incredible impact on fat loss. Fat is made up of fatty acids that combine to make adipocytes. These adipocytes are clusters of fatty acids, and unlike free fatty acids, adipocytes are not usually present in the blood.

They accumulate under the skin, in muscles, and on different organs. These adipocytes combine to make adipose tissue, full-fledged foam-shaped clusters of visible yellowish or white-colored fat in our body.

Adipose tissue is the healthiest fat to burn, but to do so, it must be broken down into adipocytes first and then into free fatty acids in a process called lipolysis. These steps are not easy as they seem, and burning extra pounds of fats can be a hard nut to crack.

The most challenging step in this cycle is breaking down the adipose tissue into adipocytes. This process is aided by compounds named polyphenols.

POLYPHENOLS ACTION

Polyphenols are well-known chemical compounds that act on an essential lean gene to activate a fat-burning action inside the human body. To be very specific, sirtfoods are foods that contain high levels of polyphenols. These compounds are present naturally in sirtfoods, and, even if they are not equally distributed, all sirtfoods contain specific amounts of different types of polyphenols.

Polyphenols are essential precursors of the fat-burning cycle of the body called lipolysis. During lipolysis, adipose tissue is broken down into free fatty acids transported by our blood and excreted from the body, thanks to the lipase enzyme. Foods rich in polyphenols increase the lipase enzyme, increasing the body's ability to burn fat.

It is fascinating to know that many sirtfoods are widespread, included in both eastern and western diets. We'll discover more about this in the next chapters.

THE ENERGY CYCLE OF THE BODY

The body's primary fuel is glucose, which is the most readily available nutrient for energy. The most significant source of glucose is carbohydrates: carbohydrates are broken down into glucose, which undergoes a series of reactions called glycolysis.

In this cycle, glucose is broken down into energy packets called ATPs produced by the mitochondria, the powerhouse of the cell. These energy packets are used to fuel the body while performing actions. High-intensity work, such as exercise, requires a much more significant amount of energy than typing on a keyboard. The higher the intensity of work, the larger number of ATPs needed.

ATPs are also used in response to stress produced in the body and are crucial for fighting infections. The higher the level of energy in the body, the greater its immune response.

The Sirtfood Diet is rich in low glycemic carbohydrates, essential for fulfilling the body's vital energy and refueling needs.

THE ESSENTIAL ROLE OF MITOCHONDRIA

When a person goes on a diet, this usually means the body will have to manage a calorie deficit. The body takes this scenario as a challenge that requires immediate action from mitochondria - the cells' powerhouses – to produce ATPs, the energy packets to supply the body with instant energy.

Energy can be produced both from glucose and fat, and when the request for energy is very high, glucose is soon depleted, and the body starts using fat as fuel. The Sirtfood Diet, with its short calorie deficit created during the first days, helps to mobilize stored fat and use it for energy, thus causing weight loss.

SIRTUINS AND THEIR ACTIVITY ON GENES

To understand how the Sirtfood Diet works and why these particular foods are necessary, we will look at their role in the human body. As already explained, Sirtfoods got their name from Sirtuins, the compounds they include in different quantities.

The activity of Sirtuins was first researched in yeast, where a mutation caused an extension in the yeast's lifespan. Sirtuins were also shown to slow aging in laboratory mice, fruit flies, and nematodes. As the research on Sirtuins showed effects also on mammals, they were examined for their use in dieting and slowing the aging process. The type of sirtuins in humans are different, but they essentially work in the same ways and for the same reasons.

There are seven "members" that make up the sirtuin family. It is believed that sirtuins play a significant role in regulating certain cell functions, including proliferation (reproduction and cell growth) and apoptosis (cell death). They promote survival and resist stress to increase longevity.

They are also believed to block neurodegeneration by removing toxic proteins and supporting the brain's ability to change and adapt to different conditions (brain plasticity). As part of this, they also help reduce chronic inflammation and reduce something called oxidative stress. Oxidative stress is when there are too many cell-damaging free radicals circulating in the body, and the body cannot catch up by combating them with antioxidants. Free radicals are linked to age-related illnesses and also weight gain.

Sirtuin labels start with "SIR," which represents "Silence Information Regulator" genes. They do precisely that, silence or regulate genes, as part of their functions. Humans work with seven sirtuins: SIRT1, SIRT2, SIRT3, SIRT4, SIRT 5, SIRT6, and SIRT7. Each of these types is responsible for protecting cells in different ways.

They work by either stimulating or turning on certain gene expressions or reducing and turning off other gene expressions. This essentially means that they can influence genes to do more or less of something, most of which they are already programmed to do.

Through enzyme reactions, each of the SIRT types affects different cells responsible for the metabolic processes, organs, and functions that help maintain life.

For example, SIRT6 causes a gene expression that affects skeletal muscle, fat tissue, the brain, and the heart, while SIRT 3 causes a gene expression that affects the kidneys, liver, brain, and heart.

If we tie these concepts together, you can see that the Sirtuin proteins can change gene expression, and the Sirtfood Diet is concerned with how sirtuins can turn off the genes responsible for speeding up aging and weight management.

Another aspect to consider is the function and the power of calorie restriction on the human body. Calorie restriction simply means eating fewer calories. Calorie restriction, coupled with exercise and stress reduction, is usually a combination that supports weight loss. Calorie restriction has also been proven to increase one's lifespan through several studies on both humans and animals.

We can look further at the role of sirtuins combined with calorie restriction by looking at the SIRT3 protein, which has a role in metabolism and aging. Amongst all of the effects of the protein on gene expression (such as preventing cells from dying, reducing tumor growth, etc.), we want to understand the impact of SIRT3 on weight.

As we stated earlier, SIRT3 has high expression in metabolically active tissues, and its ability to express itself increases with caloric restriction and exercise. On the contrary, it will express itself less when following a high fat, high-calorie diet.

The role of sirtuins in regulating telomeres and reducing inflammation is also critical, as it helps fight diseases and aging.

Telomeres are sequences of proteins at the ends of chromosomes. When cells divide, they get shorter. As we age, they get even shorter, and other stressors to the body also contribute to this. Maintaining these telomeres as long as possible is the key to slower aging. Proper diet, along with exercise and other variables, can lengthen telomeres. SIRT6 is one of the sirtuins that, if activated, can help with DNA damage, inflammation, and oxidative stress. SIRT1 also helps with inflammatory response cycles that are related to many age-related diseases.

Calories restriction, as we mentioned earlier, can extend life to some degree.

Calorie restriction, as a stressor, will stimulate the SIRT3 proteins. These will kick in and protect the body from stressors and free radicals, helping the body maintain its telomeres' length. Since this is a stressor, these factors will stimulate the SIRT3 proteins to kick in and protect the body from the stressors and excess free radicals. Again, the telomere length is affected as well.

The research on Sirt proteins shows that, contrary to popular belief that "you can't change your genes" or "my Uncle Joe has this so I will too," simple lifestyle changes can influence our gene expression.

This is quite an empowering thought and yet another reason why you should be excited to have a science-based diet such as the Sirtfood diet, available to you.

PRESERVING MUSCLE MASS

Sirtuins help the body retain muscle mass even when dieting. How does this work? SIRT1 is the protein responsible for causing the body to burn fat rather than muscle for energy, which results in weight loss. Another useful aspect of SIRT1 is its ability to improve skeletal muscle.

Skeletal muscle consists of all the muscles you voluntarily control, such as the ones in your limbs, back, shoulders, and so on. There are two other muscle types: cardiac muscle, what the heart is formed from, and smooth muscles, which are involuntary and include muscles around blood vessels, the face, and various parts of organs and other tissues.

Skeletal muscle is divided into two different groups, named type-1 and type-2. Type 1 muscle is active during continued, sustained activity, whereas type-2 muscle is active during short, intense periods of activity. So, for example, you would predominantly use type-1 muscles for jogging but type-2 muscles for sprinting.

SIRT1 protects the most important type-1 muscles, but not the type-2 muscles, which are still broken down for energy. SIRT1 also influences how the muscles work.

SIRT1 is produced by the muscle cells, but the ability to make SIRT1 decreases as the muscle ages. As a result, muscle is harder to build as you age and doesn't grow as fast in response to exercise. A lack of SIRT1 also causes muscles to fatigue quicker and gradually decline over time.

This is how the Sirtfood Diet helps keep the body supple: providing SIRT1 helps skeletal muscle grow and stay in good shape.

EFFECTS ON FAT TYPE

Not only does the body have more than one type of muscle, as we saw in the previous paragraph, it also has more than one kind of fat too: white adipose tissue and brown adipose tissue.

White adipose tissue, or WAT as it is commonly abbreviated, is the fat made for storage. It's where your extra energy goes, and having more WAT makes it easier to store and gain fat in the future.

Brown adipose tissue, or BAT, is a type of fat tissue typically associated with burning fat. BAT helps keep us warm and contains high mitochondrial levels – the part of the cell responsible for producing energy.

Leaner people have higher levels of brown fat than their overweight peers. BAT is located around the neck and back, while WAT is situated in the areas typically associated with obesity – your gut, buttocks, chest, and hips. By having higher levels of BAT, fitter people have more ability to shake off calories through exercise and thermal release, so although research on BAT is still in its early stages, higher BAT levels and activity is hypothesized as being positive.

Of course, as you might now anticipate, sirtuins also affect our WAT and BAT levels. More precisely, sirtuins help convert your WAT into BAT, changing your body and making it easier to burn calories and lose weight. Over time this will produce substantial differences in your body composition, helping you lose weight and become lean and fit.

IMPROVING THE ENERGY-BOOSTING EFFECT

The amount of energy the body requires depends on an individual's daily activities, psychological factors such as stress, and metabolic rate. Essential body cells and tissues, such as the brain, need a constant energy supply to maintain their functions. The energy-boosting effect can improve the functionality of these vital tissues and cells.

The energy-boosting effect refers to all the activities geared towards ensuring constant energy supply to body organs, tissues, and cells. Following the Sirtfood Diet is undoubtedly one of these, as it guarantees an abundance of fruits and vegetables, plant and animal proteins, whole grains, and healthy fats, which play a significant role in enhancing the energy-boosting effect for a healthy living routine.

Drinking sufficient water improves the energy-boosting effect too. Water is a significant component in every food consumed. Keeping hydrated is essential for body health. Water requirement depends on age, sex, weight, physical activity level, and environmental conditions, such as the weather.

In the Sirtfood Diet, water is a significant compound, for example, in fruits and beverages. Drinks such as unsweetened coffee or flavored water are good options for staying hydrated.

Water is crucial in all physiological processes. Thus, frequent consumption of water, and drinks containing water like the ones included in the Sirtfood Diet, reduces fatigue and boosts body energy.

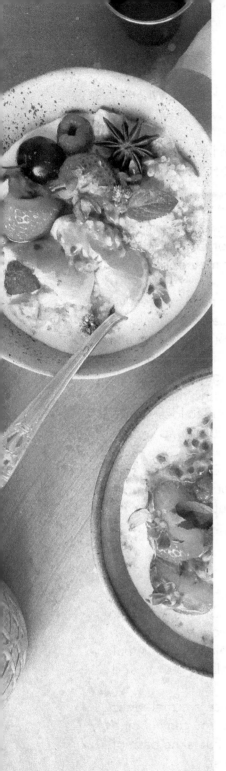

HEALTH BENEFITS
OF THE SIRTFOOD DIET

There is proof that sirtuin activators provide a wide variety of health benefits like muscle strengthening and appetite suppression. Others are improved memory, better control of blood sugar level, and the clearance of damage caused by free radical molecules that build up in cells and result in cancer and other diseases.

"The positive effects of the intake of food and beverages rich in sirtuin activators in decreasing chronic disease risks are an important observational evidence," said Professor Frank Hu, an authority on diet and epidemiology at Harvard University, in a recent paper in Advanced Nutrition. Losing weight is simply not enough nowadays, as the diet you follow needs to have plenty of health benefits as well; otherwise, you can't stick to it in the long run. Therefore, you need to see the bigger picture and not focus on losing many pounds in a short amount of time. Radical diets usually come with side effects, but if you find a meal plan that works for you in terms of weight loss and delivers plenty of health benefits, why not stick to it and make it your default diet?

The less processed food you eat, the more chances you will have to experience your meal plan's health benefits, so you don't have to see a doctor very often.

Let's have a look in detail at the main benefits the Sirtfood Diet will guarantee you for a lifetime.

IMMEDIATE WEIGHT LOSS

The most obvious of the health benefit is that you will lose weight on this diet. Whether you are exercising or not, there is no way that you can't not lose weight when you follow the diet to a T.

This diet has you restrict your calories enough so that anyone can lose weight. The average person uses around 2,000 calories per day, but during the diet, you will ingest 1,000 or 1,500 calories based on the phase you are in.

A calorie deficit causes weight loss — it is as simple as that. When you restrict your calories, but you keep your metabolism up, you will find that you will naturally lose weight. This is normal. However, usually, that weight loss is a mix of fat and muscle. As you lose weight and muscle, you would then naturally see your metabolism slow as well.

Of course, this means that over time, your weight loss plan is not nearly as effective as it was supposed to be. As a direct result, you will have to cut calories further to keep that deficit between consumed calories and the calories that your body naturally burns. This means that weight loss eventually slows or even plateaus if all you do is cut calories. You will lose muscle if you are not careful, which will work against you.

However, thanks to the fact that you do not lose muscle mass during the Sirtfood Diet, you do not have to worry about this problem; you simply continue to lose weight because you can maintain your metabolism at levels favorable to continued weight loss.

Sure enough, one remarkable observation from the Sirtfood Diet trial is that participants lost excessive weight while building muscle, contributing to a more toned body. It is the beauty of Sirtfoods: fat burning is activated, but muscle growth, maintenance, and repair are promoted as well.

POSITIVE INFLUENCE ON GENETICS

Is thinness a genetic trait? If so, how can you ever hope to lose weight?

Even if some people are blessed by activated "skinny genes" and can eat whatever they want without worrying about gaining weight, you can activate your skinny genes as well; they are inscribed in our DNA, after all! We just need to remind our cells that it's not science fiction. Our environment and our habits shape our cellular growth and gene replication: this is called epigenetics.

Every one of us has genes able to activate sirtuins or SIRTs. These are metabolic regulators that control our ability to burn fat and regenerate our cells. You can imagine them as sensors that get activated when our energy levels are low. That is the base of most fasting diets. But let's examine the drawbacks of this type of diet.

Many fasting diets have become popular in the past years. The most well-known are the variants of the intermittent fasting structure, such as the five-two diet. In the five-two diet, you fast during the weekend and usually eat during the week's working days. These diets have proven and demonstrated effects on longevity, weight loss, and overall health.

This is because these fasting diets activate the 'skinny gene' in our body. This gene causes the fat-storage processes to shut down and allows the body to enter a state of 'survival' mode, which causes the body to burn fat.

Anytime cells in your body replicate, there is a small chance of your DNA being damaged in the process. However, if your body repairs dying and older cells, there is no risk of DNA damage, which is why fasting is associated with a lower prevalence of degenerative diseases, such as Alzheimer's.

However, as the name implies, the problem with fasting diets is that you have to fast. Fasting feels awful, especially when other people with regular eating habits surround us. It also puts your diet into a social spotlight – explaining to your co-workers or your extended family why you are not eating on certain days is bound to generate doubt and challenges to your diet regime.

Furthermore, even though fasting has numerous associated benefits, there are some downsides too. Fasting is associated with muscle loss, as the body doesn't discriminate between muscle mass and fat tissue when choosing cells to burn for energy.

When fasting, you also risk malnutrition, simply by not eating enough foods to get essential nutrients. This risk can be somewhat alleviated by taking vitamin supplements and eating nutrient-rich foods. Still, fasting can also slow and halt the digestive system altogether – preventing the absorption of supplements. These supplements also need dietary fat to be dissolved, which you might also lack if you were to implement a strict fasting method.

On top of this, fasting isn't appropriate for a vast range of people. You don't want children to fast and potentially inhibit their growth. Likewise, the elderly, the ill, and pregnant women are all just too vulnerable to the risks of fasting.

Additionally, there are several psychological detriments to fasting, despite commonly being associated with spiritual revelations. Fasting makes you irritable and causes you to feel slightly on edge – your body is constantly telling you that you need to forage for food, enacting physical processes that affect your mood and emotions.

Sirtuins were first discovered in 1984 in yeast molecules. Of course, once it became apparent that sirtuin activators affected various factors, such as lifespan and metabolic activity, interest in these proteins blossomed.

Sirtuin activators boost mitochondrial activity, the part of the biological cell responsible for energy production. This, in turn, mirrors the energy-boosting effects, which also occur due to exercise and fasting. The Sirtfood Diet is thought to start a process called adipogenesis, which prevents fat cells from duplicating – which should interest any potential dieter.

The exciting part is that the sirtuin activators actually influence your genetics. The notion of the 'genetic' lottery is embedded in the public consciousness, but genes are even more changeable than you might think. You can't change your eye color or height, but you can activate or deactivate specific genes based on environmental factors. This is called epigenetics, and it is a fascinating field of study.

APPETITE UNDER CONTROL

Though your first few days on Sirtfood Diet, you may find that you are ravenous as your body adjusts to its new normal, but it will quickly adapt to the calorie restriction. You will be okay because the food you will be eating will include nutrient-dense ingredients that will help your body feel satisfied.

We'll explore the complete list of ingredients in the following chapters, but for example, lentils and buckwheat are very dense foods that are featured heavily in this diet. Adding healthy fats, such as olive oil, to your diet will make you feel content, knowing that you have given yourself enough to keep your body going. You will find that you will tolerate the lower amounts of food, which is a huge plus.

PRESERVED MUSCLE AND BONES MASS

Studies have shown that sirtuins can help boost muscle mass, especially in elderly individuals. A study done on aging mice showed that a sirtuin rich diet helped allow for the development and growth of blood vessels and muscle. This would then boost the energy that the elderly mice had by upwards of 80%. That is massive.

If you want to make sure that your metabolism stays regulated, you must ensure that your muscles are there to help you, and if they are not, you can run into all sorts of problems. This means that if you want to find a diet that will help you gain muscle and burn fat, the sirtuin-rich Sirtfood Diet is one of the best for you.

Of course, retaining muscle isn't just better from an overall fitness perspective, but also an aesthetic view.

Another critical reason why retaining muscle mass is important is your resting energy expenditure. Your muscles require energy, even when you are not using them intensely. Due to this, people with high skeletal muscle levels burn more calories than people who don't, even if both are sedentary. Being muscular allows you to eat more calories and get away with it!

Furthermore, sirtuins help improve overall heart health by protecting and strengthening the cardiac muscle (presumably similar to how SIRT1 protects skeletal muscle) and bones. They help retain precious osteoblasts, which are cells in our bones that allow more bone cells to be produced.

BLOOD SUGAR LEVELS UNDER CONTROL

Sirtuin-rich foods are known to inhibit the release of insulin improving blood sugar management. With the use of sirtuins, you can prevent your blood sugar from dropping too low. This is a great point to keep in mind as compelling for completing this diet, especially when you recognize that you ultimately want to maintain stable blood sugar to feel functional when restricting calories. When you limit calorie consumption, you run into other problems, such as not correctly managing your blood sugar. Have you ever skipped a meal or two and felt dizzy or weak? That is the impact of lower blood sugar—but the sirtuins will help you regulate your levels so that you feel strong enough to proceed until you're happy with the result.

BETTER SLEEP

Adequate sleep is essential and reduces the probability of getting certain chronic illnesses. It keeps the brain and digestion system healthy and boosts the immune system.

Sirtuin activators cause the SIR genes to activate, which in turn increases the release of SIRTs. SIRTs, or Silent Information Regulators, also help regulate the circadian rhythm, which is your natural body clock and influence sleep patterns.

Sleep is essential for many vital biological processes, including those that help regulate blood sugar (which is also crucial for losing weight). If you find yourself repeatedly stuck in a state of lag and brain fog, your circadian rhythm may be out of sync. The Sirtfood Diet can help your body regain a healthy circadian rhythm.

The Sirtfood Diet can significantly promote good sleep thanks to the introduction of ingredients like walnuts and chamomile tea, which boost relaxation and the ability to fall asleep easier.

LESS STRESS AND ANXIETY

Stress and large amounts of emotion consume a lot of energy in the body. Anxiety comes as a result of feeling anxious, sad, scared, or uncomfortable. Stress can be reduced in many ways, such as talking with friends or consulting with a psychotherapist. Sticking to regular mealtimes and planning meals can also manage some of the stress.

Additionally, stress can be managed successfully with the Sirtfood Diet. Examples of a Sirtfoods that can significantly reduce stress include Brazil nuts, fatty fish, dark chocolate, eggs, and pumpkin seeds.

ANTI-AGING EFFECT

As previously said, the Sirtfood Diet helps sustain muscle mass. This is something powerful and protective, especially against aging. Osteoporosis makes bones weak and more prone to break in older people. An overall muscle mass with good tone and volume can help fight off bone fractures that may come with osteoporosis.

Likewise, the clearing of free radicals also helps to slow down the aging process.

Anti-aging is somehow linked to autophagy, an intracellular process that repairs or replaces damaged cell parts. This rejuvenation occurs at an intracellular level. We can't mention autophagy without saying something about AMPK, an enzyme essential for cellular energy homeostasis. AMPK helps boost energy by activating fatty acid, glucose, and oxidation when cellular energy is low. It represents the body's response when facing an elevated energy demand (e.g., an intense physical exercise).

However, a part of this response is lysosomal degradation autophagy. Now you are probably wondering what sirtuins have to do with all of this. Well, SIRT1 can activate AMPK (and the other way around), so it can be considered one of the triggers of autophagy. Autophagy rejuvenates the cell, and this process can happen in all the cells of your body, from the cells of your internal organs to those of your skin.

There are a few ways to induce autophagy, and it has a very positive effect on your health and overall lifespan. Just think of the cell as a car, and autophagy is a skilled mechanic capable of fixing or replacing any broken parts in it. Obviously, the cell will have a longer life, and this extends to your overall life. If your cells are functioning correctly, then you can expect increased longevity. You can't reverse aging, as there is no such cure for it, and autophagy is not "the fountain of youth." However, this process can significantly slow down aging and its effects. The best part is that it can be activated by sirtuins, especially SIRT1, through the Sirtfood Diet.

FIGHTS FREE RADICALS

The antioxidants provided by most sirtfoods are great at defending your body from suffering the effects of cancer or other chronic diseases. They are incredibly beneficial for the body — they are designed to protect your body from free radicals that are harmful by-products of breaking down food or being exposed to radiation. Antioxidants work to protect your body against these enemies that will harm you, and because they do that, they can help reduce your risk of heart disease, cancer, and other common diseases that are suffered from today.

Essentially, antioxidants work because they protect the body; many plant-based foods are rich in antioxidants, and they are quite powerful. The body itself cannot properly remove those free radicals that you are exposed to overtime. It is impossible not to be—even the sun will leave you exposed to radiation every time you leave your house. Free radicals and oxidative stress have been linked to Parkinson's disease, arthritis, and strokes. Sirtfoods, with their antioxidant effects, protect you constantly. That's why it's essential to keep their intake up for a lifetime.

FIGHTS CHRONIC DISEASES

Medicine may be progressing, but this doesn't mean that people are getting healthier. It is quite the opposite. Around 70 percent of deaths nowadays are caused by chronic diseases.

This is indeed shocking, but the cause can be traced to the food we eat. The antidote to most of our diseases is healthy food. Processed food causes these issues, but healthy food can make it right.

Modern-day eating habits and lifestyles encourage the accumulation of fats and toxins (fat tissue protects toxins) and increased blood sugar and insulin levels. This is where the trouble starts, from a simple pre-diabetes condition to more severe diseases (eventually, even leading to cancer).

However, the antidote to many of these issues lies hidden within us. As you already know, all bodies possess sirtuin genes, and activating them is crucial to burn fat and build a stronger and leaner body.

As it turns out, the benefits of sirtuins activity extend way beyond the fat-burning process. Whether we like it or not, a lack of sirtuins can be associated with plenty of diseases and medical conditions, while activating sirtuins will have the opposite effect. For example, sirtuins can significantly improve your arteries' function, control cholesterol levels, and prevent atherosclerosis.

DIABETES

If you have diabetes, then you should know that activating sirtuins will make insulin work more effectively. Insulin is the hormone primarily responsible for controlling the levels of sugar in the blood. SIRT1 works perfectly with metformin (one of the most powerful antidiabetic drugs).

As it turns out, pharmaceutical companies are adding sirtuin activators to metformin treatments. These studies were conducted on animals, and the results were simply excellent. It was noticed that an 83 percent reduction of the metformin dose is required to achieve the same effects.

By increasing the amount of insulin that can be released, SIRT1 can help tackle diabetes by causing higher amounts of blood sugar to be converted into fat. So, as the key to diabetes and weight gain is insulin resistance, there is positive news for the waistline.

COGNITIVE IMPAIRMENT AND ALZHEIMER'S

Sirtuins have been shown to impact neurodegenerative diseases that cause cognitive impairments like Alzheimer's disease. This is because sirtuins help regulate appetite and manage other brain stimuli, enhancing the communication signals in the brain itself, improving cognitive function, and lowering brain inflammation.

Individuals with Alzheimer's have been found to have notably lower levels of sirtuins than healthy peers, although the mechanism of action between sirtuin and the disease is not fully known.

What is known is that the Sirtfood Diet helps prevent build-ups of the amyloid-B and tau protein, molecules that are responsible for the plaques in the brains of people with Alzheimer's (and similar diseases that cause cognitive impairment).

IMPROVED ENERGY

Eating frequently can boost vitality levels and give the brain a steady supply of energy for all its functions.

As we will see later in the book, the Sirtfood Diet allows you to eat five times per day: a juice, a snack, or a meal depending on the diet phase you are in.

Frequent meals help control blood sugar and hunger throughout the day, positively affecting energy levels, thanks to the sirtuins' effect. Sirtfoods that can be consumed frequently include coffee, soy, dark chocolate, and blueberries.

Consumption of food with a low glycemic index may reduce the lag in energy that occurs after eating food with fast absorption of sugars and refined starches. Sirtfood promotes foods with a low glycemic index like vegetables, nuts, and whole grains.

These foods improve the energy-boosting effect in the body.

DIFFERENT OPTIONS FOR EVERY NEED

The Sirtfood Diet, unlike fasting, doesn't involve skipping meals to experience the benefits it can offer. Therefore, you are not going through starvation to reach your weight loss and health goals. Nonetheless, the diet involves a brief period of caloric restriction that will require a bit of focus. Then you will increase calories again, going back to having breakfast, lunch, dinner, and snacks.

The Sirtfood Diet has been developed to meet the needs of the vast majority of people who need to lose weight.

Only people with serious illnesses or who are pregnant or breastfeeding should be careful and skip to the maintenance phase, avoiding caloric restriction altogether. This means that they will still include healthy Sirtfoods (with their weight loss properties) in their everyday meals. While they may not be able to take advantage of the Phase 1 boost, they will still be able to make the best choices for their health and weight loss.

Remember, even if you cannot follow through with the restrictions, there is still a great benefit to be gained from adding the sirtuin-rich foods to your diet. As we will address shortly, many of the foods rich in sirtuins are highly nutritious, and there is no doubt that they are very healthy, and they should be included in your diet whether you want to follow the Sirtfood Diet or not.

Now you are probably wondering, "How am I going to lose pounds by eating three meals a day?"

The secret lies within the meal plan, as it can seriously deliver outstanding results. Depending on the Phase you are in, you can enjoy eating dark chocolate and red wine while losing weight!

The average weight loss during the first week is proven to be around seven pounds.

Of course, not all bodies react the same to this diet so that individual weight loss can be more or less, but this diet promises to deliver outstanding results for trying it.

Once you are satisfied with the weight you have reached, you can go into the maintenance phase of this diet and then transition to a regular healthy diet, still full of sirtuin-rich food. Sounds neat, right? This is what's great about this diet — it gives you the possibility to preserve your ideal weight long term, unlike many other radical diets where most people complain that they start to gain weight immediately after quitting.

THE SIRTFOOD DIET PLAN

The Sirtfood Diet combines a short calorie restriction phase with a long-term commitment to nutrient-dense sirtuin-activating foods. Before explaining how the diet is structured in detail, let's talk about two different and fundamental subjects when trying to achieve long-lasting results.

THE DIFFERENCE BETWEEN DIET AND DIETING

How you eat every day is your "diet," restricting how you eat is "dieting."

Aside from the first week, Phase 1, the Sirtfood Diet is not a traditional diet in the sense that, instead of merely restricting calories, you focus on increasing nutrition and improving the quality of the food you eat.

There are two main phases of the Sirtfood Diet, which are three weeks long. They are designed to set the stage for incorporating sirtfoods into your lifelong diet, eliminating your need to ever resort to dieting again. A third phase is dedicated to transitioning to a regular (not restricted) healthy sirtfood-rich diet.

The average American over-consumes solid fats and sugars, refined grains, sodium, and saturated fat. They also under-consume vegetables, fruits, whole grains, and the nationally recommended intake of dairy and oils.

If this sounds like it matches your current eating patterns, don't be too hard on yourself, you're certainly not alone. You've been practically brainwashed into adopting these poor nutrition habits.

The number of fast-food restaurants continues to grow, as do options for pre-made, packaged foods full of empty calories, and misleading promises.

When you live on a diet of foods lacking nutrition for too long, you find yourself getting sick and overweight.

How many times have you found yourself dieting, starving yourself for weeks to lose 20 pounds? Maybe you've even been successful a time or two and lost weight, but within a few months, all the weight you lost had found its way home again and brought a few extra friends along.

Studies show that when you restrict your calories severely for an extended period, you will gain the weight back as quickly as it came off, and you will do additional damage to your liver, kidneys, and muscle mass as well. Short-term calorie restriction, such as the first phase of the Sirtfood Diet, doesn't have the same effect that depleting your body of nutrition for a more extended period has.

Simply put, dieting does not help you maintain results in the long term.

More to the point, dieting is completely unnecessary. Think about many regions of the world, like Japan or the Mediterranean, where people traditionally don't count calories or diet, and they live to be 100+ with their full physical and mental capacities until one night, they drift off into a peaceful, joyous slumber never to wake up again. That sounds a lot better than spending the last few months, if not years, of your life in a hospital bed, unable to wash or feed yourself, let alone walk around or remember your grandchildren.

You get to choose your future. And it begins with choosing a healthy diet rich in delicious, fortifying, and age-defying sirtfoods.

UNDERSTANDING YOUR HEALTH GOALS

You may have first heard about the Sirtfood Diet because you saw a headline about Adele's miraculous weight loss. Or perhaps you heard that scientists had discovered a "skinny gene," and the secret to accessing it was in this diet.

You want to lose weight, look great, and feel great in your skin.

That is a common and completely understandable desire, but it's not enough to get you the results you're dreaming of, at least, not in the long-term. History has proven to us many times that, even if we succeed in reaching our goal weight, we're either not satisfied, or we are, but we return to our old habits, and the weight comes back.

One of the main reasons losing weight is ineffective is because it has an end or a result that you can achieve that allows you to give up.

If you start looking deeper and making a commitment to your health, you'll find that there is never a moment that you permit yourself to stop. Even if you're relatively healthy today, you maintain a desire to stay healthy tomorrow, and the following year, and 20 years from now.

Health is a never-ending journey, and that is where your real success and results will lie. You won't have a deadline to abide by, and you can't fail, as long as you're taking actions every day that are designed to improve some aspect of your health.

Sometimes you'll see and feel the results right away. The participants in the first Sirtfood Diet trial saw weight loss results within seven days. But other times, the benefits are on a cellular level, and you won't realize they're making such a difference in your life until you're 80 years old and you the only one of your peers that haven't been forced to move into assisted living.

One of the other significant reasons dieting has a less than impressive track record is the type of weight loss that goes along with it.

The diseases associated with obesity aren't caused only by excess weight. When you spend many years eating unhealthy foods, you damage your metabolic system and the hormones that support your metabolism. Issues like insulin and leptin resistance cause you to gain weight and develop even more lethal diseases, like diabetes and heart disease.

The food you eat is the problem, and the weight is simply a by-product of a dysfunctional metabolic system.

If you heal the system by removing the foods that damage your hormones and adding foods that heal and protect your entire body, the weight will come off naturally because you have fixed the damage.

When you try to take the weight off through calorie restriction, excessive exercise, or a combination of the two, you will likely lower the numbers on your scale. There is truth to the philosophy of "calories in, calories out."

However, if you aren't considering the quality of the calories going in, you won't control what comes off. You're just as likely to lose water weight and muscle mass as you are to lose any fat.

If, on the other hand, you commit to providing your body with all the nutrition it needs to rebalance your hormones and protect your health, the weight that you lose is going to be the weight that you don't need. Visceral fat around your vital organs and abdominal fat you've been struggling to get rid of for years will go away, your muscles will be protected, and your body will stay nicely hydrated.

Losing weight due to improved health is sustainable, so you must start to adjust your mindset and your goals if you truly want to be successful.

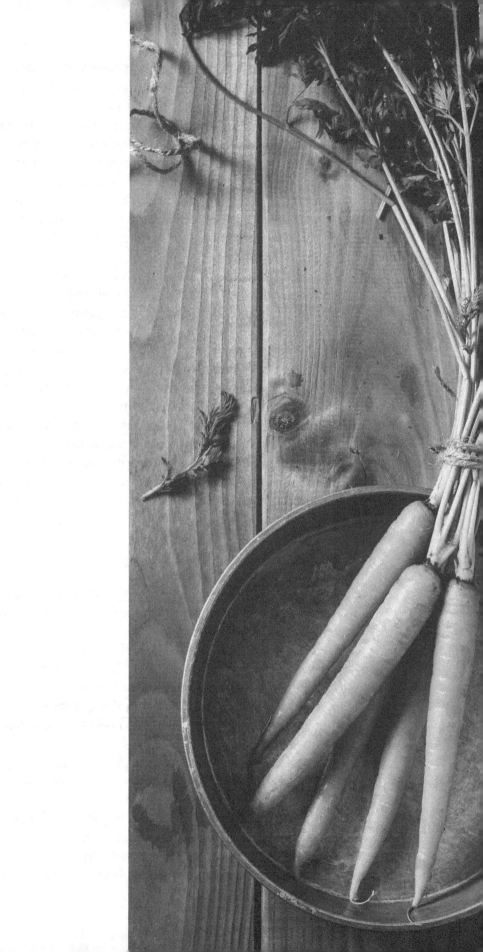

NOT ONLY WEIGHT LOSS

Your weight is not the only thing you should be focusing on. Your health is the most important aspect of your life because, without it, you will have no joy and, most likely, very little hope of ever being able to maintain your ideal body weight.

If you prioritize health goals, you will have all the motivation you need to stop damaging your body with unhealthy foods with zero nutrition. You will be excited and inspired to try the myriad of fresh new ingredients that will help you feel lighter, younger, stronger, and healthier than you can remember ever feeling.

The Sirtfood Diet is not about taking the easy route or popping a miracle cure pill. It's about finding joy in food and letting that food heal and nourish your body, allowing you to find joy in life once again. There are so many flavors waiting to be discovered; you simply need to commit to making sirtfoods the star players in your diet, with healthy proteins and fats as the phenomenal support team.

You don't have to starve yourself or even deny yourself the foods you love; you simply have to approach food with mindfulness and awareness of its consequences on your body and health.

THE DIET STRUCTURE

Phase 1: 7 Pounds in Seven Days

Phase 1 of the diet is the one that produces the most significant results. Over seven days, you will follow a simple direction to lose around 7 pounds. For the first three days, calorie intake is set to 1,000 kcal.

You will start with a lower number of calories and then gradually increase them. This will jump-start your genes and trigger the sirtuin proteins to do their job on your "skinny genes."

In the next pages, you'll find a step-by-step guide on how to plan your days during Phase 1. This will allow you the freedom to choose from existing recipes in Appendix A or even create your own using your favorite ingredients and the Sirtfoods listed in the next chapter.

Week 1: The first 3 days will include 3 juices per day; the remaining 4 days will consist of 2 juices per day.

Monday
Breakfast: Sirtfood Green juice
Snack: Two squares of dark chocolate
Lunch: Sirtfood Green juice
Snack: Sirtfood Green juice
Dinner: Sirtfood meal

Drink the juices at three different times of the day, as shown: in the morning as soon as you wake up, lunch, and mid-afternoon. For dinner, choose a recipe from Appendix A.

Tuesday
Breakfast: Sirtfood Green juice
Snack: Two squares of dark chocolate
Lunch: Sirtfood Green juice
Snack: Sirtfood Green juice
Dinner: Sirtfood meal

The formula is identical to that of the first day. The only thing that changes is the dinner recipe, as usual, selected from the recipes in Appendix A.

Wednesday
Breakfast: Sirtfood Green juice
Snack: Two squares of dark chocolate
Lunch: Sirtfood Green juice
Snack: Sirtfood Green juice
Dinner: Sirtfood meal

This is the last day you will consume three green juices a day; tomorrow, you will switch to two. Take this opportunity to browse other drinks that you can have during the diet, such as coffee, green tea, or herbal tea.
As usual, select your dinner from the recipes in Appendix A.

Thursday
Breakfast: Sirtfood Green juice
Snack: Sirtfood Green juice
Lunch: Sirtfood meal
Snack: Two squares of dark chocolate.
Dinner: Sirtfood meal

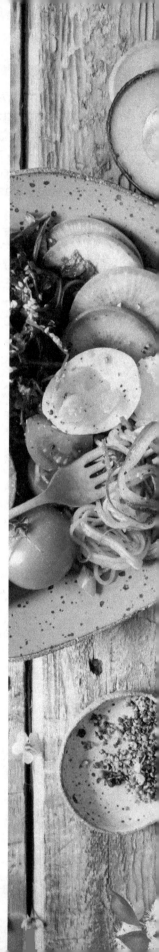

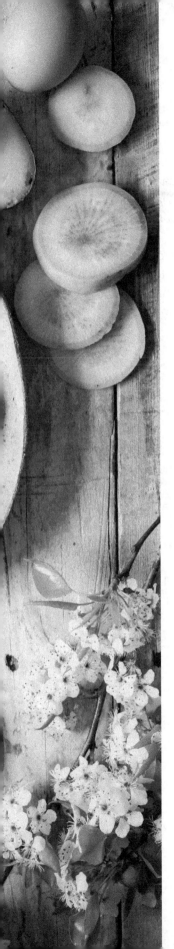

The significant change from the previous three days is that you will only drink two juices instead of three and have two meals instead of one.

As usual, select your lunch and dinner from recipes in Appendix A.

Friday
Breakfast: Sirtfood Green juice
Snack: Sirtfood Green juice
Lunch: Sirtfood meal
Snack: Two squares of dark chocolate.
Dinner: Sirtfood meal

On the fifth day, you will ingest 2 green juices and 2 meals.

As usual, select your lunch and dinner from among the recipes in Appendix A.

Saturday
Breakfast: Sirtfood Green juice
Snack: Sirtfood Green juice
Lunch: Sirtfood meal
Snack: Two squares of dark chocolate.
Dinner: Sirtfood meal

On the sixth day, you will assume 2 green juices and 2 meals

As usual, select your lunch and dinner from among the recipes in Appendix A.

Sunday
Breakfast: Sirtfood Green juice
Snack: Sirtfood Green juice
Lunch: Sirtfood meal
Snack: Two squares of dark chocolate.
Dinner: Sirtfood meal

On the seventh day, you will consume 2 green juices and 2 meals.

The seventh day is the last of phase 1 of the diet. Instead of considering it as an end, see it as a beginning because you are about to embark on a new life, in which Sirtfoods will play a central role in your nutrition. Today's menu is a perfect example of how easy it is to integrate them abundantly into your daily diet.

As usual, select your lunch and dinner from the recipes in Appendix A.

Notes

It is suggested that you should not consume any of your juices, or your main meal, after 7 pm. This is advised due to our natural circadian rhythm or our 'body clock' and how it affects our body. Generally speaking, our body wants to prepare and burn energy in the morning while storing and retaining energy during the evening. Therefore, if you eat later at night, you have a higher chance of energy in your food being stored as fat.

You should also feel free to drink non-calorie fluids. While this technically does include calorie-free fizzy drinks, green tea, black coffee, and of course, water are better choices. One surprising finding is that small doses of lemon juice can increase sirtuin absorption, so consider adding a dash to your water or green tea.

Note that only black coffee is recommended; milk, sugar, and sweeteners diminish sirtuin absorption and interfere with the calorie count. Another caveat is that you shouldn't change your coffee consumption too much from your regular habits. A sudden drop in consumption will make you feel awful; a sharp increase will make you feel jittery. Change your coffee habits gradually.

Phase 2: Maintenance

Congratulations! You have finished the first "hardcore" week. The second phase – maintenance – is more manageable. It will last two weeks, and it will keep including sirtuin-filled food selections in your everyday meals.

The calorie intake for this phase is set to 1500 kcal. This will cause your body to undergo the fat-burning stage, gain muscle, plus boost your immune system and overall health.

For this phase, you can now have 3 balanced Sirtfood-filled meals each day plus 1 green juice a day.

Try choosing healthier alternatives by adding Sirtfood in each meal as much as possible.

You should consume the same beverages you were drinking in phase 1, with a slight change, you are welcome to enjoy the occasional glass of red wine (although, don't drink more than 3 per week).

Monday to Sunday (week 2 and week 3)
Breakfast: Sirtfood meal
Snack: Sirtfood Green juice
Lunch: Sirtfood meal
Snack: Sirtfood snack or two squares of dark chocolate
Dinner: Sirtfood meal

As usual, select your lunch and dinner from the recipes in Appendix A.

You may also add a glass of red wine per day if you want to.

As far as drinks, you can have coffee, green tea, and other no-calorie beverages daily.

Phase 3: Transition to Normal Healthy Eating

After 2 weeks of mildly restricted calorie intake, you are now ready to move back up to a regular calorie intake to keep your Sirtfood intake high. You should have experienced some degree of weight loss by now, but most of all, you should also feel fitter and re-invigorated.

The suggested meal plan is:

Monday to Sunday
Breakfast: Sirtfood meal
Snack: Sirtfood Green juice or Sirtfood snack (one a day each)
Lunch: Sirtfood meal
Snack: Sirtfood Green juice or Sirtfood snack (one a day each)
Dinner: Sirtfood meal

By eating reasonable portions of balanced meals, you shouldn't feel hungry or be consuming too much. This is the main reason why the Sirtfood Diet is very sustainable. After only 3 weeks, you have changed your eating habits for the better, improving the way you nourish your body. Just keep going, without restricting portions as in the previous weeks and gradually implementing more and more sirtfoods into your lifestyle.

If you continuously try and withhold giving into temptation and always moderate your eating habits, you are bound to crack and fall off the wagon sooner or later. Instead, you should be combining your regular eating habits with the Sirtfood diet principles, slowly aligning your natural eating tendencies and taste with the Sirtfood ideal.

Remember, whenever you need a fat-burning boost, you can re-implement the three-phases of the Sirtfood Diet to speed up your weight loss and cleanse your body.

SIRTFOOD INGREDIENTS

The Sirtfood Diet has some significant advantages over other meal plans or programs designed to help you lose weight and get healthier. The ingredients are very familiar, and you can easily combine them with other healthy foods that are not rich in sirtuins.

Also, this diet is very permissive. You can try plenty of food out there, and you are not limited to just veggies and fruits.

There might be people trying sirtfoods and not losing weight. In this case, their problem lies within the form, variety, and quantity they are eating. It is tough to have a meal consisting only of sirtfoods, so you need to find the right balance between sirtfoods and everyday food.

Having regular meals is very important because if you don't have the meals within a set timeframe, the diet might not work. The general rule about not overeating at dinner or having dinner late in the evening applies.

Over the last few years, there has been an increasing and widespread aversion to grains. However, studies link whole grain consumption with decreased frequency of inflammation, diabetes, heart disease, and cancers.

While the pseudo-grain buckwheat has full Sirtfood qualification, we do see the existence of substantial sirtuin-activating nutrients in other whole grains. However, it goes without saying, the sirtuin-activating nutrient quality of whole grains is decimated when they are converted into refined "clean" forms.

We're not saying you can never eat them, but instead, you're going to be much better off sticking to the whole-grain version whenever possible.

Now, let's try to understand the secret of these sirtfoods. What exactly do they contain that activates sirtuins?

Arugula contains nutrients like kaempferol and quercetin. Buckwheat contains rutting. Capers have the same nutrients as arugula. Celery has luteolin and apigenin. Cocoa contains epicatechin.

Chilies have a higher concentration of myricetin and luteolin. Coffee contains caffeic acid. Widely used in the Mediterranean diet, extra-virgin olive oil has hydroxytyrosol and oleuropein. Kale contains the same nutrients as arugula and capers. You can find ajoene and myricetin in garlic.

In green tea, you can find EGCG epigallocatechin gallate. Medjool dates contain caffeic acid and gallic acid. Parsley has myricetin and apigenin. In red endives, you can find luteolin. Quercetin can be found in red onions.

Strawberries contain fisetin. Walnuts are a great source of gallic acid. Turmeric has curcumin. Soy contains formononetin and daidzein. Red wine has piceatannol and resveratrol.

Indeed, all these compounds have the power to trigger sirtuins, but as it turns out, a standard US diet is very poor in these nutrients. A proper Sirtfood Diet should allow you to consume hundreds of milligrams of these essential ingredients per day. If you manage to introduce most of the ingredients and sirtfoods mentioned above into your daily meal plan, you can effectively reap this diet's benefits.

ARE SUPPLEMENTS OK?

The nutrients mentioned above should be consumed in a natural state. This is how this diet works. You may not have the same effects if you take supplements, as the body absorbs and assimilates them much better in their natural form. If you take, for instance, resveratrol, this nutrient is poorly absorbed in a supplement form. However, if you consume it in a natural state, the absorption is six times higher.

Many studies suggest when specific vitamins, minerals, antioxidants, or even polyphenols are isolated and consumed outside of their natural food source, they are not metabolized effectively and, in some cases, can even be detrimental to your health.

Humans are very impressive in the field of science and medicine. Still, nature has secrets we haven't even begun to unravel, so whenever possible, it's in your best interest to find the most natural source of nutrition possible.

It is good to have as many of these sirtfoods as possible to ensure you are getting the necessary intake of sirtuin-activating nutrients. Most of them are very common or familiar. This is the beauty of the Sirtfood Diet: it is not something extraordinary to eat garlic or red onion, strawberries, blueberries, or walnuts. These are everyday ingredients. It is also highly recommended to make sure you include turmeric in your diet, as well.

When it comes to consuming fruits and veggies, most nutritionists agree that it is best to consume them fresh and raw. This is how you will get all the nutrients and vitamins from them.

However, when it comes to leafy greens, another way to reap all their benefits is to juice them. This procedure removes the low-nutrient fiber from them and allows you to have a super-concentrated dose of sirtuin-activating polyphenols.

Since this diet allows you to eat plenty of foods, it rocks when it comes to diversity. This is why you can simply feel free to consume meat, fish, and seafood if you want. As a general rule of thumb, consume less beef and pork and more poultry, fish, and seafood.

The Sirtfood Diet should slowly become your default meal plan. Therefore, you don't have to stick just to the four-week meal plan. Sirtuins need to be in your diet every day of the week, so why stop after finishing the fourth week? If you have a good thing going, you don't need to interrupt it. Plus, the longer you follow this diet, the more health benefits you will experience. This should be the ultimate motivation to make you follow the Sirtfood Diet regularly. You need to check yourself whether you want to prevent or even reverse some of the most common diseases caused by poor diet, slow down your aging process, and lose some weight while doing it.

Note

If your doctor or primary care physician has advised you to take a supplement, follow their advice. There are circumstances when supplementation is critical for your survival. There are many more circumstances when taking supplements is simply advisable.

For example, Vegans are almost always deficient in vitamin B12 and Omega 3 fatty acids because both of those nutrients are most commonly found in fatty, oily fish. If following a plant-based diet is your ethical or moral choice, you may need to supplement for your best health.

20 MAIN SIRTFOODS TO INCLUDE IN YOUR EVERYDAY MEALS

Various foods can be included in your plan of the Sirtfood Diet. This chapter is about the multiple types of sirtfoods you should include in your diet to get the best results.

The following twenty foods contain the highest amounts of sirtuin-activating polyphenols. The polyphenol levels are not uniformly distributed in all these foods, and some contain higher amounts. Moreover, different polyphenols are present in each of them, and they are associated with special effects on the sirtuin gene.

One of the most important aspects of the Sirtfood Diet is to use a variety of foods.

Each of these foods has its impressive health qualities, but nothing compares to when they are combined.

Buckwheat flour helps a lot in losing weight. The overall fat content of buckwheat is very low. In fact, the calorie count is less than that of rice or wheat. As the flour comes with a low amount of saturated fat, it can stop you from binge-eating or eating unnecessarily. Therefore, it can help in facilitating and maintaining quick digestion. The low amount of fat and a high quantity of minerals can facilitate keeping type II diabetes under control.

Arugula is an excellent sirtfood vegetable and is low in calories. It will not only help you to lose weight but also comes with several beneficial properties. Arugula is rich in chlorophyll that can help in preventing DNA and liver damage resulting from aflatoxins. For getting the best from the arugula, it is always recommended to consume this vegetable raw. It is made of 95% water, and thus it can also act as a cooling and hydrating food on summer days. Vitamin K plays an important role in maintaining bone health.

Capers are the unripe flower buds of the plant Capparis spinosa. It is rich in flavonoid compounds that also include quercetin and rutin, great sources of antioxidants. Antioxidants can act to prevent free radicals that can lead to skin diseases and even cancer. Capers can help keep a check on diabetes. It contains several chemicals that can keep blood sugar levels.

Celery is very low in calories, and that is excellent for losing weight. It can also help prevent dehydration as it contains a significant amount of water and electrolytes, which also helps eliminate bloating. It has antiseptic properties and prevents various kidney problems. Consumption of this vegetable can also help in the excretion of toxic elements from the body. Celery comes with generous amounts of vitamin K and vitamin C, along with potassium and folate.

Chilies can help burn calories. Adding a bit of spice to your daily diet, like cayenne or bird's eye chilis, can help eliminate extra calories and boost metabolism. It also helps in lowering the levels of blood sugar. It has also been found that people who have a habit of consuming chili in their diet feel fuller quickly, and thus, it can lower food cravings.

Cocoa, even in its chocolate form, can help in controlling weight. Cocoa comes with fat-burning properties and is the prime reason most trainers suggest mixing cocoa in shakes before exercising. It can help in reducing inflammation and thus can also help in proper digestion. Cocoa is rich in antioxidants like polyphenols.

Coffee is one of the most famous beverages that can be found all over the world. Coffee also has a very low-calorie count. Caffeine is a form of natural stimulant that is abundant in coffee. It increases mental functionality and alertness, making the brain alert and sharp. Caffeine can help in improving metabolism and thus can act as a great weight loss component. However, be careful not to consume it excessively, as it can affect your sleep pattern.

Garlic is one of those vegetables that can be found in every kitchen. Consumption of raw garlic can help boost energy levels that can aid in losing weight. Garlic is well known for suppressing appetite and can help you feel full longer. Thus, with the consumption of garlic, you will be able to prevent yourself from overeating. A strong relationship can be found between burning fat and the consumption of garlic. Garlic helps in stimulating the process of fat burning and removes harmful toxins from the body.

Green tea is often regarded as the healthiest type of beverage that can be found on this planet. This is mainly because green tea is full of antioxidants, along with several other plant compounds (like theine) that can provide you with several health benefits. Theine has an effect similar to caffeine and acts as a stimulant for burning fat.

It can also help boost your energy levels during exercise. Green tea comes with a high concentration of minerals and vitamins and is low calorie. It can help in improving the metabolic rate as well.

Kale is a trendy vegetable that comes with excellent weight loss properties. It is a vegetable rich in antioxidants, like vitamin C, which performs various important functions in the body's cells and improves its bone structure.

It is rich in vitamin K and helps bind calcium. Kale can provide you with 2.4 g of dietary fiber and thus reduce the feeling of hunger. It comes with compounds rich in sulfur and can help in detoxifying the liver.

Dates are rich in dietary fibers and fatty acids that can help you lose extra kilos. However, they should be consumed in moderation as they are very caloric. They allow you to stay healthy and fit, thanks to their protein content. Moderate daily consumption of dates can help boost the functioning of the immune system.

Olive oil has always been famous for cooking food. Extra Virgin olive oil can help you lose weight as it is unrefined and unprocessed. It contains a significant percentage of mono-saturated fatty acids that play an essential role in losing weight. Olive oil is also rich in vitamin E, which is good for hair and skin health. It also has excellent anti-inflammatory properties. Olive oil helps lower the absorption of fat and thus makes your food healthy and tasty at the same time.

Parsley is a common herb that can be found in every kitchen. The leaves are rich in important compounds such as vitamin A, vitamin B, vitamin C, and vitamin K. Important minerals such as potassium and iron can also be found in parsley. As it acts as a natural form of diuretic, it can help flush out toxins and any excess fluids. Parsley is rich in chlorophyll, and it can effectively aid weight. It also helps in keeping the levels of blood sugar under control. Parsley comes with certain enzymes that can help improve the process of digestion and aid in weight loss.

Endives are low-calorie and rich in fiber that can help slow down digestion and keep the energy level stable, a great combination of elements that can help promote weight loss. Thanks to their water and fiber content, you will be able to consume more volume of food without the risk of consuming extra calories. It is rich in potassium and folate as well, which are essential for proper heart health. Potassium is effective at lowering blood pressure.

Red onion is rich in an antioxidant named quercetin. Red onions can help add extra flavor to your food without piling on extra calories. Quercetin helps promote the burning of extra calories. It can also help in dealing with inflammation. Red onion is rich in fiber and can make you feel full for an extended period without the urge to consume extra calories. It can also help in improving blood sugar levels and in the maintenance of type II diabetes.

Red wine, in moderation, can help you shed extra pounds. Red wine contains a polyphenol named resveratrol that can aid in losing weight. This polyphenol can help convert white fat, the larger cells that store energy, into brown fat that can help fight obesity. It can also reduce the risk of a heart attack. In fact, serious problems like Alzheimer's disease and dementia can also be reduced by consuming two glasses of red wine daily. Red wine can also prevent the development of type II diabetes.

Soy can help in reducing your body weight thanks to its essential amino acids. It is rich in fiber that can help you to stay full for a long time. Soy can also help regulate blood sugar levels and appetite control. It can also promote better quality skin, hair, and nails, besides its weight loss benefits.

Strawberries are filled with fiber, vitamins, and polyphenols and have zero cholesterol and zero fat. They are also a great source of magnesium, potassium, and vitamin C. The high fiber content also assists in losing weight. It can help you stay full, which will reduce the chances of overeating or snacking. One hundred grams of strawberries comes with only 33 calories. Strawberries also help improve digestion and can even eliminate toxins from the body.

Turmeric is one of the primary spices in every household. It comes with an essential antioxidant called curcumin. It helps in dealing with obesity, disorders related to the stomach, and other health problems. It can help reduce inflammation linked to obesity. Remember to add some pepper when using turmeric: the absorption of curcumin will be higher.

Walnuts are rich in healthy fats and fiber that can aid in weight loss. They can provide you with a great deal of energy as well. They contain high quantities of PUFAs or polyunsaturated fats that can help keep cholesterol levels under check. At the same time, alpha-linolenic acid helps in burning body fat quickly and promotes proper heart health.

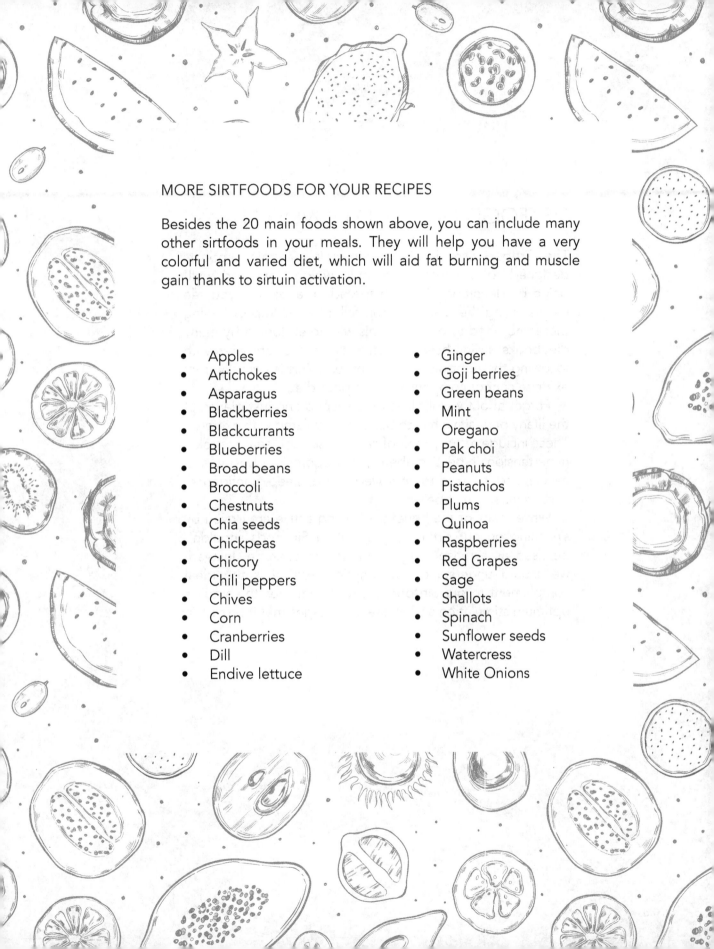

MORE SIRTFOODS FOR YOUR RECIPES

Besides the 20 main foods shown above, you can include many other sirtfoods in your meals. They will help you have a very colorful and varied diet, which will aid fat burning and muscle gain thanks to sirtuin activation.

- Apples
- Artichokes
- Asparagus
- Blackberries
- Blackcurrants
- Blueberries
- Broad beans
- Broccoli
- Chestnuts
- Chia seeds
- Chickpeas
- Chicory
- Chili peppers
- Chives
- Corn
- Cranberries
- Dill
- Endive lettuce
- Ginger
- Goji berries
- Green beans
- Mint
- Oregano
- Pak choi
- Peanuts
- Pistachios
- Plums
- Quinoa
- Raspberries
- Red Grapes
- Sage
- Shallots
- Spinach
- Sunflower seeds
- Watercress
- White Onions

SIRTFOOD DIET AND MOVEMENT

The Sirtfood Diet is about consuming certain products designed to promote sustainable weight loss and well-being by definition. But with the advantages that you see by practicing the plan, you can fall into the trap of feeling there's no need to exercise. This will be endorsed by many diet books, saying how ineffective exercise is compared with following the right diet for weight loss. This is partially true; exercise cannot compensate for a poor diet.

Forget about weight loss for a second and just glance at the litany of positive health benefits correlated with exercise. These include reduced risk of cardiovascular disease, stroke, hypertension, type 2 diabetes, osteoporosis, obesity, and cancer, and is linked to improved mood, sleep, confidence, and a sense of well-being.

While many of the benefits of being active are driven by switching on our sirtuin genes, eating Sirtfoods shouldn't be used as a reason to not engage in exercise. Instead, we should understand how physical activity is the ideal complement to our Sirtfood intake. It activates the sirtuin's optimum stimulation and all the advantages that it provides.

EXERCISE DURING PHASE 1

During phase 1, caloric intake is restricted to 1,000 calories. During this week, and this week only, you may decide to avoid exercise if you don't feel like it. It's up to you. If you are already used to training, you may want to keep going, maybe with less intensity. If you have never trained before, the suggestion is to listen to your body.

Remember that there's no need to climb a mountain during phase 1. A brisk walk will be ok, which should be suitable for everyone.

EXERCISE DURING PHASE 2 AND 3

During phases 2 and 3, you will gradually return to a regular calorie intake, and you should feel a lot more energized so, why not put the excess energy to good use?

Plenty of athletes have tried this diet, so you can easily conclude that it works perfectly fine with training and working out. To maximize the fat-burning effect, exercise while dieting is important, but it is up to you how intensely you want to train.

SUGGESTED EFFORT AND BASIC HEALTHY HABITS

It's essential to meet the 150-minute (2 hours and 30 minutes) government guidelines of moderate physical activity a week. A moderate job is the equivalent of a brisk walk.

But you don't have to be limited to this. Any sport or physical activity you love is fitting. Pleasure and exercise do not have to be mutually exclusive! The social aspect of group sports increases their enjoyment even more.

It's also about everyday changes like taking your bike instead of the car, getting off the bus one stop earlier, or just parking farther away to increase the distance you will walk.

Take the stairs and not the elevator.

Go outdoors and garden. Play in the park with your kids or get more out with the dog. Everything counts.

Everything that has you up and moving at a moderate intensity will regularly activate your sirtuin genes, enhancing the benefits of the Sirtfood Diet.

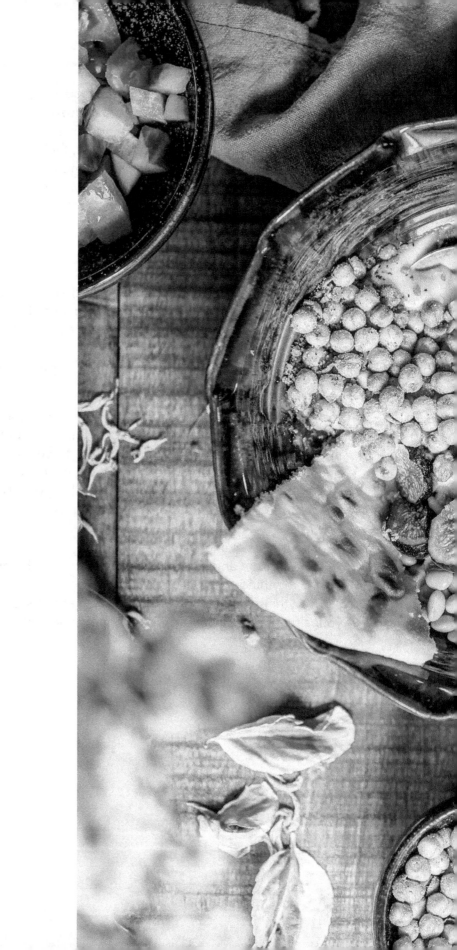

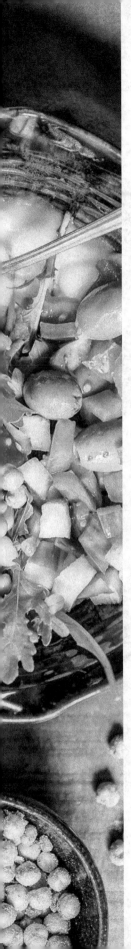

CONCLUSION

Thank you for making it to the end!

As you have now learned from this book, the key to a successful result is obtaining a perfect balance with a sustainable diet and providing all the nutrients we need that enhance our health. It's about continuing to reap the Sirtfood Diet's weight-loss rewards using the very best foods nature has to offer while getting pleasure and enjoyment from meals that include the highest range of sirtuin-activating items possible and our favorite foods. Keep following the simple rules in this book to maintain your results and live a healthy, happy life!

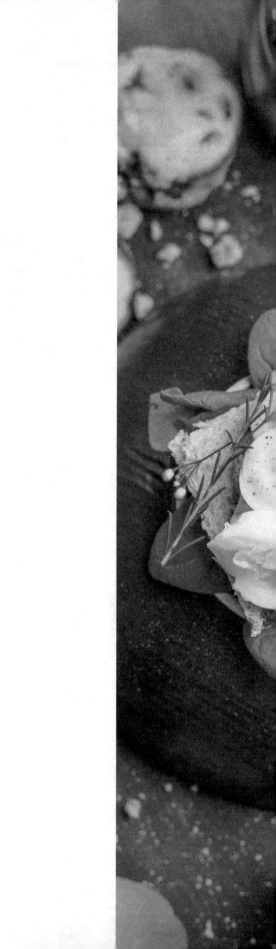

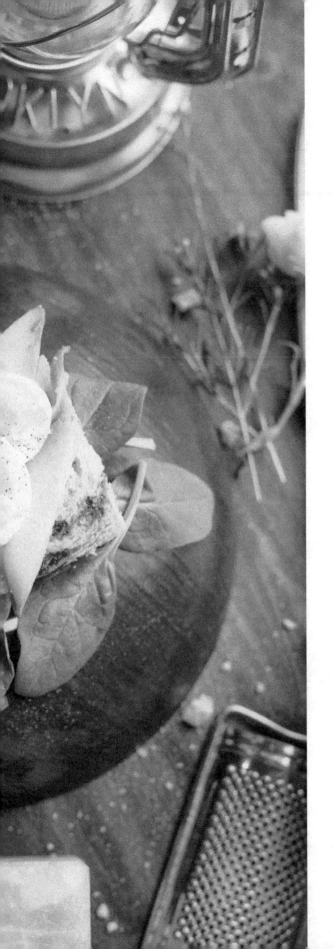

APPENDICES

APPENDIX A

SIRTFOOD RECIPE IDEAS

BREAKFAST

SIRTFOOD GREEN JUICE

 1   5 mins

Ingredients:
  Recipe 1:
    1 tbsp. parsley
    1 stalk celery
    1 apple
    ½ lemon
  Recipe 2:
    1 cucumber
    1 stalk celery
    1 apple
    3 mint leaves

Directions:
Choose one of the recipes.

Add all ingredients into a juicer and extract the juice according to the manufacturer's method.

In case you don't have one, add all the ingredients in a blender and pulse until well combined.

Filter the juice through a fine-mesh strainer and transfer it into a glass. Top with water if needed. Serve immediately.

NUTRITION FACTS: CALORIES 30KCAL FAT 0.4 G CARBOHYDRATE 4.5 G PROTEIN 1 G

CHOCOLATE DESSERT WITH DATES AND WALNUTS

 2   🕐 25 mins

Ingredients:
4 Medjool dates, pitted
2 tbsp. cocoa powder
I cup milk, skimmed
I tsp. agar powder
I tbsp. peanut butter
I pinch of salt
½ tsp. cinnamon
2 walnuts
I tsp whole wheat flour

Directions:
Blitz dates, peanut butter, and I tbsp. milk in a food processor.

Put the mix in a pan; add cocoa, cinnamon, salt, flour, agar powder. Add the remaining hot milk bit by bit and mix well to obtain a smooth mixture.

Turn the heat on, bring to a boil and cook around 6-8 minutes until dense. Divide into 2 cups, let cool, and put in the fridge. Add chopped walnuts before serving.

NUTRITION FACTS: CALORIES 326KCAL FAT 3 G CARBOHYDRATE 7 G PROTEIN 25 G

PANCAKES WITH CARAMELIZED STRAWBERRIES

 2   🕐 20 mins

Ingredients:
I egg
I ½ oz. self-raising flour
I ½ oz. buckwheat flour
I/3 cup skimmed milk
I cup strawberries
2 tsp honey

Directions:
Mix the flours in a bowl; add the yolk and form a very thick batter. Keep adding the milk bit by bit to avoid lumps.

In another bowl, beat the egg white until stiff and then mix it carefully into the batter.

Pour enough batter to make a 5-inch round pancake and cook 2 minutes per side until done. Repeat until all the pancakes are ready.

Put strawberries and honey in a hot pan until caramelized, then put half of the strawberry and honey mixture on top of each pancake serving.

NUTRITION FACTS: CALORIES 272KCAL FAT 4.3 G CARBOHYDRATE 26.8 G PROTEIN 23.6 G

MATCHA OVERNIGHT OATS

 2   10 mins +
overnight rest

Ingredients:
2 tsp. chia seeds

3 oz. rolled oats

1 tsp. matcha powder

1 tsp honey

1 ½ cups almond milk

2 pinches ground cinnamon

1 apple, peeled, cored, and chopped

4 walnuts

NUTRITION FACTS: CALORIES 324KCAL
FAT 4 G CARBOHYDRATE 37 G PROTEIN
22 G

Directions:
Place the chia seeds and the oats in a container or bowl.

In a different jug or bowl, add the matcha powder and one tablespoon of almond milk and whisk with a hand-held mixer until you get a smooth paste, then add the rest of the milk and mix thoroughly.

Pour the milk mixture over the oats, add the honey and cinnamon, and then stir well. Cover the bowl with a lid and place in the fridge overnight.

When you want to eat, transfer the oats to two serving bowls, top with the walnuts and chopped apple.

SCRAMBLED EGGS
AND RED ONION

 1   4 mins

Ingredients:
2 eggs

1 tbsp. parmesan

Salt and pepper

½ cup red onion

1 tbsp. parsley, finely chopped

Directions:
Put eggs and cheese with a pinch of salt and pepper and finely chopped onion in a bowl. Whisk quickly.

Cook the scrambled eggs in a skillet for 2 minutes, stirring continuously until done.

NUTRITION FACTS: CALORIES 278KCAL FAT 5.4 G CARBOHYDRATE 12.8 G PROTEIN 18.9 G

WALNUT DATE BANANA BREAD

🍳 8   🕐 30 mins

Ingredients:
¾ cup whole-wheat flour
¼ cup buckwheat flour
1 tbsp. cinnamon
½ tbsp. salt
¼ tbsp. baking soda
2 medium, ripe bananas, mashed
2 eggs, gently beaten
½ cup granulated sugar
⅓ cup plain nonfat yogurt
2 tbsp. vegetable oil
1 tbsp. vanilla concentrate
2 tbsp. toasted pecans, chopped
½ cups walnuts, chopped
4 dates, chopped

Directions:
Mix flour with cinnamon, baking soda, and salt in a bowl. In another bowl, whisk together bananas, eggs, sugar, yogurt, oil, and vanilla. Add flour to a greased loaf baking pan and sprinkle walnuts and dates on top.

Heat the oven to 310°F, and cook 30 to 35 minutes. Always check with a stick if the bread is well cooked through (prick the bread with the stick, that has to stay dry).

Move bread to a wire rack to cool before cutting it.

NUTRITION FACTS: CALORIES 180KCAL FAT 6 G CARBOHYDRATE 29 G PROTEIN 4 G

LUNCH & DINNER RECIPES – MAIN COURSES

AIR FRIED CHICKEN WITH SALAD SPROUTS

 1 30 mins

Ingredients:

8 oz. chicken breasts
⅛ tbsp. salt
½ tbsp. pepper,
1 tbsp. extra-virgin olive oil
1 tbsp. maple syrup
1 tbsp. Dijon mustard
6 oz. Brussels sprouts
1 garlic clove, crushed
1 handful parsley, chopped

Directions:

Spray the chicken breast with cooking spray; sprinkle with salt and 1/4 tbsp. of the pepper.

Whisk together oil, maple syrup, mustard, and 1/4 tbsp. pepper in a bowl. Add Brussels sprouts; toss to cover.

Put the chicken breast on one side of a pan, and add Brussels sprouts on the other.

Heat the oven (or air fryer) to 400°F and cook until the chicken is well colored and cooked through (15 to 18 minutes).

NUTRITION FACTS: CALORIES 337KCAL FAT 7 G CARBOHYDRATE 21 G PROTEIN 25 G

AROMATIC CURRY

 4   🕐 40 mins

Ingredients:

19 oz. garbanzo beans
2 cup vegetable broth
10 oz. spinach
7 garlic cloves, diced
3 red onions, diced
2 carrots, chopped
2 tsp. ground cumin
1 handful parsley, chopped
1 tsp. turmeric
1 tbsp. paprika
2 tsp. salt
1 tsp. ground black pepper
2 chili peppers, chopped
1/4 tsp. ginger, grated
1 yellow bell pepper, chopped
3 tbsp. extra-virgin olive oil
2/3 cup coconut milk
½ cup slivered almonds
½ cup golden raisins
2 cups cooked rice

Directions:

In a saucepan, add the spinach and cook on low heat, allowing it to thaw. Sautè garlic, onions, chili peppers in another pan with oil on medium.

Add the carrots and cook for 4 to 6 minutes, until the onions are golden brown.

Add the raisins, garbanzo beans, cumin, turmeric, ginger, paprika, and parsley and cook for 2 minutes.

Add the spinach, bell pepper, broth, and coconut milk, reduce heat to low, and simmer, covered, for 30 minutes.

Serve hot with rice.

NUTRITION FACTS: CALORIES 316KCAL FAT 5.2 G CARBOHYDRATE 13.1 G PROTEIN 6.9 G

ASIAN CHICKEN DRUMSTICKS

🍳 2   🕐 36 mins

Ingredients:
6 chicken drumsticks
¼ cup rice vinegar
3 tbsp. agave syrup
2 tbsp. chicken stock
1 tbsp. lower-sodium soy sauce
1 tbsp. sesame oil
1 tbsp. tomato paste
1 garlic clove, crushed
2 tbsp. walnuts, chopped
½ tsp. turmeric

Directions:
Put the chicken in a single layer in the oven and cook at 400°F until the skin is crispy (around 25 to 28 minutes), turning drumsticks over partway through cooking.

In the meantime, mix vinegar, stock, agave, soy sauce, oil, tomato paste, and garlic in a skillet.

Bring to a boil over medium-high. Cook for about 6 minutes until thickened.

Put the drumsticks and sauce in a bowl and toss to cover. Sprinkle with walnuts.

NUTRITION FACTS: CALORIES 388KCAL FAT 10 G CARBOHYDRATES 20 G PROTEIN 25 G

CHICKEN KOFTE WITH ZUCCHINI

 4   🕐 52 mins

Ingredients:
½ cup low-fat Greek yogurt
2 tbsp. black olives, pitted and chopped
1 handful parsley, chopped
¼ cup breadcrumbs
½ red onion, cubed
1 tbsp. ground cumin
⅛ tbsp. chili flakes
1-pound ground chicken
4 tbsp. olive oil
4 zucchini, sliced

Directions:
Mix yogurt, black olives, parsley, breadcrumbs, onion, 1/2 tbsp. salt, and 1/4 tbsp. pepper in a bowl, mixing with a whisk.

Add chicken; blend in with hands. Shape chicken mixture into 8 patties. Heat 2 tbsp. olive oil in a skillet over medium heat. Add patties; cook 4 minutes on each side or until done.

While kofte cooks, cook zucchini on a skillet. Brush them with 2 tbsp oil and season with the remaining pepper.

Cook on high heat for 5 minutes, then season with salt. Serve 2 kofte per person with zucchini on the side.

NUTRITION FACTS: CALORIES 301KCAL FAT 6.9 G CARBOHYDRATE 15 G PROTEIN 24 G

SIRT CHICKEN SOUVLAKI

 4   🕐 30mins

Ingredients:
2 cups plain yogurt
1 cucumber, cut lengthwise
1 ¼ tbsp. salt
1 clove garlic, crushed
¼ tbsp. dill
2 tbsp. extra-virgin olive oil
1 ½ tbsp. lemon juice
1 tbsp. oregano
1 ⅓ lb. chicken breasts, cubed
4 whole-wheat pitas
1 tbsp. capers
1 red onion, cut into wedges
2 tomatoes, cut into wedges
⅓ cup black olives, pitted

Directions:
Put the yogurt in a strainer lined with cheesecloth and set it over a bowl to drain some liquid. In a colander, add the cucumber with 1 tbsp. of salt; let sit for around 15 minutes.

Squeeze the cucumber and finely chop it. Put it in a bowl and add the yogurt, garlic, 1/8 tbsp. of pepper, and dill.

Warm the grill. Combine the oil, lemon juice, oregano, 1/4 tbsp. of salt, and 1/4 tbsp. of pepper.

Toss the chicken cubes in the oil blend and thread them onto skewers. Grill the chicken over high heat, turning once until done, about 10 to 12 minutes.

Grill the pitas for 1 minute per side, cut them in half. Put them on serving dishes and top them with the onion, tomatoes, and chicken skewers.

Serve with the yogurt sauce and olives on the side.

NUTRITION FACTS: CALORIES 356KCAL FAT 9 G CARBOHYDRATE 25 G PROTEIN 14 G

CHIPOTLE CITRUS-GLAZED TURKEY TENDERLOINS

🍳 4   🕐 25 mins

Ingredients:

4 5 oz. turkey breast tenderloins
¼ tsp. salt
¼ tsp. pepper
1 tbsp. extra-virgin olive oil
1 garlic clove, crushed
¾ cup orange juice
¼ cup lime juice
1 tsp. agave syrup
1 Bird's eye chili
2 tsp. minced chipotle peppers
2 tbsp. parsley, chopped

Directions:

Season turkey with salt and pepper. Cook it in a skillet with ½ tbsp. oil over high heat.

Meanwhile, in a bowl, whisk the orange juice, lime juice, agave, ½ tbsp. oil, chipotle, and chili.

Add the sauce to the skillet. Reduce heat and simmer for 14 to 16 minutes. Transfer turkey to a cutting board; let rest for 5 minutes.

Simmer glaze until thickened, about 3 minutes. Slice the turkey, top with parsley, and serve with glaze.

NUTRITION FACTS: CALORIES 294KCAL FAT 6 G CARBOHYDRATE 9 G PROTEIN 30 G

COCONUT SHRIMP

🍳 2   🕐 30 mins

Ingredients:

½ cup buckwheat flour
1 ½ tbsp. pepper
2 eggs
⅔ cup dried coconut, shredded
⅓ cup panko (Japanese-style breadcrumbs)
12 oz. deveined shrimp, tail-on
½ tbsp. salt
¼ cup agave syrup
¼ cup lime juice
1 Bird's eye chili
2 tbsp. parsley, chopped

Directions:

Mix flour and pepper in a shallow dish. Gently beat eggs in another dish and mix coconut and panko in a third one.

Holding each shrimp by the tail, dip them in flour, paing attention to not cover the tail; shake off excess. Dunk in egg, allowing any excess to trickle off.

Dip in coconut blend and coat well. Put the shrimp in oven, and cook at 400°F until golden, 5 to 6 minutes, turning them over halfway through cooking. season with 1/4 tbsp. of the salt.

While shrimp cook, whisk together nectar, lime juice, and serrano chile in a bowl. Sprinkle shrimp with parsley. Serve with sauce.

NUTRITION FACTS: CALORIES 250KCAL FAT 6 G CARBOHYDRATE 20 G PROTEIN 15 G

GARLIC CHICKEN BURGERS

 2 🕐 20 mins

Ingredients:
10 oz. chicken mince
¼ red onion, finely chopped
1 clove garlic, crushed
1 handful of parsley, finely chopped
1 cup arugula
½ orange, chopped
1 cup cherry tomatoes
3 tsp extra-virgin olive oil

Directions:
Put chicken mince, onion, garlic, parsley, salt, and pepper to taste in a bowl and mix well.

Form 2 patties and let rest 5 minutes. Heat a pan with olive oil, and when very hot, cook 3 minutes per side.

Put the arugula on two plates; add cherry tomatoes and orange, dress with salt and the remaining olive oil. Put the patties on top and serve.

These patties are delicious also when grilled. If you opt for grilling, just brush them with a bit of extra-virgin olive oil right before cooking.

NUTRITION FACTS: CALORIES 253KCAL FAT 4.8 G CARBOHYDRATE 8.1 G PROTEIN 28.3 G

LIME-PARSLEY COD

 4 🕐 15 mins

Ingredients:
4 6-oz. cod fillets
½ tsp. salt
¼ tsp. pepper
3 tbsp. extra-virgin olive oil
1 cup arugula
2 tbsp. parsley, chopped
1 tbsp. lime juice
1 tsp. lime zest

Directions:
Preheat oven to 375°F. Mix the salt, pepper, 2 tsp. olive oil, lime juice, and zest in a bowl and whisk.

Put the cod fillets on a baking dish greased with cooking spray or one drop of extra virgin olive oil.

Pour the sauce over the fish and cook 6 to 8 minutes until done. Top with parsley.

Serve with a simple side of arugula seasoned with salt, pepper, and 1 tbsp. olive oil.

NUTRITION FACTS: CALORIES 245KCAL FAT 3 G CARBOHYDRATE 5 G PROTEIN 28 G

HERBS AND CHEESE BURGERS

🍳 4   🕐 25 mins

Ingredients:

2 green onions, chopped
½ red onion, chopped
2 tbsp. parsley, chopped
4 tbsp. Dijon mustard
3 tbsp. breadcrumbs
½ tbsp. salt
½ tbsp. rosemary
¼ tbsp. sage
1 lb. lean mincemeat
2 oz. cheddar, shredded
4 buckwheat burger buns

Directions:

Preheat oven to 375°F. In a bowl, mix green onions, parsley, and 2 tbsp. mustard. In another bowl, mix breadcrumbs, red onion, sage, rosemary, and remaining 2 tbsp. mustard.

Add mincemeat and mix well using a fork or the hands. Shape into 8 patties. T

ake one patty, put a tsp. of cheddar, and a tsp. of green onion blend.

Top with another patty, and gently squeeze edges together to seal them well.

Place burgers in a baking dish and cook 6 to 8 minutes.

Serve burgers with buns, topped with arugula.

NUTRITION FACTS: CALORIES 369KCAL FAT 14 G CARBOHYDRATE 29 G PROTEIN 29 G

ITALIAN-STYLE MEATBALLS

🍳 4   🕐 45 mins

Ingredients:

2 tbsp. extra-virgin olive oil
1 medium shallot
3 cloves garlic, crushed
2-inch celery, finely diced
¼ cup buckwheat breadcrumb
2 tbsp. milk
10 oz. lean mincemeat
10 oz. turkey mincemeat
1 egg
¼ cup parsley, chopped
1 tbsp. rosemary
1 tbsp. thyme
1 tbsp. Dijon mustard

Directions:

Preheat Oven to 400°F.

Heat oil in a skillet over medium-high. Add shallot and cook until soft, about 2 minutes. Add garlic and cook 1 minute. Remove from heat. In a bowl, mix breadcrumb and milk. Add shallot and garlic, mincemeat, egg, parsley, rosemary, thyme, mustard, and salt. Mix.

Gently shape blend into small balls and put them on a tray in a single layer. Cook at 400°F until caramelized and cooked through, about 15 to 18 minutes.

Serve hot.

NUTRITION FACTS: CALORIES 322KCAL   FAT 8 G   CARBOHYDRATE 5 G   PROTEIN 17 G

KALE OMELETTE

⊙ 1   🕐 10 mins

Ingredients:
2 eggs
1 small clove garlic
2 handfuls kale
1 oz. goat cheese
¼ cup sliced onion
2 teaspoons extra virgin olive oil

Directions:
Mince the garlic and finely shred the kale. Break the eggs into a bowl, add a pinch of salt. Beat until well combined.

Place a pan over medium heat. Add 1 teaspoon of olive oil, add the onion and kale, cook for approx. 5 minutes, or until the onion has softened and the kale is wilted.

Add the garlic and cook for another 2 minutes.

Add 1 teaspoon of olive oil into the egg mixture, mix and add into the pan. Use your spatula to move the cooked egg toward the center and move the pan so that the uncooked egg mixture goes towards the edges.

Add the cheese into the pan just before the egg is fully cooked, then leave for 1 minute.

Serve immediately.

NUTRITION FACTS: CALORIES 219KCAL FAT 8 G CARBOHYDRATE 7.7 G PROTEIN 12 G

LEMON-FENNEL SPICY COD

🍳 4   🕐 15 mins

Ingredients:
1 tbsp. ground coriander
3 tbsp. extra-virgin olive oil
2 garlic cloves, crushed
4 6-ounce cod fillets
2 cups fennel, finely sliced
1/4 cup red onion, chopped
2 tbsp. lemon juice
1 tbsp. parsley, chopped
1 tbsp. thyme leaves, chopped

Directions:
Combine coriander, 2 tbsp. oil, garlic, salt, and pepper to taste in a bowl. Rub garlic blend over the cod fillets.

Warm a skillet over medium-high heat. Add the cod and cook for 5 to 6 minutes on each side. In the meantime, add fennel, onion, lemon juice, 1 tbsp.oil, thyme, and parsley in a bowl, tossing to cover.

Serve a plate of fennel salad with a cod fillet on top.

NUTRITION FACTS: CALORIES 259KCAL FAT 9.7 G CARBOHYDRATE 5.3 G PROTEIN 18 G

RED ONION FRITTATA WITH CHILI GRILLED ZUCCHINI

🍳 2   🕐 35 mins

Ingredients:
1 ½ cups red onion, finely sliced
3 eggs
3 oz. cheddar cheese
2 tbsp. milk
2 zucchini
2 tbsp. oil
1 clove garlic, crushed
½ chili, finely sliced
1 tsp. white vinegar
Salt and pepper to taste

Directions:
Heat the oven to 350°F. Cut the zucchini into thin slices, grill them, and set them aside.

Add 3 eggs, shredded cheddar cheese, milk, salt, and pepper. Whisk well and pour in a silicone baking tray and cook 25-30 minutes in the oven. Mix garlic, oil, salt, pepper, and vinegar and pour the dressing on the zucchini. Serve the frittata alongside the zucchini.

NUTRITION FACTS: CALORIES 229KCAL FAT 7.8 G CARBOHYDRATE 8.1 G PROTEIN 21.3 G

MINCE STUFFED EGGPLANTS

 6   50 mins

Ingredients:
8 oz. lean mincemeat
6 large eggplants
1 egg
3 tbsp. dry red wine
½ cup cheddar, grated
Salt and pepper, to taste
1 red onion
2 tsp. olive oil
2 tbsp. tomato sauce
2 tbsp. parsley

Directions:
Preheat oven to 350°F. Meanwhile, slice eggplants in half and scoop out the center part, leaving ½'' of meat. Place eggplants in a microwavable dish with about ½'' of water in the bottom.

Microwave on high for 4 minutes. In a saucepan, fry mince with onion for 5 minutes. Add wine and let evaporate. Add tomato sauce, salt, pepper, eggplant meat, and cook for 20 minutes

Combine mince sauce, cheese, egg, parsley, salt, and pepper in a large bowl and mix well. Pack firmly into eggplants.

Return eggplants to the dish you first microwaved them in and bake for 25 to 30 minutes, or until lightly browned on top.

NUTRITION FACTS: CALORIES 350KCAL FAT 10 G CARBOHYDRATE 22 G PROTEIN 17 G

MUSTARD SALMON WITH
BABY CARROTS

2   50 mins

Ingredients:
12 oz. salmon fillet
2 tbsp. mustard
1 tbsp. white vinegar
1 tsp parsley, finely chopped
2 cups baby carrots
4 oz. buckwheat
2 tsp. extra virgin olive oil
Salt and pepper to taste

Directions:
Heat the oven to 400°F.
Boil the buckwheat in salted water for 25 minutes then drain. Dress with 1 tsp olive oil. Set aside.
Put the salmon over aluminum foil.
Mix mustard and vinegar in a small bowl and brush the mixture over the salmon, close the foil in a packet. Cook in the oven 35minutes.
While the salmon is cooking, steam baby carrots for 6 minutes then put them in a pan on medium heat with 1tsp. olive oil, salt and pepper until light brown.
Serve the salmon with baby carrots and buckwheat on the side.

NUTRITION FACTS: CALORIES 357KCAL FAT 9.1 G CARBOHYDRATE 8 G PROTEIN 26 G

ROASTED SALMON
WITH FENNEL SALAD

 4   25mins

Ingredients:
2 tbsp. parsley
1 tbsp. thyme
1 tbsp. genuine salt,
4 6-oz. skinless salmon fillets
2 tbsp. extra-virgin olive oil
4 cups fennel, finely sliced
2/3 cup low-fat Greek yogurt
1 garlic clove, crushed
2 tbsp. orange juice
1 tbsp. lemon juice
2 tbsp. dill
½ tsp. turmeric

Directions:
Preheat oven to 200°F.
Mix parsley, thyme, and 1/2 tbsp. of the salt in a little bowl. Brush salmon with oil; sprinkle equally with herb blend.
Put salmon fillets in an oven-proof skillet, and cook at 350°F until desired doneness level, 10 minutes.
While salmon cooks, toss together fennel, yogurt, garlic, squeezed orange, lemon juice, dill, and 1/2 tbsp. salt in a medium bowl. Serve salmon ts over the fennel plate of mixed greens.

NUTRITION FACTS: CALORIES 364KCAL FAT 9 G CARBOHYDRATE 9 G PROTEIN 27 G

SALMON FRITTERS

 2   🕐 20 mins

Ingredients:

6 oz. salmon, canned
1 tbsp. flour
1 clove garlic, crushed
½ red onion, finely chopped
2 eggs
2 tsp. olive oil
Salt and pepper to taste
2 cups arugula

Directions:

Separate egg whites from yolks and beat them until very stiff. In a separate bowl, mix salmon, flour, salt, pepper, onion, garlic, and yolks.

Add egg whites and mix slowly. Heat a pan on medium-high. Add 1 tsp. oil and, when hot, form salmon fritters with a spoon.

Cook until brown (around 4 minutes per side) and serve with arugula salad seasoned with salt, pepper, and 1 tsp. olive oil.

NUTRITION FACTS: CALORIES 320KCAL FAT 7 G CARBOHYDRATE 18 G PROTEIN 27 G

SPICY CHICKEN BREASTS

 8   🕐 25 mins + 1h

Ingredients:

2 cups buttermilk
2 tbsp. Dijon mustard
1 pinch of salt
2 tbsp. hot pepper sauce
1-1/2 tbsp. garlic powder
8 chicken breast, skinless
2 cups buckwheat breadcrumbs
2 tbsp. extra-virgin olive oil
1/2 tbsp. paprika
1 pinch chili flakes
1/4 tbsp. dried oregano
1/4 tbsp. dried parsley
2 tsp. capers, finely chopped

Directions:

Preheat oven to 375°F. Marinate the chicken in buttermilk with mustard and hot sauce for at least 1 hour.

Drain the chicken. Mix garlic, salt, paprika, chili flakes, oregano, parsley, and capers with breadcrumbs and coat the chicken.

Put the chicken on a tray in a single layer. Cook for 18 to 20 minutes, turning one time halfway.

Serve hot.

NUTRITION FACTS: CALORIES 352KCAL FAT 9 G CARBOHYDRATE 11 G PROTEIN 24 G

SHRIMP SPRING ROLLS

 4   35 mins

Ingredients:
1 tbsp. sesame oil
1 tbsp. extra-virgin olive oil
½ cup cabbage, shredded
½ cup carrots
½ red pepper
½ red onion
4 oz. shrimp, finely chopped
½ cup snow peas
1/4 cup parsley, chopped
1 tbsp. lime juice
2 tbsp. fish sauce
16 (8-inch-square) phyllo batter sheets

Directions:
Cut carrots into matchsticks and finely chop snow peas, red pepper, and onion. Warm oil in a skillet over high heat.

Add cabbage, carrots, onion, snow peas, and red pepper; cook for 3 minutes. Let cool for 5 minutes. Put cabbage blend, shrimp, parsley, lime juice, fish sauce; toss to combine. Preheat the oven to 400°F.

Put one phyllo sheet on a work surface, lightly damp it with one drop of water, and cover with a second sheet.

Put 1/8 of the filling on one side, then roll the sheets to form a spring roll. Cook the spring rolls until golden, 6 to 7 minutes, turning them after 4 minutes.

NUTRITION FACTS: CALORIES 280KCAL   FAT 9 G   CARBOHYDRATE 19 G   PROTEIN 7 G

SOUTHERN STYLE CATFISH WITH GREEN BEANS

🍳 2   🕐 35 mins

Ingredients:

2 6-oz. catfish fillets
¼ cup flour
1 egg
½ cup buckwheat breadcrumbs
¼ tbsp. pepper
12 oz. green beans
2 tbsp. mayonnaise
1 ½ tbsp. dill
¾ tbsp. dill pickle relish
½ tsp. red wine vinegar
1 tsp agave syrup
1 tbsp. extra-virgin olive oil

Directions:

Steam green beans for 20 minutes. In the meantime prepare flour, egg, and breadcrumbs on three different plates.

Briefly whisk the egg; then first, coat catfish in flour, shaking excess. Then dip one piece of fish at a time in the egg and cover with breadcrumbs on all sides.

Place fish on a baking tray, drizzle olive oil on top, and cook at 400°F for 10 to 12 minutes, until crispy.

While the fish is cooking, whisk mayonnaise, dill, relish, vinegar, and agave in a bowl to form a sauce.

Serve the catfish and green beans with sauce.

NUTRITION FACTS: CALORIES 316KCAL FAT 8 G CARBOHYDRATE 11 G PROTEIN 33 G

TURMERIC COUS COUS WITH EDAMAME BEANS

🍲 2   🕐 25 mins

Ingredients:

½ yellow pepper, cubed
½ red pepper, cubed
1 tbsp. turmeric
½ cup red onion, finely sliced
¼ cup cherry tomatoes, chopped
2 tbsp. parsley, finely chopped
5 oz. couscous
2 tsp. extra virgin olive oil
½ eggplant
1 ½ cup edamame beans

Directions:

Steam edamame for 5 minutes and set aside. Add 6 oz. salted boiling water to couscous and let rest until it absorbs the water.

In the meantime, heat a pan on medium-high heat. Add oil, eggplant, peppers, onion, tomatoes, turmeric, salt, and pepper.

Cook for 5 minutes on high heat. Add the couscous and edamame.

Garnish with fresh parsley and serve.

NUTRITION FACTS: CALORIES 342KCAL FAT 5 G CARBOHYDRATE 15 G PROTEIN 32 G

TURMERIC TURKEY BREAST WITH CAULIFLOWER RICE

🍲 2   🕐 25 mins

Ingredients:

2 cups cauliflower, grated
8 oz. turkey breast, cut into slices
2 tsp. ground turmeric
1/2 pepper, chopped
1/2 red onion, sliced
2 tsp. extra virgin olive oil
1 large tomato
1 clove garlic, crushed
1 cup milk, skimmed
2 tsp. buckwheat flour
1 oz. parsley, finely chopped

Directions:

Coat turkey slices with flour. Heat a pan on medium-high with half the oil, and when hot, add the turkey.

Let the meat color on all sides, then add milk, salt, pepper, 1 tsp. turmeric. Cook 10 minutes until the turkey is soft, and the sauce has become creamy.

Warm another pan with the remaining oil over medium heat.. Add pepper, onion, and tomato, 1 tsp. turmeric, and let cook 3 minutes. Add the cauliflower and cook another 2 minutes. Add salt and pepper to taste. Let rest 2 minutes.

Serve the turkey with the cauliflower rice.

NUTRITION FACTS: CALORIES 187KCAL FAT 2.9 G CARBOHYDRATE 10.6 G PROTEIN 12.1 G

ASIAN NOODLE SOUP

🍲 2   🕐 30 mins

Ingredients:
2 cups vegetable broth
1 egg
2 cups of spinach
1 cup zucchini, chopped
6 oz. shrimp
6 oz. chicken breast
2 oz. bean sprouts
1 stalk celery, chopped
1 packet of Konjak noodles
1 tbsp. soy sauce
1 tbsp. fish sauce
1 handful fresh parsley
1-inch ginger, peel and chopped

Directions:
Boil the egg for 7 minutes, then drain it and cool it under running water.

Cook the shrimp and chicken in the broth with the spices and chopped vegetables for 15 minutes.

Wash the noodles under running water, add them to the soup and let them warm for 2 minutes.

Put the soup in a bowl, top with half egg, bean sprouts, and parsley, and serve.

NUTRITION FACTS: CALORIES 264KCAL FAT 6 G CARBOHYDRATE 19 G PROTEIN 8 G

ASPARAGUS CREAM SOUP

🍽 2   🕐 25 mins

Ingredients:
2 cups asparagus
3 cups vegetable broth
2 tbsp. extra-virgin olive oil
2 tbsp. flour
1 egg yolk
2 tbsp. cream
1 handful parsley, chopped

Directions:
Chop the asparagus. Boil the asparagus for 15 minutes in salted water. Drain them and add them back to the pot. In a pan, heat 1 tbsp. extra-virgin olive oil, add the flour, and ½ cup broth.

Whisk in the egg yolks and the cream. Add it to the pot with asparagus and the remaining broth, add the parsley and blend with a hand blender for 2 to 3 minutes until very smooth.

Divide into 2 plates, add the remaining extra-virgin olive oil on top and serve.

NUTRITION FACTS: CALORIES 253KCAL FAT 5 G CARBOHYDRATE 19 G PROTEIN 12 G

BROCCOLI AND WALNUT SOUP

 6   🕐 40 mins

Ingredients:
2 cups broccoli
½ cup walnuts
4 cups vegetable stock
2 tbsp. cream
Fresh nutmeg
1 chili, chopped

Directions:
Cut the broccoli into florets, and then boil them in vegetable stock for 8 to 10 minutes.

Blend the walnuts in a blender, then add the broccoli and broth and blend again for 2 to 3 minutes. Season it with salt and pepper to taste, nutmeg and chili, and quickly blend again.
Serve.

NUTRITION FACTS: CALORIES 264KCAL FAT 8 G CARBOHYDRATE 17 G PROTEIN 9 G

BROCCOLI, CHEDDAR AND CHICKEN SOUP 4 *39 mins*

Ingredients:

3 tbsp. extra-virgin olive oil
1 cup red onion, diced
1 cup celery, diced
½ cup flour
1 tsp. mustard
¼ tsp. salt
¼ tsp. ground pepper
4 cups chicken stock
1 cup milk
3 cups broccoli
2 cups potatoes, diced
1 lb. chicken breast, diced
1 cup cheddar, shredded

Directions:

Heat oil in a pan over medium heat. Add onion and celery, and cook 5 minutes until the onion becomes transparent.

Sprinkle flour, mustard, salt, and pepper over the vegetables and cook, for 2 minutes. Add the stock and milk; bring to a boil and add the chicken, broccoli, and potatoes.

Cook until the potatoes are soft and the chicken is done, about 12 to 14 minutes.

Add the cheddar, let melt for 2 minutes and serve.

NUTRITION FACTS: CALORIES 3144CAL FAT 3 G CARBOHYDRATE 19 G PROTEIN 21 G

CAULIFLOWER SOUP 4 30 mins

Ingredients:

2 cups cauliflower
3 oz. bacon
1 tsp. extra-virgin olive oil
2 tbsp. parmesan, grated
3 cups vegetable broth
1 pinch nutmeg
1 tbsp. capers

Directions:

Stew the cauliflower with a little water for 18 minutes.

Drain it, then blend it with warm broth until creamy. Season with nutmeg, capers., salt, and pepper to taste.

Fry the bacon in a pan. Serve the soup in a bowl, garnished with bacon, parmesan, and olive oil on top.

NUTRITION FACTS: CALORIES 289KCAL FAT 8 G CARBOHYDRATE 13 G PROTEIN 18 G

CAULIFLOWER AND
MUSHROOM SOUP

🍲 6   🕐 55 mins

Ingredients:

35 oz. chicken fillet
1 red onion
1 tbsp. olive oil
2 garlic cloves, crushed
6 sun-dried tomatoes
2 cups mushrooms, sliced
2 cups cauliflower
1 zucchini, chopped
½ cup green beans
1 cup kale, chopped
2 tbsp. red wine vinegar
1 bay leaf
1 handful parsley

Directions:

Boil the chicken in salted water with half onion and the bay leaf. Cook on low heat for 50 minutes, then remove the meat and shred it with a fork. Set aside.

While the chicken is cooking, heat the oil in a skillet, add the remaining half onion, finely chopped, garlic, sun-dried tomatoes, and mushrooms.

Add the broth, cauliflower, zucchini, and green beans and let it simmer for 15 minutes. Then add the leafy vegetables cut in pieces and let them cook for another 10 minutes.

Serve in bowls, adding the shredded chicken and parsley on top.

NUTRITION FACTS: CALORIES 236KCAL FAT 3 G CARBOHYDRATE 17 G PROTEIN 11 G

PEAR AND CELERY SOUP

🍲 6   🕐 35 mins

Ingredients:

5 cups finely chopped celery
4 onions, chopped
¼ cup chives
½ tsp. dried thyme
½ tsp. salt
¼ tsp. pepper
6 cups vegetable stock
3 ripe pears, peeled, cored, and chopped
½ cup 10% cream

Directions:

Heat extra-virgin olive oil in a saucepan.

Cook celery, onions, chives, thyme, salt, and pepper, covered and occasionally stirring, for about 10 minutes.

Pour in the stock and bring to boil. Reduce heat and simmer until the celery is tender, about 10 minutes.

Add pears; cook for 5 minutes or until pears are tender. Purée in a blender.

Return to saucepan; pour in cream and heat through without boiling.

Serve hot.

NUTRITION FACTS: CALORIES 116KCAL FAT 4 G CARBOHYDRATE 13 G PROTEIN 7 G

PUMPKIN SOUP WITH PUMPKIN SEEDS AND GINGER

🍲 4   🕐 25 mins

Ingredients:

3 cups pumpkin, chopped
2 carrots
1 shallot
1 red onion
1 ¼ in. ginger
3 cups water
2 tbsp. pumpkin seeds
1 tbsp. extra-virgin olive oil

Directions:

Peel and dice the carrots. Peel the shallot and finely chop it Sauté the shallot in a saucepan with oil.

Add the squash and carrots and sauté them for5 minutes. Pour boiling water and simmer over medium heat for 15 minutes.

Peel and grate the ginger. Add it to the soup, then blend it with a hand blender until smooth.

Season the soup with lime juice, salt, and pepper to taste. Top with pumpkin seeds and serve.

NUTRITION FACTS: CALORIES 127KCAL FAT 3 G CARBOHYDRATE 15 G PROTEIN 4 G

ROASTED CAULIFLOWER AND POTATO CURRY SOUP

 4   🕐 40 mins

Ingredients:

2 tsp. ground cumin
½ tsp. ground cinnamon
1 ½ tsp. turmeric
⅛ tsp. cayenne pepper
1 cauliflower, chopped into florets
2 tbsp. extra-virgin olive oil
1 red onion
1 cup carrot, chopped
3 cloves garlic, crushed
1 ½ tsp. ginger, grated
1 bird's eye chili, chopped
14 oz. tomato sauce
4 cups vegetable stock
1 potato, diced
1 sweet potato, diced
1 handful parsley, chopped

Directions:

Preheat the oven to 400°F. Mix parsley, cumin, cinnamon, turmeric, salt, pepper, and cayenne in a bowl.

Toss cauliflower with 1 tbsp. oil in a bowl, add the spices mix, and toss again to cover. Transfer the cauliflower to a baking dish and cook it in the oven until caramelized, about 15 to 20 minutes.

In the meantime, heat 1 tbsp.oil in a pot over medium-high heat. Add onion and carrot and cook for 5 minutes until they are both soft. Lower the heat, and add garlic, ginger, and chili.

Cook for 1 minute, then add the tomato sauce, stock, potato, and sweet potato. Bring to a boil and simmer for 20 minutes.

Mix in coconut milk and the cooked cauliflower and warm through. Trim with parsley and serve.

NUTRITION FACTS: CALORIES 120KCAL FAT 3 G CARBOHYDRATE 10 G PROTEIN 8 G

MEDITERRANEAN CHICKPEA SOUP

 6   2h + 5mins

Ingredients:
1 ½ cups dried chickpeas, soaked overnight
2 lbs. turkey breast
1 red onion, finely chopped
1 celery stalk, chopped
15 oz. tomatoes, diced
2 tbsp. tomato paste
4 cloves garlic
2 tsp. turmeric
1 tsp. sage
1 tsp. marjoram
14 oz. artichoke hearts
2 tbsp. extra-virgin olive oil
¼ cup parsley, chopped

Directions:
Drain chickpeas and put them in a pot. Add 6 cups of water, onion, tomatoes, tomato paste, garlic, turmeric. Bring to a boil.

Add the turkey and bring back to a boil, lower the heat, and cook, covered, for 75 minutes. Season with salt to taste, add artichokes, and cook for another 15 minutes.

The turkey should now be cooked. If so, remove it from the pot and set aside, if not keep cooking with the soup until done.

Chickpeas cook in about 2 hours. Shred the turkey with a fork and mix it back into the soup.

Sprinkle chopped parsley on top and serve.

NUTRITION FACTS: CALORIES 280KCAL FAT 3 G CARBOHYDRATE 26 G PROTEIN 23 G

SQUASH AND CORN SOUP

 4   50 mins

Ingredients:
3 tbsp. extra-virgin olive oil
1 cup red onion, diced
1 cup celery, diced
½ cup flour
1 ½ tsp. dried marjoram
4 cups vegetable broth
1 cup milk
3 cups summer squash, diced
2 cups red potatoes, diced
1 cup corn
¾ cup ham, diced

Directions:
Sautè the celery and onion in a skillet with oil for minutes until soft. Add flour and marjoram, season with salt and pepper to taste, and cook, mixing, for 2 minutes.

Add the broth and milk; bring to a boil, and squash, potatoes, and corn.

Stew, until the potatoes are tender, about 14 minutes.

Add ham, warm through and serve.

NUTRITION FACTS: CALORIES 285KCAL FAT 7 G CARBOHYDRATE 16 G PROTEIN 18 G

SALADS

CELERY AND RAISINS SNACK SALAD

 4   10 mins

Ingredients:
½ cup raisins
4 cups celery, sliced
¼ cup parsley, chopped
½ cup walnuts, chopped
Juice of ½ lemon
2 tbsp. extra virgin olive oil
Salt and black pepper to the taste

Directions:
In a salad bowl, mix celery with raisins, walnuts, parsley, lemon juice, oil, and black pepper, toss, divide into small cups and serve as a snack.

NUTRITION FACTS: CALORIES 120KCAL FAT 3 G CARBOHYDRATE 6 G PROTEIN 5 G

DIJON CELERY SALAD

 4   10 mins

Ingredients:
2 tsp. honey
½ lemon, juiced
I tbsp. Dijon mustard
2 tsp. extra virgin olive oil
Black pepper to taste
2 apples, cored, peeled, and cubed
I bunch celery roughly chopped
¾ cup walnuts, chopped

Directions:
In a salad bowl, mix celery and its leaves with apple pieces and walnuts.

Add black pepper, lemon juice, mustard, honey, and olive oil.

Whisk well, add to the salad, toss, and serve.

NUTRITION FACTS: CALORIES 125KCAL FAT 2 G CARBOHYDRATE 7 G PROTEIN 7 G

EASY SHRIMP SALAD

 2   5 mins

Ingredients:
2 cups red endive, finely sliced
I cup cherry tomatoes, halved
I tsp. of extra virgin olive oil
I tbsp. parsley, chopped
3 oz. celery, sliced
6 walnuts, chopped
2 oz. red onion-sliced
I cup yellow pepper, cubed
½ lemon, juiced
6 oz. steamed shrimp

Directions:
Put red endive on a large plate. Evenly distribute finely sliced onion on top, yellow pepper, cherry tomatoes, walnuts, celery, parsley, and shrimp.

Mix oil and lemon juice, with a pinch of salt and pepper, and distribute the dressing on top.

NUTRITION FACTS: CALORIES 232KCAL FAT 4.8 G CARBOHYDRATE 13 G PROTEIN 18 G

SNACKS

AVOCADO FRIES

 4   ⏱ 20 mins

Ingredients:
½ cup flour
1 ½ tbsp. pepper
2 eggs
½ cup panko (Japanese-style breadcrumbs)
2 avocados, chopped into 8 wedges each
¼ tbsp salt
2 tbsp. ketchup
2 tbsp. mayonnaise
1 tbsp. apple juice vinegar
1 tbsp. Sriracha sauce
1 tbsp. turmeric

Directions:

Mix flour, a pinch of salt, and pepper in a shallow dish. Delicately beat eggs and water in another dish and panko in a third one.

Dip avocado in flour, shaking off excess.

Dunk in egg blend, then dip in panko and coat them completely.

Put avocado wedges on a baking sheet, and cook them at 400°F until golden, 7 to 8 minutes, turning them after 4 minutes. Season with remaining salt.

While avocado wedges cook, whisk ketchup, mayonnaise, vinegar, turmeric, Sriracha, and pepper to taste in a bowl.

Serve avocado fries with sauce.

NUTRITION FACTS: CALORIES 262KCAL   FAT 8 G   CARBOHYDRATE11 G   PROTEIN 17 G

BUFFALO CAULIFLOWER BITES

 4 30 mins

Ingredients:
3 tbsp. ketchup
2 tbsp. hot sauce
2 egg whites
¾ cup panko (Japanese-style breadcrumbs)
1 lb. cauliflower, cut into florets
1 garlic clove, crushed
1 handful parsley, finely chopped
1/4 tbsp. pepper

Directions:
Whisk together ketchup, hot sauce, parsley, pepper, salt to taste, and egg whites in a bowl until smooth. Add panko to another bowl. Toss together cauliflower florets and ketchup blend in another bowl until covered. Coat the cauliflower with panko mixture.

Cook the cauliflower in the oven at 320°F until colored and firm (around 20 minutes). Serve.

NUTRITION FACTS: CALORIES 125KCAL FAT 4 G CARBOHYDRATE 7 G PROTEIN 8 G

MEDITERRANEAN TOFU SCRAMBLE SNACK

 2 18 mins

Ingredients:
1 tsp. extra virgin olive oil
½ onion, chopped
½ zucchini, chopped
1 cup baby spinach
½ cup halved cherry tomatoes
1 tbsp. sundried tomatoes in oil
4 oz. tofu crumbled

Directions:
Place a pan with oil on medium heat. When hot, add the onion and cook for 5 minutes.

Add zucchini, tomatoes, and spinach. Season with salt and pepper, and cook for 5 minutes until they are soft.

Add tofu and sun-dried tomatoes, finely sliced, and cook 2 minutes. Serve.

NUTRITION FACTS: CALORIES 134KCAL FAT 9 G CARBOHYDRATE 5 G PROTEIN 10 G

CRISPY ONION RINGS WITH SAUCE

 2   25 mins

Ingredients:

½ cup flour

1 tbsp. smoked paprika

1 egg

1 cup buckwheat breadcrumbs

1 red onion, chopped in 1/2-in thick rings

¼ cup low-fat Greek yogurt

2 tbsp. mayonnaise

1 tbsp. ketchup

1 tbsp. Dijon mustard

¼ tbsp. garlic powder

¼ tbsp. paprika

1 cup arugula

1 tsp. extra-virgin olive oil

1 tsp. lime juice

Directions:

Mix flour, smoked paprika, and 1/4 tbsp. of salt in a shallow dish. Delicately beat the egg in another dish, and put breadcrumbs and 1/4 tbsp. of salt in a third one.

Dip onion rings in flour, shaking off excess. Dip in egg, then in breadcrumbs.

Put onion rings in a single layer on a baking sheet, and cook at 375°F for about 10 minutes until crisp, turning them over halfway through cooking.

In the meantime, mix yogurt, mayonnaise, ketchup, mustard, garlic powder, and paprika in a bowl until smooth.

Serve over a simple arugula salad, dressed with 1 tsp. olive oil, 1 tsp. lime juice, salt, and pepper to taste.

NUTRITION FACTS: CALORIES 262KCAL FAT 8 G CARBOHYDRATE 9 G PROTEIN 15 G

THE SCIENCE BEHIND THE SIRTFOOD DIET

The Sirtfood Diet is based on a solid scientific foundation, which is precisely what the Sirtfood diet offers. Let's take a look at the science; I swear you won't get bored!

Scientific Studies on the Skinny Gene

Many studies have indicated that weight variation is greatly influenced by genetics.

Nowadays, lots of research has focused on obesity. A study was conducted by Professor Farooqi and his team to examine the real reason behind why some people remain thin, and others do not.

The study looked at 14,000 participants, of which 1,622 were thin men and women, 1,985 were obese, and over 10,000 people were of average weight. The study compared the DNA of the participants.

The truth is our DNA consists of proteins that are responsible for some particular functions in our bodies. Any kind of change in these genes, genetic variants, can form another protein type, altering the protein's function within the body.

Suppose it's a protein that involves metabolism. In that case, there will be changes in the way our body processes and digests food and even stores the energy.

Furthermore, the team was able to identify some genetic variants that are linked to an increased risk of becoming obese. They were also able to find a novel genetic reason that explains why some are thin (Riveros-McKay et al. 2019).

The impact these genetic variants have on an individual's weight was consolidated in a risk score. It was discovered that thin individuals have a significantly low genetic risk score. The result proved that lean individuals are lean because they possess genes that decrease their chance of becoming obese or overweight.

People believe that genetics is a causal factor of most diseases like cancer, obesity, etc. Genetics make up just 10 percent of the risk factor of these diseases, while the remaining 90 percent is dependent on environmental factors. Surprising right?

The way we sleep, eat, walk, behave, drink, reason, and talk are all factors you control.

In older adults, weight gain is a significant factor in how quickly they age. The fact that your body functions with the 90/10 rule makes it even easier for you to make good use of the genes at your disposal.

There are some genes called famine genes. These are genes that work to assist you in extracting as much energy as they can from the food you consume—thereby giving you the ability to store fat and live through a famine.

While these genes have proven useful for our ancestors at various points in history, they cause us to gain weight more easily for most of us nowadays.

There are also ways in which you can control these genes and activate them as you wish. Even though these genes are a part of you, there are ways you can control them; you have the power to decide how they interact and relate within your body.

Genes Associated with Weight Gain

There are specific genes associated with weight gain that are responsible for how people gain weight unnecessarily, mainly because of their eating habits. Some of these genes include:

The FTO gene

This is the gene that has the strongest link with your body mass index. It's your greatest risk for diabetes and obesity. There's a variant that switches on the gene, and if this variant is present in your body, you will not be able to control the hormone of satiety called leptin. Thus, making you eat unnecessarily. The FTO gene acts as a fat sensor, and people with this kind of gene tend to overeat, especially fatty foods, particularly in childhood. People who share an abnormal gene from both parents weigh more and are at a greater risk of becoming obese. At the same time, people with a normal gene have a lower risk of obesity.

The FTO gene can be switched on with the adequate physical exercise. Ensure you sleep between 7 to 8 hours at night, consume low carbohydrate food, and increase your higher fiber intake. With a proper diet and good lifestyle, your risk of obesity can be reduced.

The Melanocortin 4 Receptor

People born with this gene will consume more snacks, even if they are not hungry. They spend much of their time eating between meals, snacking on cake, chips, and so on. This gene increases cravings for fat.

If you have an increasing urge for a snack, simply learn to eat three times a day. Eat at intervals of four to six hours between each meal, with no snacking in between. Don't rush when eating. Set a boundary for your food consumption so you can easily combat food addiction.

The Adrenergic beta-2 Surface Receptor

This is a different kind of famine gene, and it's associated with the distribution of fat. When this gene is turned on, it can hinder your body fat from breaking down, resulting in a slower metabolic rate, making you store fat. This famine gene can increase your risk of obesity three times over. It can also increase your risk of type 2 diabetes. Also, people with this kind of gene find it challenging to lose weight.

How do you deal with this gene? It's simple. Exercise is one of the possible solutions. Accept that losing weight will be difficult for you so, don't feel bad when you see another person losing weight faster than you. Be disciplined in your eating habits. Eat the right kind of food with the right amount of nutrients. This is a slow and steady mission, so you mustn't rush it.

Weight Loss Regulation

Hypothalamic SIRT1 has been proven to help in weight loss. The hypothalamus is the central weight and energy balance controller. It modulates energy intake and energy consumption through neural inputs from the periphery and direct fluid inputs, which senses the body's energy status.

Leptin, an adipokine, is one of the factors that signal that sufficient energy is stored in the periphery. Leptin plasma levels are favorable for adiposity, suppressing energy intake, and stimulating energy spending.

A prolonged increase in the level of plasma leptin can cause leptin resistance. Leptin resistance, in turn, can prevent the hypothalamus from having access to leptin. This reduces leptin signals transduction in the hypothalamic neurons.

Reduced peripheral energy-sensing by leptin can lead to a positive energy balance and incremental weight gain and adiposity improvements, further exacerbating leptin resistance.

Leptin resistance causes an increase

in adiposity, associated with aging. Similar observations occur in central insulin resistance. Therefore, the improvement of humoral factors in the hypothalamus can prevent progressive weight gains, especially among middle-aged individuals.

SIRT1 is a protein deacetylase, NAD+ dependent with many substrates, such as transcription factors, histones, co-factors, and various enzymes. SIRT1 improves the sensitivity to leptin and insulin by decreasing the levels of several molecules that impair the transduction of leptin and insulin signals. Hypothalamic SIRT1 and NAD+ levels decrease with age.

An increase in the level of SIRT1 has been shown to improve the health in mice and so prevents age-related weight gain. By preventing the loss of age-dependent SIRT1's role in the, there will be a boost in the activity of humoral factors in the hypothalamus and the central energy balance control.

Sirtuins and Metabolic Activity

SIRT1, just like other SIRTUINS, is an NAD+ dependent protein deacetylase associated with cellular metabolism. All sirtuins, including SIRT1, are important for sensing energy status and in protecting against metabolic stress. They coordinate cellular response towards Caloric Restriction (CR) in an organism. SIRT1's diverse location allows cells to easily sense changes in the energy level anywhere in the mitochondria, nucleus, or cytoplasm. They are associated with metabolic health through the deacetylation of several target proteins such as muscles, liver, endothelium, heart, and adipose tissue.

SIRT1, SIRT6, and SIRT7 are localized in the nucleus where they take part in the deacetylation of cytoplasm to influence gene expression epigenetically. SIRT2 is located in the cytosol, while SIRT3, SIRT4, and SIRT5 are located in the mitochondria, where they regulate metabolic enzyme activities and moderate oxidative stress.

SIRT1 aids in mediating the physiological adaptation to diets. Several studies have shown the impact of sirtuins on Caloric Restriction. Sirtuins deacetylase non-histone proteins that define pathways involved during metabolic adaptation when there are metabolic restrictions. Caloric Restriction, on the other hand, causes the induction of expression of SIRT1 in humans. Mutations that lead to loss of function in some sirtuins genes can reduce the effects of caloric restrictions. Sirtuins, therefore, have the functions listed in the following sections.

Regulating the liver

The Liver regulates body glucose homeostasis. During fasting or caloric restriction, glucose levels become low, resulting in a sudden shift in hepatic metabolism to glycogen breakdown and gluconeogenesis to maintain glucose supply and ketone body production to mediate the energy deficit.

Also, during caloric restriction or fasting, muscle activation and liver oxidation of fatty acids are produced during lipolysis in white adipose tissue. For this switch to occur, there are several transcription factors involved to adapt to energy deprivation. SIRT1 intervenes during the metabolic switch to control the energy deficit.

At the initial stage of fasting, that is the post glycogen breakdown phase, there is the production of glucagon by the pancreatic alpha cells to active gluconeogenesis in the Liver through the cyclic amp response element-binding protein (CREB), and CREB regulated transcription coactivator 2 (CRTC2), the coactivator.

During prolonged fasting, the effect is canceled out and replaced by SIRT1 mediated CRTC2 deacetylase, resulting in targeting the coactivator for ubiquitin/proteasome-mediated destruction.

SIRT1, on the other hand, initiates the next

stage of gluconeogenesis through acetylation and activation of peroxisome proliferator-activated receptor coactivator one alpha, which is the coactivator necessary for forkhead box O1. In addition to supporting SIRT1 during gluconeogenesis, coactivator one alpha is required during the mitochondrial biogenesis needed for the liver to accommodate the reduction in energy status. SIRT1 also activates fatty acid oxidation through deacetylation and activation of the nuclear receptor to increase energy production.

SIRT1, when involved in acetylation and the repression of glycolytic enzymes, such as phosphoglycerate mutate 1, can shut down the production of energy through glycolysis. SIRT6, on the other hand, can be used as a co-repressor for hypoxia-inducible Factor 1 Alpha to repress glycolysis. Since SIRT1 can transcriptionally induce SIRT6, sirtuins can coordinate the duration for each fasting phase.

Aside from glucose homeostasis, the liver also takes over lipid and cholesterol homeostasis during fasting. When there are caloric restrictions, the liver's fat and cholesterol synthesis is turned off, while lipolysis in the white adipose tissue commences.

SIRT1, upon fasting, causes the acetylation of steroid regulatory element-binding protein (SREBP) and targets the protein to destroy the ubiquitin-proteasome system.

The result is that fat cholesterol synthesis will be repressed. During the regulation of cholesterol homeostasis, SIRT1 regulates the oxysterol receptor, thereby assisting the reversal of cholesterol transport from peripheral tissue through upregulation of the oxysterol receptor target gene ATP-binding cassette transporter A1 (ABCA1).

Further modulation of the cholesterol regulatory loop can be achieved via the bile acid receptor, necessary for the biosynthesis of cholesterol catabolic and bile acid pathways. SIRT6 also participates in regulating cholesterol

levels by repressing the expression and post-translational cleavage of SREBP1/2 into the active form. Furthermore, in the circadian regulation of metabolism, SIRT1 participates through regulating the cellular circadian clock.

Mitochondrial SIRT3 is crucial in the oxidation of fatty acid in mitochondria. Fasting or caloric restrictions can result in the up-regulation of activities and levels of SIRT3 to aid fatty acid oxidation through deacetylation of long-chain specific acyl-CoA dehydrogenase. SIRT3 can also cause the activation of ketogenesis and the urea cycle in the liver.

SIRT1 also acts in the metabolic regulation in the muscle and white adipose tissue. Fasting causes an increase in the level of SIRT1, leading to the deacetylation of coactivator one alpha, which causes the activation of genes responsible for fat oxidation.

The reduction in energy level also activates AMPK, which will activate the expression of coactivator one alpha. The combined effects of the two processes will increase mitochondrial biogenesis and fatty acid oxidation in the muscle.

Sirtuins, Muscles, and Oxidative Capacity

The expression of sirtuin in the muscle is affected by physical exercise, which controls cellular antioxidant system changes, mitochondrial biogenesis, and oxidative metabolism.

Skeletal muscles are involved in force and movement and engaged in endocrine activities by their ability to secrete cytokines and transcription factors into the bloodstream, thereby controlling other organs' functions. Furthermore, skeletal muscle is a metabolically active tissue that plays a vital role in maintaining the body's metabolism.

The skeletal muscle makes up about 40% of the entire weight of the body. The insulin-stimulated uptake of glucose and the main energy-consuming lipid catabolism is mainly at this site. For skeletal muscle, metabolic flexibility is essential to preserve physiological processes and metabolic homeostasis.

It determines the ability to switch from glucose to lipid oxidation. Advances in the understanding of the molecular mechanisms underlying skeletal muscle activity are a therapeutic benefit. Sirtuins' roles have been widely investigated in skeletal muscle, specifically concerning their role in controlling glucose and lipid metabolism, insulin functions and sensitivity, and mitochondrial biogenesis.

Cellular metabolic stress results from physical exercise, which affects the sirtuins. The most studied sirtuins in this respect are SIRT1 and SIRT3: SIRT1 is localized in the nucleus while SIRT3, in the mitochondria. SIRT3 is more expressed in type I muscle fiber.

One study showed that mouse skeletal muscle SIRT3 reacted to the six-week voluntary exercise dynamically to coordinate the downstream molecular response (Palacios et al., 2009). The result also showed that movement increases SIRT3 protein, CREB, coactivator one alpha, and citrate synthesis activity.

The downregulation of CREB, AMP-activated protein kinase (AMPK) phosphorylation, and the mRNA of PGC-1α are all symptoms of SIRT3 knockout. This shows that these key cellular molecules are essential for SIRT3 to carry out the biological signals effectively.

Palacios et al. discovered that SIRT3 responds to exercise dynamically to enhance muscular energy homeostasis through AMPK and PGC-1α. Voluntary exercise causes an increase in the SIRT3 content of skeletal muscle. Muscle Immobility can, therefore, lead to the downregulation of SIRT3.

Furthermore, SIRT1 protein content and PGC-1 in the muscle tends to increase with exercise. Bayod et al. (2012) reported that SIRT1 protein content and PGC-1 in rat's muscle increased after 36 weeks of treadmill training and enhancement in antioxidant defenses.

There's an increase in ATP demand during exercise, leading to increased NAD+ level and NAD+/NADH ratio. The result is an increase in the substrate for SIRT1 and SIRT3. SIRT3 is responsible for the increased ATP production and a reduction in protein synthesis in the mitochondria.

The ATP produced activates and deacetylases tricarboxylic acid (TCA) enzymes, electron transport chain, and β-oxidation, which maximizes the availability of reducing equivalents for ATP production. SIRT1, on the other hand, responds to exercise by contributing to mitochondrial biogenesis via independent mechanisms.

In summary, strenuous exercise activates SIRT1, which enhances biogenesis and mitochondrial oxidative capacity.

Furthermore, repeated sessions of strenuous exercise will activate both SIRT1 and SIRT3, which in turn start ATP production and the mitochondrial antioxidant function.

SIRTFOOD DIET MEAL PLAN

A Smart 4-Week Program to Jumpstart Your Weight Loss and Organize Your Meals Including the Foods You Love. Save Time, Feel Satisfied, and Reboot Your Metabolism in One Month

KATE HAMILTON

First published in the United States of America in 2020

Copyright © 2020 Kate Hamilton

Typeset by Leah Jespersen

Images from Unsplash.

ISBN 979-8668824359

SIRTFOOD DIET
MEAL PLAN

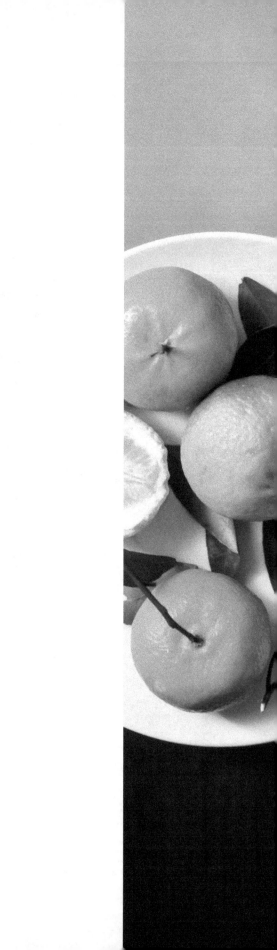

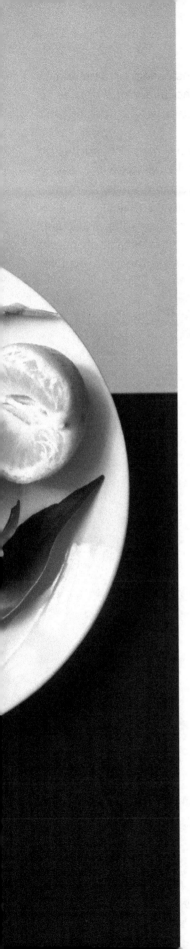

INTRODUCTION

So, you are ready to lose weight, but you are not sure how. You are looking through diets online. You see the Mediterranean Diet. You see the Keto Diet. You see the Paleo Diet. There are countless options out there, all claiming that they are the best because they will help you lose weight quickly.

Which one do you choose? You may scroll through them all without choosing one because you cannot decide which one is right for you. You see all sorts of options, but none of them speak to you.

Maybe you've tried Keto, but you missed fruits and carbs too much. Perhaps you tried the Paleo diet, but it just didn't work for you. Whether or not you have failed a diet in the past does not define your future: you can lose weight for good. You can learn how to properly shed pounds so that you will feel comfortable in your own skin and be healthier. You just need a new way of making it work for you.

The Sirtfood Diet was designed in the UK by celebrity nutritionists Aidan Goggins and Glen Matten to include certain foods that help people rapidly shed pounds without the same consequences commonly seen in other diets.

Some diets require you to starve yourself, causing you to lose muscle along with fat. Others require you to give up on foods that you enjoy, making them so restrictive that they are difficult for most people to keep up with. The Sirtfood Diet, on the other hand, encourages you to focus on sirtuin-rich foods that can be combined into delicious and satisfying meals. How does chicken curry sound? You can eat it on the Sirtfood Diet. What about a nice turmeric salmon? That is also a meal that you can enjoy while on the diet. You can even dig into blueberry pancakes for breakfast.

The Sirtfood Diet results from extensive studies on a group of proteins called sirtuins, which are metabolic regulators. They control our body's ability to burn fat and allow our bodies to remain healthy. They are active participants in many body functions, help us live longer, and prevent many pathologies.

The diet was created in 2016. Since then, it has been supported by several research studies on the benefits of sirtuin rich foods and by many epic transformations like Adele losing an impressive 66 lbs. in just a few months. After her reappearance in the newspapers, the same singer admitted that her miraculous weight loss came from following a carefully planned Sirtfood Diet.

This diet is a real revolution for those seeking to stay healthy and maintain results. It focuses on eating real food, capable of helping us lose weight without suffering. This is why doctors and nutritionists around the world have approved it. Let's dive in and analyze what the Sirtfood Diet exactly is and why it is effective.

WHAT IS THE SIRTFOOD DIET?

The Sirtfood Diet regime takes its name from SIRT1, a protein that positively impacts fat metabolism. In particular, certain foods high in sirtuins can speed up weight loss, allowing followers of the diet to lose up to three and a half pounds a week.

Unlike many other diets, it is not based on fasting, which in many cases, is responsible for feelings of hunger, irritability, and the loss of muscle mass.

The Sirtfood Diet introduces a group of nutrient-rich foods, named sirtuins, into daily meals. These can activate the skinny genes triggered when you fast, without actually forcing a person to fast for real.

Sirtuins became quite well-known thanks to research conducted in 2013. In that year, it was seen that resveratrol, a substance in grapes and red wine, can have the same effects obtained by calorie restriction. As a result of this study, researchers decided to further investigate the topic and find other foods with the same properties.

The scientific basis behind the Sirtfood Diet lies in the fact that sirtuin activators have several health benefits, including building muscles, suppressing appetite, improving memory, and controlling blood sugar levels, while cleansing cells of free radicals that accumulate.

Resveratrol is an excellent example of an antioxidant with anti-inflammatory and vasoprotective properties. Other similar plant pigments have a chemical substance that prevents liver damage and antioxidant actions.

When Goggins and Matten got together to study sirtfoods, they tested them and designed a diet to maximize their intake while encouraging a mild calorie restriction.

In their test group, they found that, on average, participants who consumed sirtuin-rich foods and restricted their calories to between 1000 and 1500 kCal for a short period saw impressive weight loss, even without any increase in exercise or physical activity.

On average, during that first week, subjects lost 7 pounds without doing much else other than changing their diet. Does that sound promising to you?

Even better, these people reported that they gained muscle rather than losing it—something that is practically unheard of in the diet world.

Typically, weight loss comes with muscle loss, but these individuals were able to build muscle. They also reported that they were happier and healthier in general—their mental health and general well-being increased.

Overall, those are some pretty compelling reasons to start considering the Sirtfood Diet—if you want to lose weight, gain muscle, and be healthier; this is a great way to do this.

Of course, it will take some diligence and dedication, but if you can commit to this process, you, too, can reap these benefits. You can begin to be a healthier individual, inside and out.

The Diet is designed to last three weeks. At the end of these three weeks, you are encouraged to continue consuming sirtfoods and drinking the green juice. You may also decide to repeat the plan if you feel the need to.

This book is structured to guide you through the three weeks of the Sirtfood Diet. It also offers a fourth transitional week to show you how sirtuin rich foods can be included in an everyday eating plan without effort for tasty, pleasant, and fulfilling results.

Whether you are vegetarian, vegan, or meat-lover, this diet can work for you. All you have to do is follow the guidelines provided in the following sections.

MAIN BENEFITS OF THE DIET

While it is still being researched, current research shows a wide range of benefits from sirtuin activation.

The most exciting fact is that those benefits derive from everyday diet foods that are easy to find. Most people already enjoy consuming these foods, so it's just a matter of adding them to your diet in the right proportions to give you the body and health you need.

Appreciating these benefits doesn't require you to implement extreme calorie restrictions for long periods, nor does it require grueling exercise regimens (although staying consistently active is a good thing, of course).

Let's go over some of the most common benefits now.

YOU WILL LOSE WEIGHT

The most obvious of the benefits is that you will lose weight on this diet. Whether you are exercising or not, there is no way you can't lose weight when you follow the diet to the letter.

This diet will have you restrict your calories enough so that anyone would lose weight. The average person uses around 2000 calories per day, and this diet will work to have you cut that in half; you will be consuming just 1000 or 1500 calories depending on the phase you are in.

Weight loss is caused by a calorie deficit—it is as simple as that. When you restrict your calories, but you keep your metabolism up, you will find that you will naturally lose weight. This is normal. However, usually, that weight loss is a mix of fat and muscle. As you lose weight and muscle, you would then naturally see your metabolism slow as well. Of course, this means that your weight loss plan is not nearly as effective over time as it was supposed to be. As a direct result, you would have to cut calories further to maintain a deficit between calories consumed and the calories that your body naturally burns. This means that weight loss will eventually slow or even plateau if all you do is use a weight-loss regimen that only cuts calories. You will lose muscle if you are not careful, and that will work against you.

However, thanks to the fact that you do not lose muscle mass during the Sirtfood Diet, you do not have to worry about this problem. You will simply continue to lose weight because you can maintain your metabolism at levels that will aid your weight loss.

YOUR APPETITE WILL SLOW

You may find that you are ravenous as your body adjusts to its new standard in the first few days, but this sensation will decrease over time.

Your body will adjust to the calorie restriction, and you will be okay with the lower calorie days, mainly because the food you will be eating will include nutrient-dense food that will help your body feel more satisfied.

Veggies and buckwheat are very nutritious foods that are featured heavily in this diet. You can also add healthy fats, such as olive oil, to give your body enough to keep going. You will find that you will tolerate the lower amounts of food, which is a huge plus.

SIRTFOODS HAVE AN ANTI-AGING EFFECT

Anti-aging is linked to autophagy, an intracellular process of repairing or replacing damaged cell parts. This is rejuvenation at an intracellular level. We can't mention autophagy without saying something about AMPK, an enzyme essential for cell energy stability. This enzyme boosts energy by activating fatty acid, glucose, and chemical reactions when cell energy is low. It represents the body's response when facing an elevated energy demand (e.g., intense physical exercise).

However, a part of this response is the lysosomal degradation pathway autophagy. Now, you are probably wondering what sirtuins have to do with this. SIRT1 can activate AMPK (and the other way around), so it can be considered one of the autophagy triggers. Autophagy rejuvenates the cell, and this process can happen in all the cells of your body: from those of your internal organs to those of your skin.

There are a few ways to induce autophagy, and it obviously has a very positive effect on your health and overall lifespan.

Just think of the cell as a car, and autophagy is a skilled mechanic capable of fixing or replacing any broken parts. Obviously, the cell will have a longer life, and this will impact your overall life. If your cells are functioning correctly, like a Swiss watch, then you can expect increased longevity.

You can't reverse aging, as there is no cure, and autophagy is not "the fountain of youth." However, this process can significantly slow down aging and its effects. The best part is that sirtuins, especially SIRT1, can activate the process.

Up till now, people were not aware of how to best trigger autophagy. Some were doing it the hard way through intermittent fasting. Others were trying to induce it through an LCHF diet, like the keto diet. Now there is a better way to activate it, which is through the Sirtfood Diet.

STRUCTURE OF THE SIRTFOOD DIET

The Sirtfood Diet is made of two different phases, and we are going to analyze them below. This book also includes a third phase to help you effortlessly transition back to a regular everyday sirtuin-rich diet.

PHASE 1: THE 7 DAY 'HYPER SUCCESS PHASE'

Phase 1 will take you through a process of hyper-success, where you will take a massive step towards achieving a slimmer, leaner body.

Duration: 7 days

WHAT TO EXPECT

This Phase is famous for being a clinically proven method to lose 7 pounds in 7 days. This is what is experienced by the vast majority of people following the Phase 1 guidelines.

Since all people are different, though, it's very important to specify that you shouldn't rely only on the number on the scale during this part of the process. You may find that you look slimmer and that your clothes are looser, or even too big, without seeing a real difference on the scale. This may depend on several factors, such as your starting point (if you only have a few pounds to lose, you may not see immediate results on the scale) and how much muscle mass you build (which may balance any fat loss leading to a stable weight).

Be mindful of other improvements, such as your general well-being, energy levels, and how clear your skin appears.

At your local pharmacy, you can get your general cardiovascular and metabolic well-being tested to see improvements. These tests will look at your blood pressure, blood sugar levels, and blood fats, like cholesterol and triglycerides.

Remember, weight loss aside, introducing sirtfoods into your diet is a massive step in making your body fitter and more disease resistant, setting you up for an exceptionally healthy lifetime.

HOW TO FOLLOW PHASE 1

We already said that Phase 1 is 7 days long. The week is divided into two parts: days 1-3 and days 4-7.

Days 1 to 3: These are the only days where a significant caloric restriction occurs. You are limited to 1,000 calories for the whole day. To put this into perspective, an average person should consume 2,000 calories per to maintain her current weight, but if she wants to lose about 1 pound per week, the calorie limit drops to 1,500 calories.

To stay within the given parameters for the first three days, the ideal daily menu includes:

- 3 servings of green juice
- 1 light snack (optional)
- 1 balanced meal

Days 4 to 7: Calories increase to 1,500 calories per day. To meet this requirement, the ideal daily menu includes:

- 2 servings of green juice
- 1 light snack (optional)
- 2 balanced meals

The green juices and meals should include as many sirtfoods as possible while keeping recipe options very tasty and enjoyable.

The recommended snacks for each day can be eaten either in the morning or in the afternoon. Early risers tend to consume their snack in the morning because of the long period between breakfast and lunch.

On the other hand, people who have heavier workloads later in the day prefer to consume their snack in the afternoon for an energy boost. Feel free to pick the meal schedule that works for you.

WHAT TO DRINK

As shown above, 2 or 3 daily servings of green juices are included in the Meal Plan, but of course, they are not the only thing you can drink.

The most important rule is that the beverages you consume should be no-calorie drinks like water, black coffee, and green tea, which are also great for boosting the activation of sirtuin in your body.

One thing you ought to be mindful of is that we don't suggest changing your usual coffee drinking habits. Cutting down coffee will give you caffeine withdrawal symptoms, which may make you feel lousy for a few days. Likewise, large increases in coffee consumption may be unpleasant, especially for those sensitive to caffeine's effects. As some researchers have found that adding milk reduces the absorption of beneficial nutrients that activate sirtuin, we recommend drinking coffee black. The same results have been found for green tea, although adding lemon juice increases nutrient absorption for sirtuin activation.

If you prefer herbal or teas, do not hesitate to add these to your diet.

Store-bought juices and soft drinks are forbidden during this Phase. Instead, consider adding a few sliced strawberries, cucumber, or mint to still or sparkling water to make a sirtfood-infused health cocktail if you want to spice things up.

Refrigerate for a few hours, and you will have a surprisingly cooling alternative to soft drinks and juices.

Remember that this is the period of hyper-success. While you can be comforted by the fact that it is just for a week, you need to be careful and consistent. The only alcohol included in this week is red wine; however, it can only be used as a cooking ingredient. Alcoholic drinks of any kind are not allowed during this phase.

SIRTFOOD GREEN JUICE

Green juice is an essential component of the Sirtfood Diet. In every juice recipe, you get a potent cocktail of compounds like apigenin, kaempferol, luteolin, quercetin, and EGCG that work together to switch on your sirtuin and encourage fat elimination.

We have also added lemon to the recipes, as it has been shown that its natural acidity stabilizes and improves the absorption of the sirtuin-activating nutrients. In some recipes, we added a touch of apple and ginger too. You will find a collection of 24 recipes to choose from so that you will never get bored.

PHASE 2: MAINTENANCE

By the beginning of week 2, you should be already noticing a radical change in how you feel and most probably in how you look. However, feeling revived and reenergized is just as important as looking slimmer and more toned.

Phase 2 is designed to keep you on the right track, help you lose more weight (we should say fat!), and stabilize the diet's positive effects on your body.

Remember that most of the weight that individuals lose is from fat and that many put on some muscle. So, once again, don't use your scale as the only measure of progress and use other tools to understand how things are proceeding. Pay attention to how your clothes fit or use a measuring tape to measure yourself. Probably, you will begin receiving compliments on your progress. Use the compliments as a booster to keep you focused on your journey to get even more significant results.

Remember, your health is improving as you keep going and that you're planting the seeds for a healthy lifestyle.

Duration: 14 days

HOW TO FOLLOW PHASE 2

The caloric restriction is now very moderate, and you shouldn't even notice it. This is because the long-term goal of the diet is not on calorie counting.

For the average person, calorie counting is not a practical or successful approach long term. Instead, the Sirtfood Diet concentrates on healthy servings, well-balanced meals, and as the name implies, including more sirtfoods in your diet so that you can start to benefit from their fat-burning and health-promoting effects.

We've designed the meals in the plan to be satiating and to help you feel fuller longer. This, coupled with sirtfoods natural appetite-regulating powers, means you're not going to spend the next 14 days feeling hungry, but instead, you will feel happily relaxed, well-fed, and well-nourished. Just like in Phase 1, remember to listen and be guided by your appetite. When preparing meals according to our guidelines, you may find that you are full before you finish them. If that happens, make sure to stop eating when you feel full.

The meal plan includes:

- 1 serving of green juice
- 2 snacks (optional)
- 3 balanced meals

As already said, the meals will have to fit around your schedule, so arrange them to make your life easier. Maybe one day you are particularly busy at work, or at the gym, or running around with your children. Perhaps it would be easier that day to switch a snack with a meal, just to have something quick and easy to hold you over to the next meal. That is perfectly fine; the plan is designed to be flexible and easy to follow.

Genuine progress goes past total control. Total control is not sustainable. Your eating habits must be adapted to your life and not incur extra stress.

During Phase 1, you consumed 1 to 2 meals daily, which gave you heaps of adaptability over when you ate your meals. In Phase 2, there are 3 meals a day. This is why we highly suggest eating breakfast to start the day in the best way possible.

Having a healthy breakfast gets us ready for the day, raising our levels of vitality and focus. Eating earlier keeps our blood sugar and fat levels in check. Many studies point out that eating breakfast is a good idea, usually finding that people who eat breakfast are often less likely to be overweight.

Since this is an important meal, we kept breakfast recipes quick and straightforward so that everyone will be able to prepare them, regardless of their crazy busy life. Some meals can also be prepared in advance, the day before, or in batches to freeze or keep handy.

Dedicating at least a few minutes every morning to breakfast will yield rewards not only for your day but also for your weight and well-being in the longer term. Sirtfoods ability to supercharge our energy levels is considerably more powerful in the early morning.

WHAT TO DRINK

As in Phase 1, you will keep having a green juice every day all throughout the Phase. This is to keep your sirtuin levels high. Keep in mind that you can have your daily green juice whenever is best for you.

You can have it as soon as you get up, 30 minutes before breakfast, or as a mid-morning or mid-afternoon snack. The green juice will help you feel fuller longer and keep you from getting too hungry before lunch or dinner whenever you drink it. Simply go with whatever works for you.

The other drinks allowed are water, black coffee, and tea (preferably matcha green tea).

You will also be allowed one glass of wine per day (optional). This is because red wine is rich in sirtuin-initiating polyphenols, particularly resveratrol and piceatannol. One glass is the perfect amount to get benefits without prompting weight gain from the extra calories.

No other alcoholic beverages are allowed.

PHASE 3: TRANSITION TO NORMAL HEALTHY EATING

Phase 3 will go back to a standard caloric intake while continuing to encourage the consumption of sirtfoods throughout the day.

The Meal plan will include healthy and delicious recipes to show how effortless it is to eat sirtuin-rich foods every day. The plan is stress-free and offers and mouthwatering dishes for every meal of the day.

Duration: 1 week

HOW TO FOLLOW PHASE 3

Simply cook the suggested recipes. As usual, you can switch lunch and dinner if it's best for you and arrange meal times to fit your needs.

WHAT TO DRINK

We suggest staying healthy and avoiding sugary drinks and alcoholic beverages, limiting them to special occasions. Red wine can be consumed daily in moderate quantities.

Water, coffee, green tea, and other no-calorie beverages can be consumed as you wish.

IS THE SIRTFOOD DIET RIGHT FOR YOU?

You may be wondering if the Sirtfood Diet is right for you. If you are currently pregnant or breastfeeding, you may want to postpone this diet because of your condition.

If you are already following a restricted plan due to a physical condition, remember to talk to your doctor before making any changes.

Even if you cannot strictly follow the Meal plan in this book, adding sirtuin-rich foods to your diet will still benefit you. As we will address shortly, many foods rich in sirtuins are highly nutritious and healthy, and they should be included in your diet whether you want to follow the Sirtfood Diet or not.

This diet should be a perfect fit for nearly everyone else.

OBESITY

Sirtuins burn fats quickly, and that's what makes this diet great for weight loss. When we study all the successful Sirtfood Dieters' cases, we can see how well they fought against obesity. Adele is just one example; she amazed the world with her 66-pound weight loss achieved following the Sirtfood Diet. Anyone struggling to lose extra pounds can switch to the Sirtfood Diet and try a carefully made plan approved by doctors and nutritionists, like the one in this book.

STRESS

There is another advantage to higher sirtuin levels, and that is the reduction in stress and depression. Research is still being conducted on the relationship between sirtfoods and stress. However, sirtuins can enable quick brain cell recovery and boost brain activity by eliminating all unwanted metabolic waste. Efficient brain function reduces stress, which is, therefore, how the Sirtfood Diet can also help with stress relief.

INFLAMMATION

Often weight gain and metabolic inactivity are connected to the inflammation of both cells and organs. This inflammation is both the result and cause of several health problems. Sirtfoods contrast inflammation at cellular levels and effectively prevents it at the level of tissues and organs.

AGING

Aging seems like a threat. When those wrinkles start appearing on the skin, it can make you feel weak inside and out! Sirtuins can play their part in countering the effects of aging. They help prolong the life of DNA and also aid in the repair process. Sirtuins are also responsible for apoptosis and lead to the formation of new healthy cells. This is why people entering middle age should consider following the Sirtfood Diet to fight aging signs in the years to come effectively.

NO WORKOUTS

Working out is an excellent way to lose some pounds, but not all people invest the required time and energy to train properly. Individuals who, for whatever reason, struggle or are unable to maintain a regular exercise routine can follow the Sirtfood Diet. This diet will help them manage their weight, even while doing only basic physical activities.

LOW OR POOR METABOLIC ACTIVITY

Since sirtuins are mainly responsible for better cell metabolism, lower sirtuin levels in the body can hamper natural cell activities and hinder metabolism. Insufficient metabolic activity results in less physical strength, obesity, hormonal imbalance, low enzyme activity, and several other related problems. Therefore, the Sirtfood Diet is suggested to boost the body's metabolic rate and revitalize both body and mind with better energy levels.

FULL SIRTUIN INGREDIENT LIST

Sirtuin activating compounds tend to elevate insulin sensitivity and reduce blood sugar levels. The main ones are:

Polyphenols – Present in turmeric, or curcumin. A moderate amount is needed to have a beneficial effect on the body.

Resveratrol – Present in blueberries, red grapes, raspberries, and peanuts. It helps in contrasting inflammation and improving heart health.

Quercetin – Available in apples, kale, capers, berries, onions, and citrus fruits. It helps fight inflammation.

Piceatannol – Popularly used as an herbal medicine in Asian countries. It's present in red wine.

Oligonol – Rich in anti-inflammatory properties and present in lychees.

Fisetin – Improves long term memory and is present in strawberries.

Omega-3 – Present in flaxseeds and fish like salmon, catfish, tilapia, etc.

Melatonin

These compounds are found in the 20 main sirtfoods at the base of the Sirtfood Diet. They are:

ARUGULA

This green salad leaf (also known as rocket) is very common in the Mediterranean diet. It has a peppery taste and is useful for digestive and diuretic purposes. It contains nutrients like quercetin and kaempferol, which can activate sirtuins. This combination of nutrients has very positive effects on the skin as it can moisturize it and improve collagen synthesis.

BUCKWHEAT

This crop, excellent for ecological and sustainable farming, is a fruit seed and not a grain. Rich in calcium and other essential minerals, it is also one of the best sources for rutin, a sirtuin-activator nutrient.

CAPERS

Capers are the flower buds of the caper bush, a plant that grows abundantly in the Mediterranean region. Usually handpicked and preserved, they have some interesting antidiabetic, anti-inflammatory, antimicrobial, antiviral, and immunomodulatory properties. Capers are also rich in sirtuin-activating nutrients, and they are included in some of the recipes for their rich taste.

CELERY

Celery is a plant that has been used for thousands of years. In ancient Egypt, people were already aware of its detoxing and cleansing properties. Celery consumption is perfect for your gut, kidney, and liver health.

CHILIES

Thes veggies should be in your diet, whether you like eating spicy food or not. They contain capsaicin, which makes them even more savory. Consuming chilies is excellent for activating sirtuins, and they speed up your metabolism. The spicier the chili is, the more powerful it is when it comes to activating sirtuins. A recent study showed that people who eat spicy foods three or four times per week have a 14 percent lower death rate than people who eat them less than once a week. Bird's eye chilies are very spicy, meaning they have a high sirtuin-activating effect.

COCOA AND DARK CHOCOLATE

Cocoa was considered sacred by the Aztecs and Mayans, and it was a food type reserved only for the warriors or the elite. While back then, it was mostly used as a drink, you don't have to dilute it with milk or water to reap its full benefits. The best way to consume cocoa and get the sirtuin-activating flavonols is by eating dark chocolate. Your choice of chocolate should have at least 85% cocoa solids to be considered a sirtfood.

COFFEE

This is a drink enjoyed by most adults worldwide, and it is considered indispensable by many. Caffeine is known to activate sirtuins, so there's more to drinking coffee than it being a popular and enjoyable social activity. It is no secret that coffee is perfect for giving your metabolism and energy levels a boost.

EXTRA-VIRGIN OLIVE OIL

This oil is perhaps the healthiest form of fats you can think of, and you will find it all over salads in the Mediterranean diet. The health benefits of consuming this oil are countless. It prevents and fights diabetes, different types of cancers, osteoporosis, and many more conditions. Plus, extra-virgin olive oil can be associated with increased longevity, as it also has anti-aging effects. This oil has the right nutrients to activate the sirtuin gene in your body.

GARLIC

Garlic has a potent antifungal and antibiotic effect and has been successfully used to treat stomach ulcers. Plus, it can be used to remove waste products from your body. It has an incredible impact on your blood pressure, blood sugar levels, and heart health. Garlic contains allicin, a nutrient capable of triggering sirtuins, but this nutrient can only be accessed if the garlic clove is crushed or finely chopped. This is the primary way to use garlic in the Sirtfood Meal plan included in this book.

GREEN TEA

This sirtuin-filled beverage is a popular choice for health buffs, making it the world's most consumed beverage after water. It is known to help boost weight loss, prevent Alzheimer's disease, reduce cholesterol build-up, and combat heart disease. Some of the essential vitamins and minerals it contains are folate, vitamin b, magnesium, and other antioxidants. It also contains EGCG (epigallocatechin), which is known to be a potent sirtuin activator. The most powerful version of green tea is matcha.

KALE

This is a popular "superfood" since it is filled with antioxidants (beta-carotene, kaempferol, quercetin, and more). This veggie has one of the highest oxygen radical absorbance capacity, or ORAC, ratings. It is known to be nutrient-dense – it has omega 3 fatty acids, vitamins A, K, C, B6, calcium, potassium, and magnesium. It can also lower cholesterol levels, has anti-cancer effects, and can help you lose weight.

MEDJOOL DATES

If you have the chance to go to any country in the Middle East or on the Arabian Peninsula, you will find that dates are a very common snack. Dehydrated, covered in chocolate, or in a fresher form, dates are perhaps the most common snack you can find there.

You are probably wondering if it has any health benefits, especially considering Medjool dates are about 66 percent sugar. However, naturally occurring sugar is a lot less harmful than processed or refined sugar, which doesn't have any sirtuin-activating properties and is linked to weight gain (even obesity), heart disease, and diabetes.

PARSLEY

Parsley leaves are included in many of the recipes in this book; they are an easy way to add sirtfoods to your diet. Just chop them and toss them in your meal. With their refreshing and vibrant taste, they will complete any meal and make it tasty.

This sirtuin food has vitamins A, C, and K (it is the richest herbal source for vitamin K) and contains essential oil and flavonoids. It is also said to help promote osteotropic activity in our bones. It is an excellent source of apigenin, which is a sirtuin-activating nutrient. This nutrient is rarely found in such large quantities, and it can help you relax and quickly fall asleep.

RED ENDIVE

This recently popularized lettuce is grown all over the world. It plays a major role in the Sirtfood Diet because of its high luteolin concentration, a sirtuin-activating nutrient.

A great way to raise the quantity of luteolin in your diet is to add red endive to your salad. Naturally, pour some extra-virgin olive oil on it to make it more sirtuin-activating. Endives can come in different colors. Red ones are considered the best, but you can settle for yellow if you cannot find red endive.

RED ONIONS

Aside from adding flavor to our dishes, onion is a popular component for different home remedies. It is known to heal infections, reduce inflammation, and regulate sugar. It also has a high polyphenol content, contains essential oil and organic sulfur compounds. It has plenty of antioxidants, and it is known to fight against inflammation, heart diseases, and diabetes. It is an excellent source of quercetin, an amazing sirtuin-activating nutrient that is believed to enhance sports performance.

RED WINE

The Mediterranean diet encourages the consumption of red wine, and there are plenty of reasons why you should consider moderate consumption of it. We won't focus on its effects on your blood sugar or how moderate consumption can decrease heart disease-related deaths but on its sirtuin-activating nutrients. Red wines like Merlot, Cabernet Sauvignon, or Pinot Noir have an incredible polyphenol concentration to activate your sirtuins.

SOY

Soy contains formononetin and daidzein, two great sirtuin-activating nutrients. This book's meal plan includes it in two different forms: tofu (the vegan protein boost) and miso (a Japanese fermented paste with an intense umami flavor). You can experiment with its many forms in your everyday meals after completing the 4-week plan.

STRAWBERRIES

Of all the fruits out there, strawberries are among the ones with the most health benefits. For example, they have a very high concentration of fisetin, a nutrient that can activate sirtuins.

Consumption of this fruit can lower insulin demand, basically turning the food into a sustainable energy releaser. Research claims that eating strawberries has similar effects on diabetes as drug therapies.

TURMERIC

Curcumin, a substance found in turmeric, has potent anti-inflammatory effects and is an antioxidant. It is also known to help with liver problems, arthritis, heartburn, kidney problems, and even depression. To boost curcumin absorption, cook it in liquid and add some fat and black pepper. This is how it has been frequently added to the recipes in this book.

WALNUTS

Without a doubt, walnuts are the best nuts when it comes to health. They have a high concentration of good fats, and moderate consumption (they are very caloric, so eating too many is not recommended) is associated with a lowered risk of diabetes, the prevention of cardiovascular diseases, and weight loss. Walnuts are also known for their anti-aging effects, and their nutrients are known to activate sirtuins.

Besides the 20 main foods shown above, you can include many other sirtfoods in your meals. This will help you have a very colorful and varied diet, which will aid in fat burning and muscle gain thanks to sirtuin activation.

Apples
Artichokes
Asparagus
Beans
Blackberries
Blackcurrants
Blueberries
Bok Choi
Broccoli
Chestnuts
Chia seeds
Chickpeas
Chicory
Chili peppers
Chives
Corn
Cranberries
Dill
Endive lettuce
Ginger
Goji berries
Green beans
Mint
Oregano
Peanuts
Pistachios
Plums
Quinoa
Raspberries
Red Grapes
Sage
Shallots
Spinach
Sunflower seeds
Watercress
White Onions

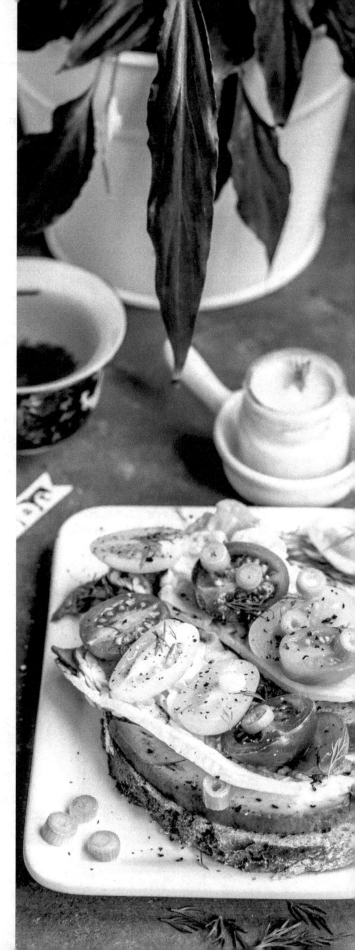

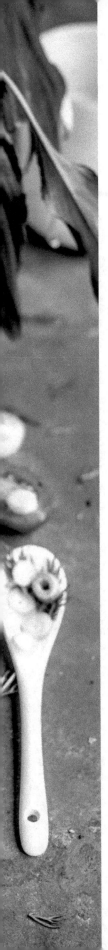

MEAL PREP SUGGESTIONS

In this Book, the Meal plan provided includes many different recipes to let you enjoy as much variety as possible. As you know, after week 4, you transition to normal, healthy eating, and you may need to experiment less because you will already know what recipes you like. This is when Meal prepping will come in handy.

Meal prepping is cooking and packing in individual servings of weekly meals and snacks in advance. Meal prep can be done one or two days a week, depending on your individual needs and schedule. The same recipe will be divided and boxed for several meals and can be frozen (if needed) or ready to heat-and-eat, like a casserole, or to eat cold, like a salad. There are more benefits to meal prepping than just convenience.

MEAL PREP DOS AND DON'TS

Developing smart meal prep habits is part of the learning process. Here are some meal prep dos and don'ts worth keeping in mind as you get started:

○ DO Select one or two days a week to meal prep. Sundays work best for many folks, but another day during the week might work better for you. For example, if you work over the weekend, then a day off during the week will probably be a better day for you to meal prep. You can also choose two days each week to prep food.

○ DO flag healthy recipes you love. After trying healthy recipes, keep the ones you love in a folder or mark them in this book or other cookbooks you already have that you may want to use as inspiration. This way, when you go back to normal healthy eating, you will have plenty of ideas to choose from.

○ DO keep variety in mind when it comes to protein, whole grains, and veggies as you decide which recipes to swap into your meal prep schedule. Nutritionally, this will allow you to take in a broader range of nutrients. Suppose one meal for the week is fish with asparagus. In that case, you'll probably want to select a chicken, beef, pork, or vegetarian recipe with a different vegetable to rotate with during the week. At the same time, you can try to keep some of the ingredients between recipes the same, which can help you decrease your grocery spending and help reduce waste. For example, if you have a meal for breakfast, plan to use the remaining ingredients for one of the other meals.

○ DO go at your own pace. You can successfully meal prep with three recipes or six recipes. You don't need to prepare 10 or more recipes for the week. Start slowly and build your way up.

○ DO make the most of your time and money. After selecting your recipes, go through the ingredients, and check if you have them. List the ingredients you need to purchase according to the flow of your market. For example, if you shop at a traditional supermarket, produce is usually by the entrance. Categorize your shopping list in this order: fruits, vegetables and herbs, milk and dairy, proteins (like meat, chicken, and fish), packaged goods, and frozen items. Note how much you need of each ingredient to avoid buying too much.

○ DO work with your schedule. Some weeks you'll be able to prepare more recipes than other weeks. Does whatever work for you and your schedule.

○ DO freeze extras. Some weeks you will have a few extra meals. Freezer-friendly meals can be frozen and kept for up to a few months, as noted in the recipes.

○ DO make cleanup easy. You'll have many vegetable scraps, eggshells, and empty containers to toss, so keep your recycling, compost bin, and trash nearby for easy cleanup.

○ DON'T wait too long. Plan ahead for the best results. Meal prepping is about scheduling your time in advance, so you can get to the market, buy the ingredients you need, and then cook and pack them without too much effort.

○ DON'T divide meals later. The last step of meal prepping is to divide recipes into individual portions and pack them into containers. Don't skip this step or divide meals right before digging into one. Dividing meals upfront helps maintain reasonable portion control, prevents last-minute scrambling, and ensures your meals will last through the week.

○ DON'T over prep. The last thing you want to do is prep meals that will go uneaten unless, of course, you can freeze them. To get into the meal prepping jive, start slow and get to know your meal prepping needs.

WHY AREN'T YOU LOSING WEIGHT?

Let's clarify a common doubt. You feel that you are already eating some sirtfoods you read about in this book. So why haven't you lost weight already? Here's why.

HITTING YOUR QUOTA

Most people just don't eat nearly enough sirtfoods to enjoy intense fat-burning and fitness-boosting effects. For Americans, the average intake of the five basic sirtuin-activating compounds (quercetin, luteolin, myricetin, kaempferol, and apigenin) is a miserable 13mg a day.

To give perspective, Japanese daily consumption is more than 5 times greater, and the Japanese are among the best consumers in the world of sirtuin-rich foods.

This book is designed to drastically improve your intake (in some cases up to 50 times) in a way that fits your busy schedule. You can efficiently and cheaply reach the level of consumption needed to gain all of the benefits.

THE POWER OF SYNERGY

The smartest way to guarantee our body the correct intake of nutrients is by eating a wide variety of whole foods (organic, where possible).

Along with the primary nutrients we all know, whole foods contain dozens of lesser-known compounds that work together in synergy to increase our well-being.

It has been proven by several studies that single nutrient supplementation does not give the same permanent effect as the same component ingested in the form of whole food.

Take, for example, the component resveratrol, which activates sirtuin. This can be consumed in supplementary form, but its bioavailability (how well it can be absorbed) is at least 6 times higher if consumed in the form of red wine.

This is because red wine includes resveratrol and a complete variety of sirtuin-activating polyphenols, like myricetin, piceatannol, quercetin, and epicatechin, which work together to provide positive effects.

Another example is curcumin, which is the main sirtuin-activating ingredient in turmeric. It has been proven that turmeric has a much stronger PPAR action to enhance fat burning and is much more capable of suppressing cancer and decreasing blood glucose levels than isolated curcumin.

This is why, unlike many other diets, supplements are not recommended: supplementing a single nutrient is nowhere near as impactful as eating it.

Combining multiple sirtfoods is what truly makes this book and its 4-week Meal plan unique. For example, introducing quercetin-rich sirtfoods boosts the benefits of resveratrol contained in other foods. Resveratrol effectively promotes the deterioration of mature fat cells, while quercetin prevents new fat tissue from developing.

Foods that are high in apigenin boost quercetin absorption and increase its function.

Quercetin has been proven to work in synergy with epigallocatechin gallate (EGCG). EGCG's work with curcumin has also proven to be complementary. In conclusion, whole food products are more effective than single nutrient supplements, and combining several sirtuin-rich foods gives even more benefits thanks to the synergy between the compounds.

JUICING AND FOOD: GET THE BEST OF BOTH WORLDS

As explained, the Sirtfood Diet combines freshly made juices and whole food products. For some people, that may sound counterintuitive, based on the fact that the fiber is lost when ingredients are juiced. Yet this is just what we need, especially from leafy green vegetables.

This is because they contain sirtuin-activating polyphenols and non-extractable polyphenols (or NEPPs) bound to the food's fibrous portion. NEPPs cannot be processed by the body and are simply eliminated as waste.

So, by juicing them and eliminating the low-nutrient material, we obtain an amazingly concentrated dose of sirtuin-activating polyphenols, with no trace of the harmful components which undermine our health.

There is yet another benefit of eliminating the fiber. The type of fiber in green leafy vegetables contain is called non-soluble fiber, and it has a gastrointestinal scrubbing action. When we consume too much of it, we disrupt the digestive lining, possibly aggravating or even inducing IBS (irritable bowel syndrome) and obstructing nutrient intake.

Without fiber, the digestion of ingredients (like matcha tea, for example) has been proven much more successful when combined with a green juice, which is true for many essential nutrients, like magnesium and folic acid.

A NUTRITIONIST'S TIPS TO GET TOP RESULTS

Here some common tips from Nutritionists worldwide to help you get the most from the Sirtfood Diet.

DRINK WATER

Thirst can be confused with hunger cravings. In case you're feeling a sudden craving, try drinking a massive glass of water and then waiting a couple of minutes. You might discover that the craving disappears as your body was actually only thirsty.

Moreover, drinking a lot of water can have many health benefits. For example, water before meals can lower hunger and help with weight reduction.

EAT EARLY

It has been proven that it is best to eat your last meal of the day before 7 p.m. for several reasons. First of all, the sirtfoods' natural satiating powers starting early in the morning. Having food that will leave you feeling full, happy, and energetic as you go about your day is more effective than spending the whole day feeling hungry.

Plus, eating most of your food late means you won't have enough time to digest it before going to bed, which negatively impacts your sleep.

EAT THE RIGHT AMOUNT OF PROTEIN

Sirtfoods are proven to work best with the correct amount of protein per meal. In particular, protein leucine helps SIRT1 to enhance fat loss and boost blood sugar regulation.

Leucine also has another role: inducing anabolism (building things) in our cells, especially muscle. Anabolism is an activity that requires a great deal of energy and ensures that our energy producers (called mitochondria) have to work extra hours.

Sirtfood supports this activity, increasing the growth of more mitochondria, boosting their efficiency, and making them burn fat as fuel. As you can see, there is a synergetic action between sirtuins and proteins like leucine, and this synergy helps you to lose fat to support muscle development.

PLAN MEALS

If possible, attempt to organize your diet daily or weekly. This Book gives you an example of what a month of good planning could be, offering many solutions for your meals.

By understanding what you will consume, you eliminate the spontaneity and doubt that can result in cravings and poor choices.

AVOID GETTING TOO HUNGRY

Hunger is one of the primary reasons why people experience cravings. To avoid becoming too hungry, the best things to do are eat regularly and have healthy snacks at hand. By being ready and preventing hunger, you will protect yourself against cravings.

FIGHT STRESS

Stress may cause food cravings and influence eating behaviors. Unfortunately, it has been shown that, under stressful situations, people are more likely to eat more calories and experience more significant cravings than non-stressed people.

Try to minimize stress in your environment by addressing it early, meditating, and generally slowing down.

GET ENOUGH SLEEP

Your appetite is affected by hormones that change throughout the day. Studies support this, revealing that sleep-deprived men and women are up to 55 percent more likely to gain weight in comparison to folks who get enough sleep.

Sleep deprivation might interrupt ordinary changes in desire hormones, resulting in cravings and inadequate appetite control. Put your phone down at least 2 hours before going to bed to avoid disrupting your sleep.

EAT PROPER MEALS

The scarcity of essential nutrients may cause cravings. It is critical to eat proper healthy foods so that the body gets the nutrients it needs to avoid hard-to-manage cravings.

DON'T SHOP HUNGRY

Grocery stores are one of the most challenging places to be when you're hungry. Have a light snack and a big glass of water before going, prepare a complete shopping list, including all the items you need, and stick to it. This way, you won't have to think much about other foods and spend less time in a place that may cause you to fall off the wagon.

DISTANCE YOURSELF FROM THE CRAVING

When you feel a craving, make an effort to distance yourself from it. For example, take a brisk walk or perhaps a shower to focus your mind on something else. A significant change in environment and thought patterns can help block the craving.

EXERCISE MINDFUL EATING

Mindful eating is all about practicing mindfulness, a kind of meditation, around eating, and food. Mindful eating teaches us how to distinguish between cravings and actual hunger. It makes it possible to consciously think about the process, rather than eating thoughtlessly or impulsively. It works by helping you deepen your understanding of meal planning and your feelings, appetite, cravings, and bodily senses.

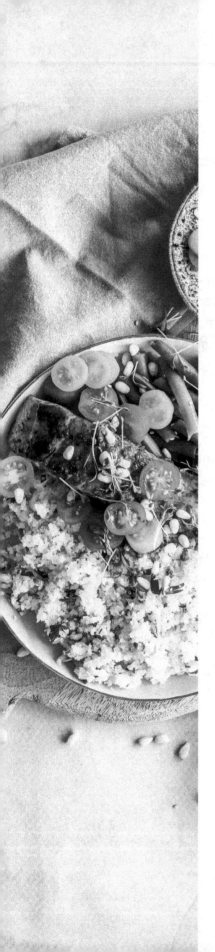

4-WEEK MEAL PLAN

This is, without a doubt, the most important section of this Book. You will learn about the new healthy way you will be eating over the next 4 weeks.

Here you will fully understand what following a Sirtfood Diet means, how easy it is to reach your goals while making significant, lifelong changes that will guarantee weight loss results that last and improve health conditions. Just follow the instructions, and the month will fly by without you even noticing.

Note: Plant based 4-week mean plan is on page 186.

But before starting, let's talk about pantry basics.

PANTRY BASICS

The following ingredients are probably already in your pantry. If not, buy them <u>once</u> to have them handy over the next 4 weeks (but most of them will last much longer, even months).

COOKING BASICS:

Agave Syrup, Arrowroot, Baking powder, Basmati rice, Breadcrumbs, Brown Rice, Capers, Chickpea flour, Cocoa powder, Canned Tomatoes, Coconut Oil, Cooking Spray, Cornstarch, Cranberries, Dark chocolate, Dark chocolate chips, Dates, Extra-virgin Olive Oil, Flour, Honey, Nutritional Yeast, Raisins, Red wine, Rolled oats, Sesame oil, Stock cubes, Tomato sauce, Vegetable Stock Powder.

DRESSINGS:

Balsamic Vinegar, Mustard, Red Wine Vinegar, Salt, Soy Sauce, Tamari, Teriyaki sauce, Worcestershire sauce.

HERBS AND SPICES:

Bay, Basil, Cayenne, Chili, Cinnamon, Cumin, Curry, Dill, Garam Masala, Garlic, Ginger, Marjoram, Nutmeg, Oregano, Paprika, Pepper, Rosemary, Sage, Thyme, Turmeric, Vanilla Extract.

NUTS AND SEEDS:

Almonds, Flax seeds, Pecans, Pumpkin seeds, Sesame seeds, Tahini, Walnuts

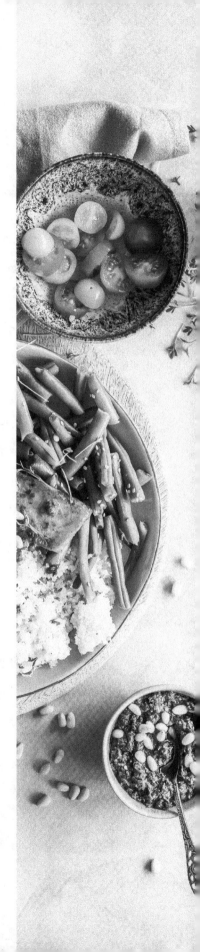

WEEK I – PHASE I

Quick Recap of the 7 day 'Hyper success Phase'

This week is divided into two moments:
Day 1-3 with 3 juices a day, 1 optional snack, and a full meal.
Day 4-7 with 2 juices a day, 2 optional snacks, and a full meal.

WEEK I – PHASE I – SHOPPING LIST

- Artichokes
- Arugula
- Avocado
- Baby Spinach
- Bird's eye chili
- Broccoli
- Buckwheat
- Buckwheat flour
- Carrots
- Celeriac
- Celery
- Chicken Breast
- Chicken Thighs

- Chicken Wings
- Chicory
- Coconut cream
- Dates
- Goat Cheese
- Kale
- Lettuce
- Leeks
- Lemons
- Orange
- Parmesan
- Parsley
- Red Onions

- Red Peppers
- Salmon
- Shrimps
- Smoked Salmon
- Spinach
- Sweet potatoes
- Tomatoes
- Tuna Steak
- Turkey Breast
- Turnips
- Yellow Peppers

<u>Important:</u> The Plan lets you choose your favorite Sirtfood Green Juices Recipes each week. Remember to add the ingredients to this list.

DAY	BREAKFAST	SNACK	LUNCH	SNACK	DINNER
MON	Sirtfood Green Juice (page 127)	2 squares of dark chocolate	Sirtfood Green Juice (page 127)	Sirtfood Green Juice (page 127)	Sweet Potato and Salmon Patties Raw Artichoke Salad (pages 136/34)
TUE	Sirtfood Green Juice (page 127)	2 squares of dark chocolate	Sirtfood Green Juice (page 127)	Sirtfood Green Juice (page 127)	Lemon Paprika Chicken with Vegetables (page 133)
WED	Sirtfood Green Juice (page 127)	2 squares of dark chocolate	Sirtfood Green Juice (page 127)	Sirtfood Green Juice (page 127)	Tomato Soup with Meatballs (page 137)
THU	Sirtfood Green Juice (page 127)	Sirtfood Green Juice (page 127)	Chicken with Kale and Chili Salsa (page 130)	2 squares of dark chocolate	Seared Tuna in Soy Sauce and Black Pepper (page 134)
FRI	Sirtfood Green Juice (page 127)	Sirtfood Green Juice (page 127)	Sirt Salmon Salad (page 135)	2 squares of dark chocolate	Green Veggies Curry (page 132)
SAT	Sirtfood Green Juice (page 127)	Sirtfood Green Juice (page 127)	Shrimp Tomato Stew (page 135)	2 squares of dark chocolate	Turkey Breast with Peppers (page 137)
SUN	Sirtfood Green Juice (page 127)	Sirtfood Green Juice (page 127)	Goat Cheese Salad with Cranberries and Walnut (page 131)	2 squares of dark chocolate	Spicy Chicken Stew (page 136)

WEEK 2 AND 3 – PHASE 2:

Quick Recap of the 'Maintenance Phase'

This week is divided into two parts:
Week 2 with 1 juice a day, 2 optional snacks, and 2 full meals.
Week 3 with 1 juice a day, 2 optional snacks, and 2 full meals.

WEEK 2 – PHASE 2 – SHOPPING LIST

- Almond Milk, unsweetened
- Arugula
- Asparagus
- Avocado
- Baby Spinach
- Banana
- Bird's eye chili
- Blueberries
- Broccoli
- Buckwheat, puffed
- Carrots
- Cauliflower
- Celeriac
- Celery
- Cherry tomatoes
- Chicken Wings
- Chicory
- Chocolate, 85%

- Coconut milk, full fat
- Cucumber
- Eggs
- Greek yogurt
- Kale
- Lean Mince
- Lettuce
- Lemons
- Lentils, canned
- Lime
- Milk, skimmed
- Mixed Berries, frozen
- Mozzarella
- Mushrooms
- Oats
- Orange
- Parmesan
- Parsley

- Parsnip
- Red Onions
- Red Peppers
- Salmon fillets
- Scallions
- Shrimps
- Sirloin
- Strawberries
- Tomatoes
- Trout fillets
- Turkey Breast
- Turnips
- Yellow Peppers

<u>Important:</u> The Plan lets you choose your favorite Sirtfood Green Juices Recipes each week. Remember to add the ingredients to this list.

DAY	BREAKFAST	SNACK	LUNCH	SNACK	DINNER
MON	Fluffy Blueberry Pancakes (page 146)	Sirtfood Green Juice (page 127)	Caprese Skewers (page 144)	2 squares of dark chocolate	Baked Salmon with Stir-Fried Vegetables (page 142)
TUE	Kale and Mushroom Frittata (page 147)	Sirtfood Green Juice (page 127)	Trout with Roasted Vegetables (page 154)	Banana Strawberry Smoothie (page 142)	Mince Stuffed Peppers (page 150)
WED	Vanilla Parfait with Berries (page 154)	Sirtfood Green Juice (page 127)	Arugula Salad with Turkey and Italian Dressing (page 141)	2 squares of dark chocolate	Creamy Mushroom Soup with Chicken (page 145)
THU	Super Easy Scrambled Eggs and Cherry Tomatoes (page 152)	Sirtfood Green Juice (page 127)	Lemon Ginger Shrimp Salad (page 149)	Blueberry Smoothie (page 143)	Lemon Chicken Skewers with Peppers (page 149)
FRI	Overnight Oats with Strawberries and Chocolate (page 151)	Sirtfood Green Juice (page 127)	Spicy Salmon with Turmeric and Lentils (page 153)	2 squares of dark chocolate	Chicken and Broccoli Creamy Casserole (page 144)
SAT	Sautéed Mushrooms and Poached Eggs (page 151)	Sirtfood Green Juice (page 127)	Asian Beef Salad (page 141)	Chocolate Mousse (page 145)	Creamy Turkey and Asparagus (page 146)
SUN	Banana Vanilla Pancake (page 143)	Sirtfood Green Juice (page 127)	Shredded Chicken Bowl (page 152)	2 squares of dark chocolate	Indian Vegetarian Meatballs (page 148)

WEEK 3 – PHASE 2 – SHOPPING LIST

- Almond Milk, unsweetened
- Artichokes
- Arugula
- Avocado
- Banana
- Bird's eye chili
- Blueberries
- Brussels Sprouts
- Buckwheat
- Carrots
- Celery
- Cheddar
- Cherry tomatoes
- Chicken Breast
- Chickpeas, canned

- Cilantro
- Eggplants
- Eggs
- Feta cheese
- Greek yogurt
- Kale
- Lettuce
- Lemons
- Milk, skimmed
- Mint
- Mixed Berries, frozen
- Miso Paste
- Mozzarella
- Mushrooms
- Oats
- Orange

- Parmesan
- Parsley
- Plain Yoghurt
- Red Onions
- Ricotta cheese
- Salmon fillets
- Scallions
- Sirloin
- Spinach
- Sweet potatoes
- Tomato paste
- Tomatoes
- Tortillas, wholegrain
- Tuna Steak
- Turkey Bacon
- Turkey Breast

Important: The Plan lets you choose your favorite Sirtfood Green Juices Recipes each week. Remember to add the ingredients to this list.

WEEK 3 – PHASE 2 – MEAL PLAN

DAY	BREAKFAST	SNACK	LUNCH	SNACK	DINNER
MON	Blueberry and Walnut Bake (page 157)	Sirtfood Green Juice (page 127)	Shrimp Tomato Stew (page 135)	Buckwheat Granola (page 158)	Turkey Bacon Fajitas (page 165)
TUE	Brussels Sprouts Egg Skillet (page 158)	Sirtfood Green Juice (page 127)	Orange Cumin Sirloin Simple Arugula Salad (pages 161/65)	2 squares of dark chocolate	Garlic Salmon with Brussels Sprouts and Rice (page 160)
WED	Banana Vanilla Pancake (page 143)	Sirtfood Green Juice (page 127)	Indian Vegetarian Meatballs (page 148)	Blueberry Smoothie (page 143)	Sesame Glazed Chicken with Ginger and Chili Stir-Fried Greens (page 163)
THU	Super Easy Scrambled Eggs and Cherry Tomatoes (page 152)	Sirtfood Green Juice (page 127)	Brussels Sprouts and Ricotta Salad (page 157)	2 squares of dark chocolate	Sesame Tuna with Artichoke Hearts (page 162)
FRI	Fluffy Blueberry Pancakes (page 146)	Sirtfood Green Juice (page 127)	Baked Salmon with Stir-Fried Vegetables (page 142)	Chocolate Mousse (page 145)	Spicy Stew with Potatoes and Spinach (page 164)
SAT	Sautéed Mushrooms and Poached Eggs (page 151)	Sirtfood Green Juice (page 127)	Roasted Butternut and Chickpeas Salad (page 162)	2 squares of dark chocolate	Eggplant Pizza Towers (page 159)
SUN	Vanilla Parfait with Berries (page 154)	Sirtfood Green Juice (page 127)	Arugula Salad with Turkey and Italian Dressing (page 141)	Mango Mousse with Chocolate Chips (page 161)	Greek Frittata with Garlic Grilled Eggplant (page 160)

WEEK 4 – PHASE 3

Quick Recap of the 'Transition Phase'

After completing successfully Phase 1 and 2, Phase 3 helps you transition to a normal healthy eating plan that continues to include a variety of sirtfoods in daily meals.

Week 4: 1 juice a day, 2 snacks, and 3 full meals.

WEEK 4 – TRANSITION – SHOPPING LIST

- Almond Milk, unsweetened
- Almond Flour
- Arugula
- Avocado
- Baby potatoes
- Baby Spinach
- Banana
- Blueberries
- Broccoli
- Brussels sprouts
- Buns, whole wheat
- Butternut Squash
- Buckwheat
- Cheddar

- Chicken Breast
- Chicken Mince
- Chickpeas, canned
- Chicory
- Coconut, shredded
- Dates
- Eggs
- Lamb, shoulder
- Lean Mince
- Lettuce
- Lentils, canned
- Mozzarella
- Mushrooms
- Oats
- Parmesan

- Parsley
- Peanut Butter
- Potatoes
- Red Onions
- Red Peppers
- Ricotta cheese
- Shrimps
- Spinach
- Strawberries
- Sweet potatoes
- Tomatoes
- Tuna Steak
- Wine

Important: The Plan lets you choose your favorite Sirtfood Green Juices Recipes each week. Remember to add the ingredients to this list.

WEEK 4 – PHASE 3 – MEAL PLAN

DAY	BREAKFAST	SNACK	LUNCH	SNACK	DINNER
MON	Brussels Sprouts Egg Skillet (page 158)	Chocolate Mousse (page 145)	Creamy Turkey and Asparagus (page 146)	Sirtfood Green Juice (page 127)	Spicy Indian Dahl with Basmati Rice (page 173)
TUE	Vanilla Parfait with Berries (page 154)	Sirtfood Green Juice (page 127)	Lemony Chicken Burgers (page 172)	Walnut Energy Bar (page 175)	Sesame Tuna with Artichoke Hearts Baked Sweet Potato (page 162/169)
WED	Blueberry and Walnut Bake (page 157)	Mango Mousse with Chocolate Chips (page 161)	Shredded Chicken Bowl (page 152)	Sirtfood Green Juice (page 127)	Creamy Broccoli and Potato Soup (page 170)
THU	Chickpea Fritters (page 169)	Sirtfood Green Juice (page 127)	Lemon Tuna Steaks with Baby Potatoes (page 172)	Chocolate Mousse (page 145)	Lamb, Butternut Squash and Date Tagine (page 171)
FRI	Fluffy Blueberry Pancakes (page 146)	2 squares of dark chocolate	Lemon Ginger Shrimp Salad (page 149)	Sirtfood Green Juice (page 127)	Mince Stuffed Peppers (page 150)
SAT	Overnight Oats with Strawberries and Chocolate (page 151)	Sirtfood Green Juice (page 127)	Chicken and Broccoli Creamy Casserole Baked Sweet Potato (page 144/169)	Buckwheat Granola (page 158) ½ cup plain yogurt	Spinach Quiche (page 174)
SUN	Banana Vanilla Pancake (page 143)	Sirtfood Green Juice (page 127)	Brussels Sprouts and Ricotta Salad (page 157)	Energy Cocoa Balls (page 170)	Mexican Chicken Casserole (page 173)

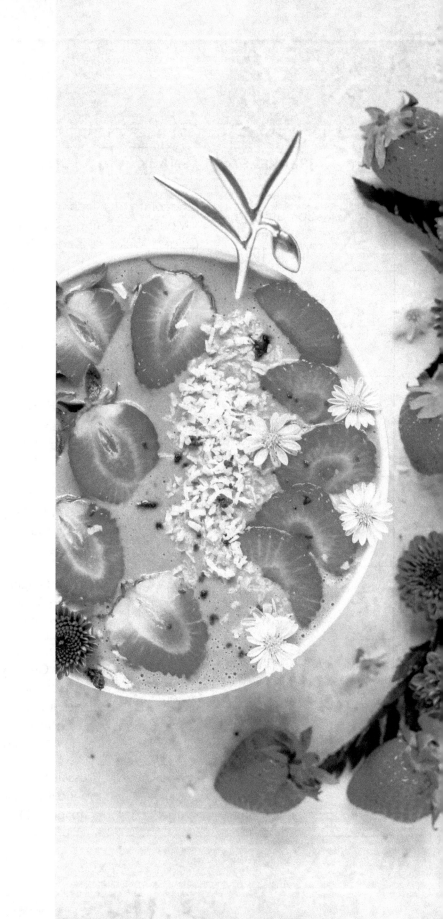

RECIPES

SIRTFOOD GREEN JUICE COLLECTION

Below, you can find a collection of 24 different recipes to choose from for your daily Green Juice. Simply go for your favorite one or try them all! It's up to you.

1 grapefruit ½ lemon ½ spirulina sparkling water	2 apples ¼ white cabbage ½ fennel 3 mint leaves	2 apples 1 cucumber 1-inch ginger 3 mint leaves
2 apples ¼ lettuce ½ lemon ½ tsp matcha tea	2 apples 2 kale leaves 1 stick celery 1/3 cucumber ½ beetroot	1 cucumber 2 apples 1-inch ginger 2 mint leaves
1 cucumber 2 pears ½ lemon handful lovage	1 cucumber 3 tomatoes handful parsley ½ lemon	1 cucumber 1 apple 1 stick celery ½ lemon
1 handful parsley ½ apple 4 broccoli florets ½ grapefruit	8 broccoli florets handful parsley 3 apples	8 broccoli florets 2 sticks celery 2 pears
2 cups spinach 2 stick celery 2 oranges	8 broccoli florets 2 grapefruit ½ tsp matcha tea	2 kale leaves 2 apples ½ cucumber
handful parsley ¼ white cabbage ½ cucumber ½ melon	½ lettuce 2 apples ½ lemon ½ cup spinach	handful parsley 1 lemon 5 tomatoes
1 cup spinach 2 mint leaves ½ pineapple	2 grapefruits ¼ red cabbage ½ tsp matcha tea	2 grapefruits ½ fennel 1 apple 3 mint leaves
1 grapefruit ½ cucumber 1 celery 2 mint leaves	1 orange 1 carrot 1 cucumber 1 stick celery	1 orange 1 carrot 1 stick celery 1-inch ginger

SIRTFOOD GREEN JUICE

2   5 mins

Directions:

Choose one of the recipes in the table opposite.

Add all ingredients into a juicer and extract the juice according to the manufacturer's method.

In case you don't have one, add all the ingredients in a blender and pulse until well combined.

Filter the juice through a fine-mesh strainer and transfer it into two glasses.

Serve immediately.

NUTRITION FACTS: CALORIES 32KCAL FAT 0.5 G CARBOHYDRATE 6.5 G PROTEIN 1 G

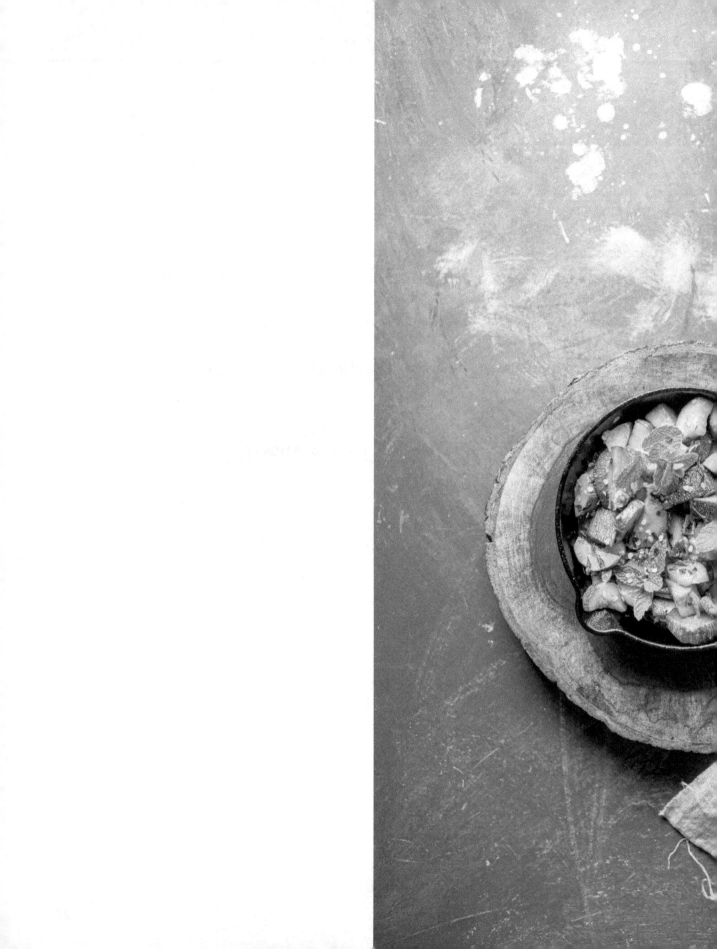

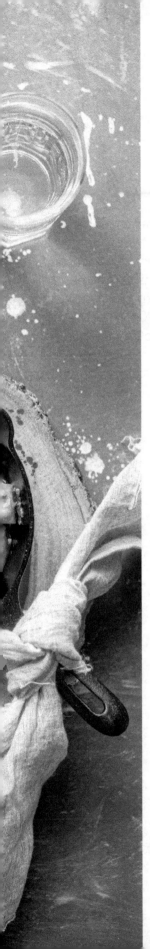

WEEK I – PHASE I RECIPES

CHICKEN WITH KALE AND CHILI SALSA

🍳 2   🕐 45 mins

Ingredients:
3 oz. buckwheat
1 tsp. fresh ginger
½ lemon, juiced
1 tsp. turmeric
2 cups kale, chopped
1 oz. onion, sliced
8 oz. chicken breast
3 tsp. extra-virgin olive oil
1 tomato
1 handful parsley
1 bird's eye chili, chopped
1 tsp. paprika

Directions:
Cook the buckwheat in salted water for 25 minutes. In the meantime, finely chop the tomato and parsley, mix them with chili, lemon juice, 1 tsp. olive oil, salt, and pepper to taste. Drain the buckwheat, dress it with the chili tomato sauce, and set aside. Preheat the oven to 400°F. Marinate the chicken with 1 tsp. oil, turmeric, paprika, and let it rest for 10 minutes. Warm a pan over high heat, and when hot, add marinated chicken and allow it to cook for 2 minutes per side until golden. Transfer the chicken to the oven, and bake it for 8 to 10 minutes until it is cooked. Fry the ginger and red onions with 1 tsp. oil until they are soft, then add in the kale and sauté it for 10 minutes. Serve the buckwheat with kale and chicken.

NUTRITION FACTS: CALORIES 290KCAL FAT 3.8 G CARBOHYDRATE 24.3 G PROTEIN 22 G

GOAT CHEESE SALAD WITH CRANBERRIES AND WALNUT

 2 10 mins

Ingredients:

2 tbsp. dried cranberries
10 walnuts, chopped
1 cup lettuce
½ cup arugula
½ cup baby spinach
1 tbsp. balsamic vinegar
1 tsp mustard
4 oz. goat cheese
2 tsp extra virgin olive oil
Salt and pepper to taste

Directions:

Mix lettuce, arugula, and baby spinach in a bowl. Whisk oil, mustard, salt, pepper, and vinegar, put the dressing on the salad, and mix well.

Transfer to a serving plate. Crumble goat cheese over the top.

Add cranberries and walnuts on top and serve.

NUTRITION FACTS: CALORIES 250KCAL FAT 20.9 G CARBOHYDRATE 3.4 G PROTEIN 20.3 G

GREEN VEGGIES CURRY

 2   40 mins

Ingredients:
2 tsp. coconut oil
¼ small red onion, chopped
1 tsp. garlic, minced
1 tsp. fresh ginger, minced
1 cup broccoli florets
1 tbsp. red curry paste or powder
2 cups spinach
½ cup coconut cream
2 tsp. low-sodium soy sauce
½ Bird's eye chili
1 tsp. fresh parsley, chopped finely

Directions:
Melt coconut oil in a skillet over medium heat, and sauté the onion for 5 minutes. Add the garlic, chili, curry, and ginger and stir to combine. Add the broccoli, reduce the heat to low, and cook for 5 minutes. Add the soy sauce and coconut cream and simmer for 10 minutes. Add in the spinach, and cook until curry reaches the desired thickness, about 8 to 10 minutes. Remove from the heat and serve hot, topped with parsley.

NUTRITION FACTS: CALORIES 324KCAL FAT 24.5 G CARBOHYDRATE 8 G PROTEIN 17.5 G

LEMON PAPRIKA CHICKEN WITH VEGETABLES

 2   55 mins

Ingredients:
2 carrots, chopped
2 bay leaves
2 tbsp. red wine
Juice of 1 lemon
½ celeriac, peeled and chopped
3 turnips, peeled and chopped
8 oz. of chicken wings
3 tbsp. extra virgin olive oil
2 tbsp. paprika
2 cups stock
Sprigs of rosemary and thyme
2 cups kale, chopped

Directions:
Heat a pan with oil and, when hot, add the carrots, paprika, celeriac, turnips, and chicken wings and cook over medium-high heat for 6 minutes. Add the wine over the chicken and let it evaporate. Add the stock, bay leaves, rosemary, thyme, lemon juice, salt, and pepper to taste. Bring to the boil, turn the heat down, cover it with a lid, and gently simmer for 25 minutes. Add the kale and cook for another 10 minutes, until the kale and the chicken are done.

NUTRITION FACTS: CALORIES 154KCAL   FAT 2.2 G   CARBOHYDRATE 32.1 G   PROTEIN 21.4 G

RAW ARTICHOKE SALAD

 2   20 mins

Ingredients:

2 Roman artichokes
1 lemon, juiced
1 tsp. extra virgin olive oil
Salt and pepper

Directions:

Wash and peel the artichokes by removing the outer leaves. Cut them in two and gently remove the hair inside.

Cut them very finely (using a mandolin if you have one)

Put them in water and lemon so that they do not turn brown.

When ready to serve, drain the artichokes, mix them with olive oil, a few drops of lemon, salt, and pepper, and put them on a serving plate.

NUTRITION FACTS: CALORIES 100KCAL FAT 10.9 G CARBOHYDRATE 3.4 G PROTEIN 13.3 G

SEARED TUNA IN SOY SAUCE AND BLACK PEPPER

 1   23 mins

Ingredients:

5 oz. tuna, 1-inch thick
1 red onion, chopped
2 tbsp. soy sauce
¼ tsp. ground black pepper
½ tbsp. grated ginger
1 tsp. sesame seeds
2 tsp. extra virgin olive oil
2 cups baby spinach
1 tbsp. orange juice

Directions:

Marinate tuna with 1 tbsp. soy sauce, oil, and black pepper for 30 minutes. Place a skillet over high heat and, when very hot, add tuna and quickly cook 1 minute per side.

Cut the tuna into slices, dress them with 1 tbsp. soy sauce mixed with grated ginger. Add green onion and sesame seeds on top.

Serve with a baby spinach salad dressed with 1 tsp olive oil, salt, pepper, and orange juice.

NUTRITION FACTS: CALORIES 154KCAL FAT 4.1 G CARBOHYDRATE 3 G PROTEIN 15 G

SHRIMP TOMATO STEW

 2   ⏱ 40 mins

Ingredients:
8 oz. shrimps
1 tbsp. extra virgin olive oil
2 leeks, finely chopped
1 large carrot, finely chopped
1 celery stick, finely chopped
1 Garlic clove, finely chopped
1 Bird's eye chili, thinly sliced
2 tbsp. wine
2 cups tomatoes
2 cups stock
1 tbsp. parsley, chopped
Salt and pepper to taste

Directions:
Fry garlic, onion, celery, carrot, and chili in oil over low heat for 5 minutes. Add the leeks. Turn up the heat to medium, add the wine, and let evaporate.

Add tomatoes and cook for 5 minutes, then add the stock and let simmer for 20 minutes.

Add shrimps and let cook for 4-5 minutes until they become opaque. Don't overcook it.

Serve warm.

NUTRITION FACTS: CALORIES 213KCAL FAT 13.1G SUGAR 51.67 G PROTEIN 80.62 G

SIRT SALMON SALAD

2   ⏱ 15 mins

Ingredients:
1 large Medjool date, thinly chopped
1 cup endive leaves
½ cup arugula
1 tsp. of extra virgin olive oil
1 tbsp. parsley, chopped
3 oz. celery, sliced
6 walnuts, chopped
1 tbsp. capers
2 oz. red onion, sliced
½ avocado, sliced
Juice of ½ lemon
6 oz. smoked salmon

Directions:
Mix endive and arugula and put them on a large plate. Evenly distribute on top finely sliced onion, avocado, walnuts, capers, celery, and parsley.

Mix oil, lemon juice with a pinch of salt and pepper and distribute the dressing on top.

NUTRITION FACTS: CALORIES 353KCAL FAT 4.8 G CARBOHYDRATE 28.1 G PROTEIN 28.3 G

SPICY CHICKEN STEW

 2   40 mins

Ingredients:
2 red peppers, chopped
2 large onion, sliced
2 garlic cloves, minced
1 ½ cups vegetable broth
3 tsp. extra virgin olive oil
½ tsp. ground nutmeg
1 tbsp. paprika
1 Bird's eye chili, sliced
1 tomato, chopped
4 chicken thighs
4 oz. buckwheat
1 tbsp. parsley

Directions:
Boil the buckwheat for 25 minutes, then drain it and set it aside.

Put the oil in a pan and heat, add onion, garlic, chili and spices and cook for 5 minutes until soft. Add the chicken and let it turn golden brown on medium-high heat for 5 minutes.

Add the peppers and the tomato, salt, and pepper and cook another 3-5 minutes until they start softening. Add the stock, turn the heat down and let simmer for 25 minutes. Add the buckwheat and let it absorb all the spicy flavors for 2-3 minutes. Serve hot.

NUTRITION FACTS: CALORIES 305KCAL FAT 9.5 G CARBOHYDRATE 14.2 G PROTEIN 3.7 G

SWEET POTATO AND SALMON PATTIES

 2   40 mins

Ingredients:
3 tbsp. buckwheat flour
8 oz. wild salmon, cooked or tinned
8 oz. sweet potato cooked and mashed
1 tbsp. dill
1 head red endive
1 tbsp. extra virgin olive oil
1 tbsp. balsamic vinegar

Directions:
Preheat the oven up to 325°F.

Mix the sweet potato, salmon, dill, salt, and pepper. Take a small handful of the mixture and shape it into a ball. Flatten into the shape of a burger, then dip into the flour on each side. Place it on a lined baking tray. Repeat until the blend is used up.

Bake only turning once for 20 minutes. Serve with a salad made with finely sliced red endive seasoned with a vinaigrette made with olive oil, salt, pepper, and vinegar.

NUTRITION FACTS: CALORIES 316KCAL FAT 6.3 G CARBOHYDRATE 18.3 G PROTEIN 19.2 G

TOMATO SOUP WITH MEATBALLS

🍳 2   🕐 45 mins

Ingredients:
8 oz. lean mince
1 egg
1 tbsp. parmesan
1 tbsp. breadcrumbs
2 tsp. of extra virgin olive oil
1 red onion finely chopped
1 yellow pepper, chopped
1 red pepper, chopped
1 can tomatoes or 3 ripe large tomatoes
2 cups stock
1 clove of garlic, crushed
1 Bird's eye chili, finely sliced
4 oz. buckwheat
salt and pepper to taste

Directions:
Put mince, egg, breadcrumbs, parmesan, salt, and pepper in a bowl and mix well, then create small meatballs.

Heat a pan, add oil and gently sauté onion and garlic until transparent.

Add the meatballs and cook another 5 minutes.

Add peppers and chili, let flavors mix, add the tomatoes (canned or roughly chopped if fresh), add the broth, and let it simmer for 20-25 minutes.

While the soup cooks, boil buckwheat for 25 minutes, drain it, and add it to the soup right before serving it.

NUTRITION FACTS: CALORIES 348KCAL FAT 7.6 G CARBOHYDRATE 28.4 G PROTEIN 23.2 G

TURKEY BREAST WITH PEPPERS

🍳 2   🕐 30 mins

Ingredients:
4 oz. buckwheat
8 oz. turkey breast
1 tsp. ground turmeric
2 peppers, chopped
2 oz. red onion, sliced
1 oz. celery
1 tsp. chopped fresh ginger
1 lemon, juiced
2 tsp. extra virgin olive oil
1 large tomato
1 Bird's eye chili, finely sliced
1 oz. parsley, finely chopped

Directions:
Boil the buckwheat for 25 minutes, then drain. Set aside. In the meantime, marinate the turkey breast with turmeric, 1 tsp oil, lemon juice, celery, and ginger.

Cook the marinated chicken in the oven for 10 to 12 minutes. Remove from the oven, cover with foil, and leave to rest for 5 minutes before serving. Meanwhile, fry the red onions and the ginger in a 1 tsp oil until they become soft, then add peppers and fry on high heat for 6 minutes. They have to stay crunchy. Serve buckwheat alongside chicken and peppers.

NUTRITION FACTS: CALORIES 107KCAL FAT 2.9 G CARBOHYDRATE 20.6 G PROTEIN 2.1 G

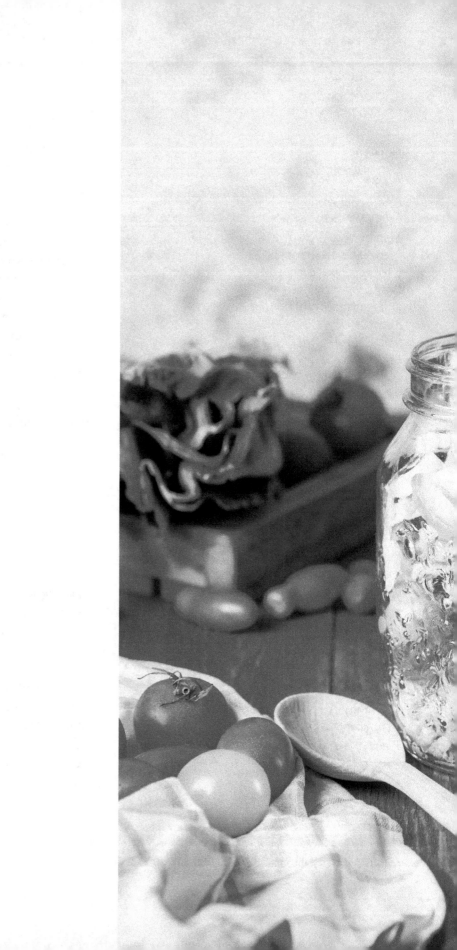

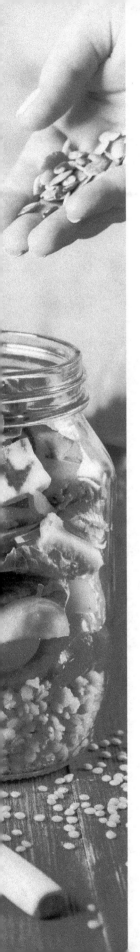

WEEK 2 – PHASE 2 RECIPES

ARUGULA SALAD WITH TURKEY AND ITALIAN DRESSING

2   20 mins

Ingredients:

8 oz. turkey breast
1 cup arugula
1 cup lettuce
2 tsp. Dijon mustard
½ cup celery, finely diced
2 tsp. oregano
¼ cup scallions, sliced
2 tsp. extra virgin olive oil
Salt and pepper to taste

Directions:

Grill the turkey and shred it. Set aside.

Mix lettuce and arugula on a plate. Evenly distribute shredded turkey, celery, and scallions.

In a small bowl, mix all dressing ingredients: mustard, oil, lemon juice, oregano, salt, and pepper and pour it over the salad just before serving.

NUTRITION FACTS: CALORIES 165KCAL FAT 2.9 G CARBOHYDRATE 13.6 G PROTEIN 26.1 G

ASIAN BEEF SALAD

2   23 mins

Ingredients:

3 tsp. extra virgin olive oil
8 oz. sirloin steaks
½ red onion, finely sliced
½ cucumber, sliced
½ cup cherry tomatoes, halved
2 cups lettuce
1 handful parsley
1 tbsp. soy sauce
½ Bird's eye chili
3 tbsp. lemon juice
2 cloves of garlic

Directions:

Crush the garlic, mix it with finely sliced chili and parsley, 2 tsp olive oil, and soy sauce. This will be the dressing.

Prepare the salad in a bowl placing lettuce on the bottom, then onion, cherry tomatoes, and cucumber. Heat a skillet until very hot. Brush the steaks with remaining oil, season them with salt and pepper and cook them to your taste.

Transfer the steaks onto a cutting board for 5 minutes before slicing. Drizzle the dressing on the salad and mix well. Place steak slices on top and serve.

NUTRITION FACTS: CALORIES 262KCAL FAT 12 G CARBOHYDRATE 15.2 G PROTEIN 25.2 G

BAKED SALMON WITH STIR-FRIED VEGETABLES

 2 50 mins

Ingredients:
Zest and juice of 1 lemon
1 tsp. sesame oil
2 tsp. extra virgin olive oil
2 carrots cut into matchsticks
1 bunch of kale, chopped
2 tsp. of root ginger, grated
8 oz. wild salmon fillets
Salt and pepper to taste

Directions:
Mix ginger lemon juice and zest together. Place the salmon in an ovenproof dish and pour over the lemon-ginger mixture. Cover with foil and leave for 30-60 minutes to marinate.

Bake the salmon at 375°F in the oven for 15 minutes. While cooking, heat a wok or frying pan, then add sesame oil and olive oil. Add the vegetables, and cook, constantly stirring for a few minutes.

Once the salmon is cooked, spoon some of the salmon marinades onto the vegetables and cook for a few more minutes. Serve the vegetables onto a plate and top with salmon.

NUTRITION FACTS: CALORIES 458KCAL FAT 13.2 G CARBOHYDRATE 15.3 G PROTEIN 21.4 G

BANANA STRAWBERRY SMOOTHIE

 1 5 mins

Ingredients:
1 cup strawberries
½ banana
½ cup almond milk, unsweetened
½ tsp cocoa powder
3 cubes ice (optional)

Directions:
Blend all ingredients and serve immediately.

NUTRITION FACTS: CALORIES 92KCAL FAT 1.3 G CARBOHYDRATE 12.8 G PROTEIN 3.6 G

BANANA VANILLA PANCAKE

 2   🕐 15 mins

Ingredients:
1 egg
1 egg white
1 banana
2 tsp. honey
1 cup rolled oats
¼ tsp. baking powder
A pinch of salt
1 tsp. vanilla extract
½ cup almond milk, unsweetened

Directions:
Put half of the banana, eggs, oats, vanilla, baking powder, salt, and almond milk in a blender and blend until smooth.

Heat a skillet, and when hot, pour the batter in to form pancakes. Cook 2 minutes per side until done. Repeat until all the pancakes are ready.

Top with honey and the other half banana.

NUTRITION FACTS: CALORIES 232KCAL FAT 5.3 G CARBOHYDRATE 22.8 G PROTEIN 18.6 G

BLUEBERRY SMOOTHIE

🥛 1   🕐 5 mins

Ingredients:
1 cup blueberries
½ banana
½ cup orange juice
3 cubes ice (optional)

Directions:
Blend all ingredients and serve immediately.

NUTRITION FACTS: CALORIES 87KCAL FAT 1.1 G CARBOHYDRATE 11.8 G PROTEIN 1.6 G

CAPRESE SKEWERS

 2 🕐 15 mins

Ingredients:
4 oz. cucumber, cut into 8 pieces
8 cherry tomatoes
8 small balls of mozzarella or 4 oz. mozzarella cut into
8 pieces
1 tsp. of extra virgin olive oil
8 basil leaves
2 tsp. of balsamic vinegar
salt and pepper to taste

Directions:
Use 2 medium skewers per person or 4 small ones. Alternate the ingredients in the following order: tomato, mozzarella, basil, yellow pepper, cucumber, and repeat.

Mix oil, vinegar, salt, and pepper and pour the dressing over the skewers.

NUTRITION FACTS: CALORIES 280KCAL FAT 8.6 G CARBOHYDRATE 14.4 G PROTEIN 17.2 G

CHICKEN AND BROCCOLI CREAMY CASSEROLE

 2 🕐 45 mins

Ingredients:
3 cups broccoli
8 oz. chicken breast, cubed
½ white onion
1 cup mushrooms
½ cup broth
2 tbsp. wine
1 tbsp. flour
2 tbsp. parmesan

Directions:
Heat the oven to 350°F. Steam the broccoli for 5 minutes, drain and cool in water and ice to set the bright green color.

Cut the chicken breast into medium-sized cubes. Mix chicken and broccoli and put them in a baking tray.

Prepare the creamy sauce. Sauté the onion with olive oil on low heat, then set to high heat. Add in the mushrooms, a pinch of salt and pepper, flour, and mix.

Add the wine and mix until it has evaporated. Add the broth, cook for 5 minutes, then hand blend until smooth.

Pour the sauce over the chicken and broccoli, spread 2 tbsp. of parmesan and cook in the oven for 30-35 minutes. Turn on the broiler for the last 5 minutes.

NUTRITION FACTS: CALORIES 30KCAL FAT 0.4 G CARBOHYDRATE 4.5 G PROTEIN 1 G

CHOCOLATE MOUSSE

 1    5 mins

Ingredients:
½ avocado
1 tsp cocoa powder
1 tsp honey

Directions:
Blend all ingredients and serve immediately.

NUTRITION FACTS: CALORIES 87KCAL FAT 1.1 G CARBOHYDRATE 11.8 G PROTEIN 1.6 G

CREAMY MUSHROOM SOUP WITH CHICKEN

 2   30 mins

Ingredients:
2 cups vegetable stock
8 oz. mixed mushrooms, sliced
1 red onion, finely diced
1 carrot, finely diced
1 stick celery, finely diced
4 oz. chicken breast, cubed
1 tbsp. extra virgin olive oil
3 sage leaves

Directions:
Put 1 tbsp. oil in a skillet and cook chicken until lightly brown. Set aside.

Put the mushrooms in a hot pan with 1 tbsp. oil, celery, carrot, onion, and sage. Cook for 3 to 5 minutes.

Add the stock and let it simmer for another 5 minutes. Then using a hand blender, blend the soup until smooth.

Add the chicken and cook for another 8 to 10 minutes until creamy.

NUTRITION FACTS: CALORIES 302KCAL FAT 3.5 G CARBOHYDRATE 16.3 G PROTEIN 15 G

CREAMY TURKEY AND ASPARAGUS

 2 40 mins

Ingredients:
8 oz. turkey breast
2 cups asparagus
2 cloves garlic
½ red onion
½ Bird's eye chili
2 tsp. extra virgin olive oil
½ cup full fat coconut milk
Salt and pepper

Directions:
Heat a skillet over medium-high heat, add the oil, onion, garlic, chili, and cook for 5 minutes.

Add turkey, cut in strips, and cook it another 5 minutes until golden on all sizes. Add the asparagus, cut into 2-inch pieces, and after 2 minutes, add the coconut milk.

Let it simmer for 25 minutes until the sauce is creamy.

NUTRITION FACTS: CALORIES 353KCAL FAT 4.8 G CARBOHYDRATE 28.1 G PROTEIN 28.3 G

FLUFFY BLUEBERRY PANCAKES

 2 20 mins

Ingredients:
1 egg
2 oz. self-raising flour
1 oz. buckwheat flour
1/3 cup almond milk, unsweetened
1 cup blueberries
2 tsp. honey

Directions:
Mix the flours in a bowl, add the yolk, and mix in a very thick batter. Keep adding the milk bit by bit to avoid lumps.

In another bowl, beat the egg white until stiff and then mix it carefully to the batter.

Pour enough batter on the skillet to make a 5-inch round pancake to cook 2 minutes per side until done. Repeat until all the pancakes are ready.

Put 1 tsp. honey and ½ cup blueberries on top of each serving.

NUTRITION FACTS: CALORIES 272KCAL FAT 4.3 G CARBOHYDRATE 26.8 G PROTEIN 23.6 G

KALE AND MUSHROOM FRITTATA

🍳 4   🕐 35 mins

Ingredients:
8 eggs
½ cup unsweetened almond milk
Salt and ground black pepper, to taste
1 tbsp. extra virgin olive oil
1 red onion, chopped
1 garlic clove, minced
1 cup fresh mushrooms, chopped
1 ½ cups fresh kale, chopped

Directions:
Preheat oven to 350°F. In a large bowl, place the eggs, almond milk, salt, and black pepper and beat well. Set aside. In a large ovenproof pan, heat the oil over medium heat and sauté the onion and garlic for about 3–4 minutes. Add the kale salt and black pepper, and cook for about 8–10 minutes.

Stir in the mushrooms and cook for about 3–4 minutes. Place the egg mixture on top evenly and cook for about 4 minutes without stirring. Transfer the pan to the oven and bake for about 12–15 minutes or until desired doneness.

Remove from the oven and let rest for about 3–5 minutes before serving.

NUTRITION FACTS: CALORIES 151KCAL FAT 10.2 G CARBOHYDRATE 5.6 G PROTEIN 10.3 G

INDIAN VEGETARIAN MEATBALLS

 2   ( ) 35 mins

Ingredients:
1 cup cauliflower
1 cup brown rice
¼ cup breadcrumbs
1 egg
½ tsp. turmeric
1 tsp. smoked paprika
1 tsp. of extra virgin olive oil
2 cloves garlic crushed
1 cup tomato sauce
Broth (if needed)
Cooking spray
1 tbsp. extra virgin olive oil
1 ½ tbsp. garam masala
1 tsp ginger
1 tbsp. parsley, chopped
1 red onion, diced
6 oz. full-fat coconut milk

Directions:
Steam cauliflower for 5 minutes, then blend it with rice. Use pulse to get a result similar to mince. Add egg, breadcrumbs, 1 clove garlic, salt, pepper, turmeric, paprika, and finely chopped parsley.

Mix well until you can form meatballs. Note: if it's too dry, add 1 tbsp. egg white and mix. If it's too runny, add 1 tbsp. breadcrumbs and mix. Spray a pan with cooking spray, heat it, and gently cook the meatballs for 5 minutes until golden. Be careful when you turn them so that they don't break. Put them aside

In a different pan, put oil, onion, ginger, garlic, salt, and pepper and cook on low heat until the onion is done. Add tomato sauce and coconut milk and let it simmer around 15 minutes until thickened. Put the meatballs in the sauce and cook another 5 minutes before serving.

NUTRITION FACTS: CALORIES 412KCAL FAT 7.8 G CARBOHYDRATE 39.1 G PROTEIN 18.3 G

LEMON CHICKEN SKEWERS WITH PEPPERS

 2   60 mins

Ingredients:
8 oz. chicken breast
2 cups peppers, chopped
1 cup tomatoes, chopped
3 tsp. extra virgin olive oil
1 garlic clove
½ lemon, juiced
½ tsp. paprika
½ tsp turmeric
1 handful parsley, chopped
Salt and pepper

Directions:
Cut the breast into small cubes and let it marinate with oil and spices for 30 minutes.

Prepare the skewers and set aside.

Heat a pan with oil. When hot, add garlic and cook 5 minutes, then remove the clove.

Add peppers, tomatoes, salt, and pepper and cook on high heat for 5-10 minutes.

Heat another pan to high heat. When very hot, put the skewers in and cook 10-12 minutes until golden on every side. Serve the skewers alongside the peppers.

NUTRITION FACTS: CALORIES 315KCAL FAT 20.9 G CARBOHYDRATE 5.4 G PROTEIN 15.8 G

LEMON GINGER SHRIMP SALAD

 2   20 mins

Ingredients:
1 cup chicory leaves
½ cup arugula
½ cup baby spinach
2 tsp. of extra virgin olive oil
6 walnuts, chopped
1 avocado, sliced
Juice of ½ lemon
8 oz. shrimp
1 pinch chili

Directions:
Mix chicory, baby spinach, and arugula and put them on a large plate.

Heat a skillet on medium-high, add 1 tbsp. oil and cook shrimp with garlic, chili, salt, and pepper until they are no longer transparent (5 minutes).

Blend avocado with oil, lemon juice with a pinch of salt and pepper and distribute the dressing on top. Chop the walnuts, put them on the plate as the last ingredient, and serve.

NUTRITION FACTS: CALORIES 353KCAL FAT 4.8 G CARBOHYDRATE 28.1 G PROTEIN 28.3 G

MINCE STUFFED PEPPERS

 4 75 mins

Ingredients:
4 oz. lean mince
¼ cup brown rice, cooked
2 large yellow
2 red bell peppers
1 tbsp. parmesan
2 tbsp. breadcrumbs
3 oz. mozzarella
1 egg
¼ cup walnuts, chopped
Salt and pepper, to taste
2 cups arugula
2 tsp. extra virgin olive oil
A few drops of lemon juice
Cooking spray

Directions:
Preheat oven to 350 degrees F.

In a bowl, mix the mince, parmesan, brown rice, egg, and mozzarella. Mix well and set aside.

Cut peppers lengthwise, remove the seeds, fill them with the mince mix, and put them on a baking tray. Distribute breadcrumbs on top and lightly spray with cooking spray to have a crunchy top without adding calories to the recipe.

Cook for 50-60 minutes until peppers are soft. Let cool for a few minutes.

Serve stuffed peppers with an arugula salad dressed with olive oil, salt, and a few lemon drops.

NUTRITION FACTS: CALORIES 375.1KCAL FAT 8.2 G CARBOHYDRATE 24.7 G PROTEIN 15.1 G

OVERNIGHT OATS WITH STRAWBERRIES AND CHOCOLATE

 2   5 mins + 8h

Ingredients:
2 oz. rolled oats
4 oz. almond milk, unsweetened
2 tbsp. plain yogurt
1 cup strawberries
1 tsp honey
1 square 85% chocolate

Directions:
Mix the oats and the milk in a jar and leave overnight. In the morning, top the jar with yogurt, honey, strawberries, and chocolate cut into small pieces.

It can be prepared in advance and left for up to 3 days in the fridge.

NUTRITION FACTS: CALORIES 258KCAL FAT 3.3 G CARBOHYDRATE 29.8 G PROTEIN 13.6 G

SAUTÉED MUSHROOMS AND POACHED EGGS

 2   25 mins

Ingredients:
2 eggs
1 onion, sliced
1 tsp. extra virgin olive oil
10 oz. mushrooms, sliced
10 oz. tomatoes, chopped
1 tsp. marjoram (or thyme)

Directions:
Sauté the onions in a frying pan with the oil for 5 minutes. Add mushrooms, tomatoes, herbs, and season with salt and pepper to taste.

While the mushrooms are cooking, bring some water to a boil, crack one egg at a time and poach it. Put the poached egg on top of mushrooms and serve.

NUTRITION FACTS: CALORIES 270KCAL FAT 4.3 G CARBOHYDRATE 19.8 G PROTEIN 22.8 G

SHREDDED CHICKEN BOWL

 2   45 mins

Ingredients:
8 oz. chicken breast
1 tsp. onion powder
1 tsp. garlic powder
2 cups broth
2 cups baby spinach
½ lime
2 tsp. extra virgin olive oil
2 ripe avocados
1 cup cherry tomatoes

Directions:
Put the chicken breasts in a saucepan with salt, pepper, onion, and garlic powder. Add the broth, bring to a boil, and cook 30-40 minutes with a lid until the meat starts to shred.

Remove the chicken from the broth, and shred it with a fork. Place the baby spinach as a base in a serving bowl.

Add the shredded chicken into the bowl, with sliced avocado and cherry tomatoes.

Prepare the dressing with lime, oil, salt, and pepper and drizzle it over the salad just before serving.

NUTRITION FACTS: CALORIES 420KCAL FAT 5.6 G CARBOHYDRATE 12.5 G PROTEIN 21.4 G

SUPER EASY SCRAMBLED EGGS AND CHERRY TOMATOES

 1   4 mins

Ingredients:
2 eggs
1 tbsp. parmesan or other shredded cheese
Salt and pepper
½ cup cherry tomatoes

Directions:
Put eggs and cheese with a pinch of salt and pepper in a jar. Microwave for 30 seconds, then quickly stir with a spoon.

Put back in the microwave for 60 seconds, and they are ready to eat with cherry tomatoes.

In case you don't own a microwave, cook the scrambled eggs in a skillet for 2 minutes, stirring continuously until done.

NUTRITION FACTS: CALORIES 278KCAL FAT 5.4 G CARBOHYDRATE 12.8 G PROTEIN 18.9 G

SPICY SALMON WITH TURMERIC AND LENTILS

⊙ 2   🕐 35 mins

Ingredients:

12 oz. salmon fillet
1 tsp. extra virgin olive oil
1 tsp. turmeric
¼ juice of a lemon
½ red onion, finely chopped
3 oz. lentils, canned
1 garlic clove, finely chopped
1 bird's eye chili, finely chopped
5 oz. celery cut into 2cm sticks
1 tsp. Mild curry powder
1 large tomato, cut into 8 wedges
1 cup chicken or vegetable stock
1 tbsp. parsley, chopped

Directions:

Heat the oven to 400°F. Heat a frying pan over medium-low heat; add the olive oil, then onion, garlic, ginger, chili, and celery. Fry gently for 2–3 minutes or until softened, then add the curry powder and cook for another minute.

Add the tomatoes, then stock and lentils, and simmer gently for 10 minutes. You may want to increase or decrease the cooking time, depending on how crunchy you like your celery.

Meanwhile, mix the turmeric, oil, and lemon juice and rub over the salmon. Place on a baking tray and cook for 8–10 minutes. To finish, spread parsley on top of the celery and serve with the salmon.

NUTRITION FACTS: CALORIES 177KCAL CARBOHYDRATE 4 G PROTEIN 12 G

TROUT WITH ROASTED VEGETABLES

 2 45 mins

Ingredients:
2 turnips, chopped
2 tsp.extra-virgin olive oil
1 tsp. dill
1 lemon, juiced
2 carrots, cut into sticks
2 parsnips, chopped
2 tbsp. tamari
10 oz. trout fillets

Directions:
Preheat the oven to 400°F. Put the turnips, carrots, and parsnips on a baking tray. Drizzle tamari and olive oil, season with salt and pepper to taste, and mix well. Cook for 25 minutes, then add the trout fillets on top of the vegetables. Season with salt, pepper, dill, and lemon juice. Cover with foil, and put the tray back in the oven. Lower the temperature to 375°F and cook for 20 minutes until the fish is done.

NUTRITION FACTS: CALORIES 154KCAL FAT 2.2 G CARBOHYDRATE 14.5 G PROTEIN 23.6 G

VANILLA PARFAIT WITH BERRIES

 1 5 mins

Ingredients:
4 oz. Greek yogurt
1 tsp honey or maple syrup
1 cup mixed berries, frozen is perfect
1 tbsp. buckwheat granola
½ tsp vanilla extract

Directions:
Mix yogurt, vanilla extract, and honey. Alternate yogurt and berries in a jar and top with granola.
Frozen berries are perfect if the parfait is made in advance because they release their juices in the yogurt. As far as granola, you can use one of the recipes on this book.

NUTRITION FACTS: CALORIES 318KCAL FAT 5.4 G CARBOHYDRATE 22.8 G PROTEIN 21.9 G

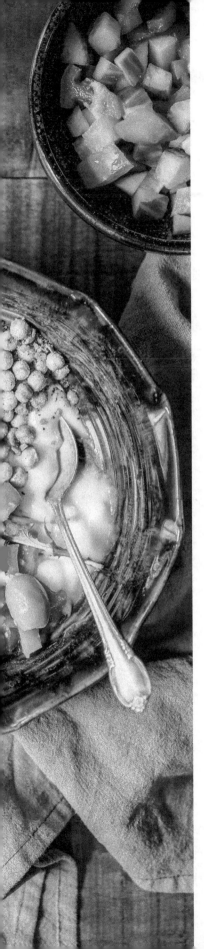

WEEK 3 – PHASE 2 RECIPES

BLUEBERRY AND WALNUT BAKE

 2   35 mins

Ingredients:
4 oz. rolled oats
12 oz. almond milk, unsweetened
1 banana, ripe and mashed
½ tsp. vanilla extract
1 oz. walnuts, chopped
1 cup blueberries
To serve: ½ cup plain yogurt

Directions:
Heat the oven to 400°F.

Mix the oats, milk, vanilla, banana, blueberries, and walnuts in a bowl. Put on a baking tray lined with parchment paper and cook around 30 minutes.

It can be eaten alone or served with ½ cup of plain yogurt.

NUTRITION FACTS: CALORIES 308KCAL FAT 5.3 G CARBOHYDRATE 35.8 G PROTEIN 15.6 G

BRUSSELS SPROUTS AND RICOTTA SALAD

2   15 mins

Ingredients:
1 ½ cups Brussels sprouts, thinly sliced
1 green apple cut "à la julienne."
½ red onion
8 walnuts, chopped
1 tsp. extra virgin olive oil
1 tbsp. lemon juice
1 tbsp. orange juice
4 oz. ricotta cheese

Directions:
Put the red onion in a cup and cover it with boiling water. Let it rest 10 minutes, then drain and pat with kitchen paper. Slice Brussels sprouts as thin as you can, cut the apple à la julienne (sticks).

Mix Brussels sprouts, onion, and apple and season them with oil, salt, pepper, lemon juice, and orange juice and spread it on a serving plate.

Spread small spoonfuls of ricotta cheese over Brussels sprouts mixture and top with chopped walnuts.

NUTRITION FACTS: CALORIES 353KCAL FAT 4.8 G CARBOHYDRATE 28.1 G PROTEIN 28.3 G

BRUSSELS SPROUTS EGG SKILLET

 2   35 mins

Ingredients:
½lb Brussels sprouts, halved
1 small red onion, chopped
10 cherry tomatoes, halved
4 eggs
1 tsp. extra virgin olive oil

Directions:
In an 8 inch cast iron skillet, heat olive oil over medium heat.

Add in onion and sauté for 1-2 minutes.

Add in Brussels sprouts and tomatoes and season with salt and pepper to taste.

Cook for 3-4 minutes, then crack the eggs, cover, and cook until egg whites have set, and egg yolk is desired consistency.

NUTRITION FACTS: CALORIES 194KCAL FAT 11.4 G CARBOHYDRATE 18.2 G PROTEIN 7.1 G

BUCKWHEAT GRANOLA

 8   35 mins

Ingredients:
2 cups buckwheat, puffed
¾ cup pumpkin seeds
¾ cup walnuts, chopped
1 tsp. ground cinnamon
1 ripe banana, mashed
2 tbsp. honey
2 tbsp. coconut oil

Directions:
Preheat your oven to 350°F. Place the buckwheat groats, pumpkin seeds, walnuts, cinnamon, and vanilla in a bowl and mix well. Add banana, honey, and coconut oil to the buckwheat mixture and mix until well combined.

Transfer the mixture onto a baking tray and spread it in an even layer. Bake for about 25–30 minutes, stirring once halfway through.

Remove the baking tray from the oven and set aside to cool.

NUTRITION FACTS: CALORIES 252KCAL FAT 14.3 G CARBOHYDRATE 27.6 G PROTEIN 7.6 G

EGGPLANT PIZZA TOWERS

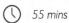 2   55 mins

Ingredients:
1 ½ eggplant
1 tbsp. tomato paste
2 cups tomato sauce
½ red onion
1 clove garlic
½ cup mozzarella
4 basil leaves
1 tsp. extra virgin olive oil
1 tbsp. parmesan
Salt and pepper

Directions:
Cut the eggplants into thick slices, add some salt and let them rest so that they let their bitter water out. In the meantime, prepare the salsa. Heat a pan with oil added, when hot add onion and garlic and cook 5 minutes.

Add tomato sauce, tomato paste, salt, and pepper and cook on low heat for about 15-18 minutes. Add a few leaves of basil. Pat the eggplants with kitchen paper and grill them. Heat the oven to 350°F.

Compose the towers: put a slice of eggplant, sauce, a few dices of mozzarella and again eggplant, sauce, mozzarella. Three layers per tower are best. Sprinkle parmesan on top.

When done, put the tray in the oven for about 10 minutes until the mozzarella is melted.

NUTRITION FACTS: CALORIES 353KCAL FAT 4.8 G CARBOHYDRATE 28.1 G PROTEIN 28.3 G

GARLIC SALMON WITH BRUSSELS SPROUTS AND RICE

 2   🕐 35 mins

Ingredients:
8 oz. salmon fillet slices
1 clove garlic, crushed
2 tbsp. wine
1 cup Brussels sprouts
1 cup cherry tomatoes
1 tsp. extra virgin olive oil
3 oz. basmati rice
3 tbsp. stock (or water), if needed

Directions:
Boil the basmati rice until tender and set aside.

Crush the garlic and coat the top of the salmon. Put a skillet on medium-high heat, and when hot, put the salmon fillets skin down. Cook for 5 minutes, then turn them. Cook them until it becomes brown and crispy (around 5-6 more minutes).

Remove the salmon from the pan and add Brussels sprouts, tomatoes, wine, and salt and cook them around 10 minutes. Add stock or water if needed. When done, add the basmati rice and mix to combine the flavors. Add the parmesan and serve, putting the salmon on top.

NUTRITION FACTS: CALORIES 353KCAL FAT 4.8 G CARBOHYDRATE 28.1 G PROTEIN 28.3 G

GREEK FRITTATA WITH GARLIC GRILLED EGGPLANT

  2   🕐 45 mins

Ingredients:
1 ½ cups shredded zucchini
3 eggs
3 oz. feta cheese
2 tbsp. milk
2 leaves mint, finely chopped
1 eggplant
2 tbsp. oil
1 clove garlic, crushed
1 tsp. balsamic vinegar
Salt and pepper to taste

Directions:
Heat the oven to 350°F. Cut the eggplant into thin slices; mix with a pinch of salt and let rest.

Mix the shredded zucchini with a pinch of salt and let it rest in a colander until some water has drained. After 10 minutes, squeeze the rest of the water out and put zucchini in a bowl.

Add 3 eggs, crushed feta cheese, milk, salt, pepper, mint, whisk well and pour in a silicone baking tray and cook 25-30 minutes in the oven. Pat the eggplant slices dry and grill them.

Mix garlic, oil, salt, pepper, and balsamic vinegar and pour the dressing on the eggplants. Serve the frittata alongside the eggplant.

NUTRITION FACTS: CALORIES 359KCAL FAT 7.8 G CARBOHYDRATE 18.1 G PROTEIN 21.3 G

MANGO MOUSSE WITH CHOCOLATE CHIPS

 1   5 mins

Ingredients:
1 cup mango
½ cup Greek yogurt
¼ tsp. vanilla extract
2 squares dark chocolate, chopped

Directions:
Blend mango, yogurt, and vanilla together. Add chocolate chips, and serve immediately.

NUTRITION FACTS: CALORIES 87KCAL FAT 1.1 G CARBOHYDRATE 11.8 G PROTEIN 1.6 G

ORANGE CUMIN SIRLOIN

 2   15 mins + 8h

Ingredients:
8 oz. sirloin
2 cloves garlic, crushed
2 tbsp. extra virgin olive oil
Juice of ½ a lime
Juice of ½ an orange
¼ cup parsley
½ tsp cumin
½ bird's eye chili
2 tbsp. soy sauce
Salt and pepper

Directions:
Prepare the marinade combining all the ingredients, reserve 2 tbsp. for later and put the rest on the sirloin in a small tray. Turn the meat several times so that the marinade covers it completely. Cover with aluminum foil and put it in the fridge for 8 hours.

Drain the meat from the marinade; pat it with kitchen paper to dry it.

Heat the grill or a skillet until very hot and cook to your taste. Let the cooked meat sit on a plate for 5 minutes, slice it and dress it with the 2 tablespoons of marinade you kept aside.

NUTRITION FACTS: CALORIES 353KCAL FAT 4.8 G CARBOHYDRATE 28.1 G PROTEIN 28.3 G

ROASTED BUTTERNUT AND CHICKPEAS SALAD

 2   40 mins

Ingredients:
1 cup chickpeas, drained
2 cups kale
2 tsp. oil
½ lemon, juiced
2 cloves of garlic
1 green apple
½ tsp. honey
Salt and pepper to taste

Directions:
Heat the oven to 400°F.

Cut the squash into medium cubes, put them in a baking tray, add drained chickpeas, garlic, 1 tbsp. oil, salt, and pepper and mix. Cook for 25 minutes.

Mix the kale with the dressing: salt, pepper, lemon, olive oil, and honey so that while the squash is cooking, it becomes softer and more pleasant to eat.

When squash and chickpeas are done, put them aside 10 minutes, and in the meantime, chop the apple and mix it with kale.

Add squash and chickpeas on top and serve warm.

NUTRITION FACTS: CALORIES 353KCAL FAT 4.8 G CARBOHYDRATE 28.1 G PROTEIN 28.3 G

SESAME TUNA WITH ARTICHOKE HEARTS

 2   20 mins

Ingredients:
8 oz. tuna steaks
2 tbsp. white sesame
2 tbsp. black sesame
1 tsp. sesame oil
2 artichokes
2 tsp. extra virgin olive oil
½ lemon, juiced
1 clove garlic
1 handful parsley

Directions:
Discard the outer leaves, and then slice artichokes very fine. Heat a pan with olive oil, add garlic and cook for a couple of minutes, then remove the clove. Add artichokes, lemon, salt, and pepper. Cook 5-10 minutes until tender. Set aside.

Mix sesame seeds and press them on tuna until it is completely covered.

Heat a pan and add sesame oil. When the oil is very hot, cook tuna for 1-2 minutes per side.

Serve tuna alongside artichokes.

NUTRITION FACTS: CALORIES 353KCAL FAT 4.8 G CARBOHYDRATE 28.1 G PROTEIN 28.3 G

SESAME GLAZED CHICKEN WITH GINGER AND CHILI GREENS

 4   🕐 35 mins

Ingredients:

1 tbsp mirin
1 tbsp. miso paste
6 oz. chicken breast
1 oz. celery
2 oz. red onion
2 zucchini
1 bird's eye chili
2 garlic cloves
1 tsp. fresh ginger
1 cup spinach
2 tsp. sesame seeds
3 oz. buckwheat
1 tsp. ground turmeric
1 tsp. extra virgin olive oil
1 tsp. tamari

Directions:

Heat the oven to 400 F. Line a roasting pan with parchment-paper Mix in the mirin and the miso. Cut the chicken lengthwise and marinate it with the miso mix for 15 minutes.

Place the chicken in the roasting pan, sprinkle it with the sesame seeds, and roast in the oven for 15-20 minutes until it has been beautifully caramelized.

Wash the buckwheat in a sieve, and then place it along with the turmeric in a saucepan of boiling water. Cook 25-30 minutes until done, and then drain. Chop celery, red onion, and zucchini into medium pieces. Chop the chili, garlic, and ginger very thinly, and set aside.

Heat the oil in a frying pan; add the celery, onion, zucchini, chili, garlic, and ginger. Fry over high heat for 1-2 minutes, then reduce to medium heat for 3-4 minutes until the vegetables are cooked through but are still crunchy.

If the vegetables begin to stick to the pan, you can add a cup of water. Add the tamari and spinach, and cook for 2 minutes. Serve with chicken and buckwheat.

NUTRITION FACTS: CALORIES 417KCAL   FAT 6.5 G   CARBOHYDRATE 34.8 G   PROTEIN 32.1 G

SPICY STEW WITH POTATOES AND SPINACH

 2 40 mins

Ingredients:
2 sweet potatoes
2 tsp. extra virgin olive oil
1 red onion, finely chopped
½ bird's eye chili
2 tbsp. paprika
1 cup tomatoes, chopped
1 cup stock
1 cup spinach
8 oz. chicken breast
Salt and pepper to taste

Directions:
Peel and cut sweet potatoes into 1-inch cubes and boil them for 12 minutes. Drain and set aside.

Heat a pan with oil on medium-high heat, add onion and cook for 5 minutes.

Add chicken cubes and spices and let the meat color on all sides for 5 minutes.

Add tomatoes and stock and let cook 15 minutes on low heat.

Add sweet potatoes and spinach, let the flavors mix for 5 minutes, then turn the heat off.

Let rest 10 minutes, then serve.

NUTRITION FACTS: CALORIES 213KCAL FAT 13.1 G SUGAR 51.7 G PROTEIN 80.6 G

SIRTFOOD GREEN JUICE

 1 5 mins

Ingredients:
Recipe 1:
1 tbsp. parsley
1 stalk celery
1 apple
½ lemon
Recipe 2:
1 cucumber
1 stalk celery
1 apple
3 mint leaves

Directions:
Choose one of the recipes.

Add all ingredients into a juicer and extract the juice according to the manufacturer's method.

In case you don't have one, add all the ingredients in a blender and pulse until well combined.

Filter the juice through a fine-mesh strainer and transfer it into a glass. Top with water if needed. Serve immediately.

NUTRITION FACTS: CALORIES 30KCAL FAT 0.4 G CARBOHYDRATE 4.5 G PROTEIN 1 G

SIMPLE ARUGULA SALAD

 2   10 mins

Ingredients:

1 white onion, sliced
1 tbsp. vinegar
1 cup arugula
¼ cup walnuts, chopped
2 tbsp. fresh cilantro, chopped
2 garlic cloves, peeled and minced
2 tbsp. extra virgin olive oil
1 tbsp. lemon juice

Directions:

In a bowl, mix the water and vinegar, add the onion, set aside for 5 minutes, and drain well. In a salad bowl, combine the arugula with the walnuts and onion, and stir.

Add the garlic, salt, pepper, lemon juice, cilantro, and oil, toss well, and serve.

NUTRITION FACTS: CALORIES 200KCAL FAT 2 G CARBOHYDRATE 5 G PROTEIN 7 G

TURKEY BACON FAJITAS

 2   25 mins

Ingredients:

3 eggs, lightly beaten
2 whole-grain tortillas
½ cup cherry tomatoes
1 red onion
2 turkey bacon slices
2 oz. cup shredded cheddar
1 tsp extra virgin olive oil

Directions:

Sauté the onion with olive oil on medium heat for 5 minutes, add the eggs and stir continuously until they are done.

Add turkey bacon, finely sliced, and cheddar cheese on top so that it starts to melt.

Quick heat the tortillas on a pan (keep them soft), divide the egg mixture between them, and serve immediately.

NUTRITION FACTS: CALORIES 353KCAL FAT 4.8 G CARBOHYDRATE 28.1 G PROTEIN 28.3 G

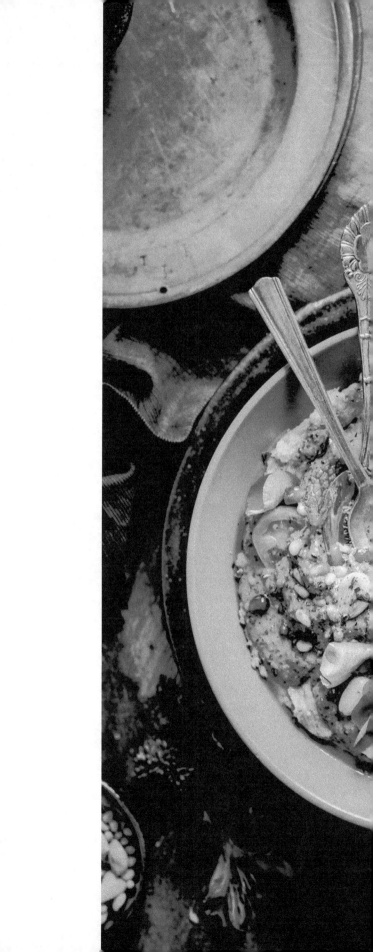

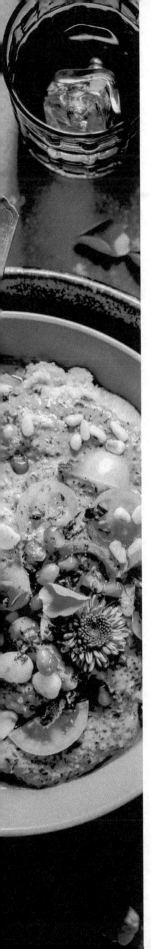

WEEK 4 – TRANSITION – RECIPES

BAKED SWEET POTATO

 1   55 mins

Ingredients:
1 medium sweet potato
1 tsp. butter

Directions:
Heat the oven to 425°F.

Clean the potato very well under running water to get rid of the dirt.

Prick it several times and put it in the oven for 50 minutes. Always remember to test if it's done using a stick.

Cut the upper part and pour the butter over the sweet potato.

NUTRITION FACTS: CALORIES 353KCAL FAT 4.8 G CARBOHYDRATE 28.1 G PROTEIN 28.3 G

CHICKPEA FRITTERS

 2   20 mins

Ingredients:
1 can chickpeas, drained
6 oz. chicken breasts, cooked and shredded
2 egg whites
½ cup fresh parsley leaves, very finely chopped
1 tsp. ginger
½ tsp. salt and pepper, to taste
2 tbsp. coconut oil, for frying

Directions:
Blend the chickpeas in a food processor, mix them with the chicken, egg whites, parsley, ginger, salt, and pepper into a smooth batter.

Heat the oil in a frying pan over medium heat. Using a large spoon, scoop the batter into fritters.

Cook each one for 2-3 minutes each side or until golden and cooked through.

NUTRITION FACTS: CALORIES 207KCAL FAT 3.1 G NET CARBOHYDRATE 35.6 G PROTEIN 10.3 G

CREAMY BROCCOLI AND POTATO SOUP

 4   ⏱ 4h + 30 mins

Ingredients:
3 cups broccoli, chopped
2 potatoes, peeled and chopped
1 large onion, chopped
3 garlic cloves, minced
1 cup raw cashews
3 cups vegetable broth
3 tsp. extra virgin olive oil
½ tsp. ground nutmeg

Directions:
Soak cashews in a bowl with boiling water and let rest for at least 4 hours.

Drain them and blend them with 1 cup of vegetable broth until smooth. Set aside. This will make the soup super creamy.

Gently heat olive oil in a large saucepan over medium-high heat. Cook onion and garlic for 3-4 minutes until tender. Add in broccoli, potato, nutmeg, and water.

Cover and bring to boil, then reduce heat and simmer for 20 minutes, stirring from time to time. Remove from heat and stir in cashew mixture.

Blend until smooth, return to pan and cook until heated through.

NUTRITION FACTS: CALORIES 305KCAL FAT 9.5 G CARBOHYDRATE 14.2 G PROTEIN 3.7 G

ENERGY COCOA BALLS

 2   ⏱ 35 mins + 4h

Ingredients:
4 dates, pitted
1 tbsp. peanut butter
20 almonds
Cocoa powder for coating

Directions:
Blend all the ingredients, then put the mix in the refrigerator for 30 minutes. Form the balls and coat them with cocoa powder. Put them back in the refrigerator for 4 hours before eating.

NUTRITION FACTS: CALORIES 132KCAL FAT 5.3 G CARBOHYDRATE 22.8 G PROTEIN 4.6 G

LAMB, BUTTERNUT SQUASH AND DATE TAGINE

 4   🕐 1h 20 mins

Ingredients:

2 tbsp. extra virgin olive oil
1 red onion, chopped
1-inch ginger, grated
3 garlic cloves, crushed
1 tsp. chili flakes
2 tsp. cumin seeds
1 cinnamon stick
2 tsp. ground turmeric
20 oz. lamb shoulder, cut into pieces
½ tsp. salt
2 oz. dates, pitted and sliced
2 cups tomatoes
1 cup broth
2 cups butternut squash, cubed
1 can chickpeas, drained
2 tbsp. fresh coriander
1 cup basmati rice

Directions:

Heat the oven to 325°F. Add oil into a tagine pot or an ovenproof saucepan with a lid, heat on the stove on low heat, and when hot, gently cook the onions until they are soft.

Add the grated ginger and garlic, chili, cumin, cinnamon, and turmeric. Stir well and cook 1 minute. Add a dash of water if it becomes too dry. Add the lamb and stir to coat it with spices and onions. Add dates, tomatoes, and 1 cup broth.

Bring the tagine to the boil, set the lid, and place on your preheated oven for about 1 hour and 15 minutes. Steam the basmati rice and put aside. After 45 minutes, add butternut squash and drained chickpeas to the tagine. Stir everything together, place the lid back on and return to the oven for 30 minutes.

Serve with basmati rice on the side.

NUTRITION FACTS: CALORIES 380KCAL FAT 13.1 G SUGAR 51.67 G PROTEIN 80.62 G

LEMON TUNA STEAKS WITH BABY POTATOES

 2 35 mins

Ingredients:
10 oz. tuna steaks
12 oz. baby potatoes, chopped
1 garlic clove, crushed
1 tbsp. thyme
½ tbsp. oregano
1 tbsp. rosemary
1 lemon
2 tsp. extra virgin olive oil
Salt and pepper to taste

Directions:
Heat the oven to 400°F. Marinate the tuna for 20 minutes with 1 tsp. oil, herbs, salt, pepper, and the juice of a half lemon. Chop the baby potatoes and season them with oil, salt, pepper, and rosemary.

Put potatoes in a baking tray, spreading the potatoes so that they are in a single layer. Cook them for 12 minutes. Cut the remaining half lemon in slices and put them on the tuna steaks. Take the tray out of the oven and add tuna steaks. Cook for another 10 minutes and serve immediately.

NUTRITION FACTS: CALORIES 305KCAL FAT 5.5 G CARBOHYDRATE 34.2 G PROTEIN 23.7 G

LEMONY CHICKEN BURGERS

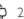 2 20 mins

Ingredients:
8 oz. chicken mince
¼ onion, finely chopped
1 clove garlic, crushed
1 handful of parsley, finely chopped
Juice and zest of ¼ lemon
2 leaves lettuce
½ tomato
2 tsp. extra virgin olive oil
2 whole-wheat buns

Directions:
Put chicken mince, onion, garlic, parsley, salt pepper, lemon zest, and juice in a bowl and mix well. Form 2 patties and let rest 5 minutes.

Heat a pan with olive oil, and when very hot, cook 3 minutes per part. They are also delicious when grilled. If you opt for grilling, just brush the patties with a bit of oil right before cooking.

Put the patties in the buns with lettuce and tomato and enjoy.

NUTRITION FACTS: CALORIES 353KCAL FAT 4.8 G CARBOHYDRATE 28.1 G PROTEIN 28.3 G

MEXICAN CHICKEN CASSEROLE

 2 45 mins

Ingredients:
½ cup buckwheat
½ red onion
8 oz. chicken mince
1 tbsp. paprika
½ bird's eye chili
1 clove garlic
4 oz. black beans, rinsed
2 cups spinach
1 cup shredded cheddar

Directions:
Boil buckwheat for 25 minutes, then rinse and put aside.

Heat a pan with oil. When hot, add onion, garlic, and chili, and cook for 5 minutes. Add mince and spices and cook for 10 minutes, stirring repeatedly. Add spinach and cook another 3 minutes.

Take a baking dish and put buckwheat as the first layer, then add chicken mince.

Spread the cheese on top and bake for 10 minutes until the cheese is melted

NUTRITION FACTS: CALORIES 353KCAL FAT 4.8 G CARBOHYDRATE 28.1 G PROTEIN 28.3 G

SPICY INDIAN DAHL WITH BASMATI RICE

 1   25 mins

Ingredients:
1 tsp. of extra virgin olive oil
2 oz. onion, nicely chopped
2 garlic cloves, nicely chopped
1 tsp. fresh ginger
1 bird's eye chili, finely sliced
1 tsp. of mild curry powder
1 tsp. of ground turmeric
1 tsp. cinnamon stick
½ tsp. cardamom seeds
½ tsp. cumin seeds
1 cup red lentils
1 medium tomato, chopped
1 oz. basmati rice
1 tsp. extra virgin olive oil

Directions:
Cook the lentils in boiling water for 20 to 25 minutes until almost done. In the meantime, cook the rice in a separate pot for 20 minutes and drain.

Put cinnamon, onion, garlic, ginger, and chili in a hot pan with olive oil. Cook until tender, for about 5 minutes, then discard the cinnamon stick. Drain the lentils and put them in the pan.

Add tomato, turmeric, curry, cardamom, and cumin and cook for a few minutes until all the flavors have mixed.

Serve Dahl with steamed rice.

NUTRITION FACTS: CALORIES 272KCAL FAT 4.3 G CARBOHYDRATE 26.8 G PROTEIN 23.6 G

SPINACH QUICHE

 4   50 mins

Ingredients:
5 oz. all purposes flour
2 oz. buckwheat flour
3 oz. almond flour
½ cup water
2 tbsp. extra virgin olive oil
1 small pinch of baking soda
6 cups spinach
3 eggs
1 cup ricotta cheese
1 tbsp. parmesan

Directions:
Mix the flours, salt, and baking soda. Add the water and mix until you get a dough. If needed, add some more water. Let the dough rest for 30 minutes.

Heat the oven to 350°F. Heat a pan with oil, put spinach and salt, and cook 5 minutes on low heat. Set aside.

When the dough is ready, roll the dough to 1/8 inch thickness and put it in a baking tin. Mix ricotta, eggs, salt, pepper, and spinach and put the filling in the tin.

Remove the excess dough with a knife. Bake 35 minutes. Let cool 10 minutes and serve.

The remaining dough can be stored in the fridge or freezer in an airtight container.

NUTRITION FACTS: CALORIES 353KCAL FAT 4.8 G CARBOHYDRATE 28.1 G PROTEIN 28.3 G

SIRTFOOD GREEN JUICE

 1   5 mins

Ingredients:
Recipe 1:
   1 tbsp. parsley
   1 stalk celery
   1 apple
   ½ lemon
Recipe 2:
   1 cucumber
   1 stalk celery
   1 apple
   3 mint leaves

Directions:
Choose one of the recipes above.

Add all ingredients into a juicer and extract the juice according to the manufacturer's method.

In case you don't have one, add all the ingredients in a blender and pulse until well combined.

Filter the juice through a fine-mesh strainer and transfer it into a glass. Top with water if needed. Serve immediately.

NUTRITION FACTS: CALORIES 30KCAL FAT 0.4 G CARBOHYDRATE 4.5 G PROTEIN 1 G

WALNUT ENERGY BAR

🍲 4   🕐 35 mins

Ingredients:
4 oz. rolled oats
1 oz. shredded coconut
8 walnuts, chopped
½ cup almond milk, unsweetened
3 tbsp. agave syrup
1 pinch salt
½ tsp vanilla extract
1 tbsp. peanut butter

Directions:
Mix all the ingredients, put them on a baking tin lined with parchment paper, and cook 20-25 minutes at 325°F until golden and crisp.

NUTRITION FACTS: CALORIES 192KCAL FAT 4.3 G CARBOHYDRATE 32.8 G PROTEIN 6.6 G

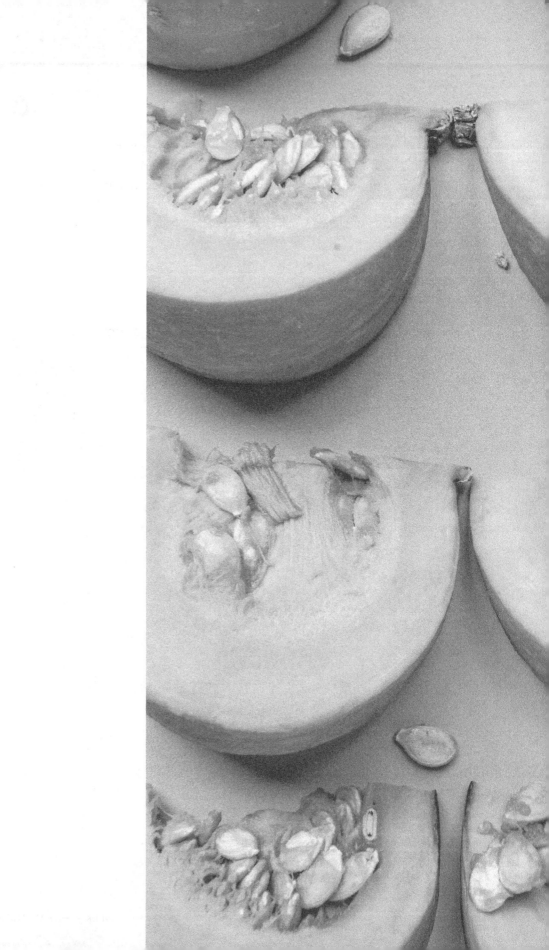

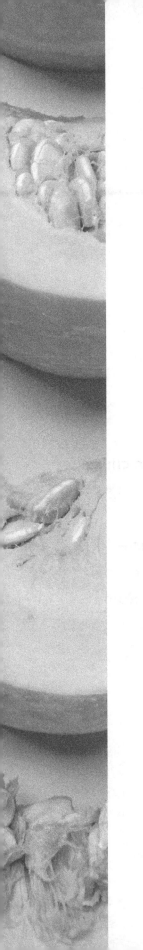

PLANT-BASED 4-WEEK MEAL PLAN AND PLANT-BASED RECIPES

WEEK 1 – PHASE 1

Quick Recap of the 7 day 'Hyper success Phase'

This week is divided into two moments:
Day 1-3 with 3 juices a day, 1 optional snack, and a full meal.
Day 4-7 with 2 juices a day, 2 optional snacks, and a full meal.

WEEK 1 – PHASE 1 – SHOPPING LIST

- Artichokes
- Asparagus
- Avocados
- Basil
- Beet
- Bird' eye chili
- Black olives
- Bread
- Broccoli
- Brown rice
- Buckwheat
- Butternut squash
- Carrots
- Celery
- Chick peas
- Coconut cream
- Garlic
- Ginger
- Green peppers
- Leek
- Lemons
- Mushrooms
- Oranges
- Parsley
- Peas
- Pecans
- Potatoes
- Red endive
- Raspberries, frozen
- Red onions
- Red peppers
- Red quinoa
- Romaine
- Scallions
- Shallot
- Soy protein chunks
- Spinach
- Tofu, firm
- Tomato paste
- Tomatoes, canned
- Tomatoes, Roma and cherry

<u>Important:</u> The Plan lets you choose your favorite Sirtfood Green Juices Recipes each week. Remember to add the ingredients to this list.

WEEK 1 – PHASE 1 – PLANT-BASED MEAL PLAN

DAY	BREAKFAST	SNACK	LUNCH	SNACK	DINNER
MON	Sirtfood Green Juice (page 127)	2 squares of dark chocolate	Sirtfood Green Juice (page 127)	Sirtfood Green Juice (page 127)	Squash and Peppers Soup (pages 194)
TUE	Sirtfood Green Juice (page 127)	2 squares of dark chocolate	Sirtfood Green Juice (page 127)	Sirtfood Green Juice (page 127)	Colorful Quinoa Salad (page 190)
WED	Sirtfood Green Juice (page 127)	2 squares of dark chocolate	Sirtfood Green Juice (page 127)	Sirtfood Green Juice (page 127)	Crispy Tofu Cubes Raw Artichoke Salad (page 190/134)
THU	Sirtfood Green Juice (page 127)	Sirtfood Green Juice (page 127)	Grilled Asparagus with Tapenade Toast (page 191)	2 squares of dark chocolate	Mushrooms and Buckwheat Soup (page 184)
FRI	Sirtfood Green Juice (page 127)	Sirtfood Green Juice (page 127)	Romaine Hearts with Tofu and Candied Pecans (page 193)	2 squares of dark chocolate	Green Veggies Curry (page 132)
SAT	Sirtfood Green Juice (page 127)	Sirtfood Green Juice (page 127)	Avocado with Raspberry Vinegar Salad (page 188)	2 squares of dark chocolate	Irish Cabbage Soup (page 192)
SUN	Sirtfood Green Juice (page 127)	Sirtfood Green Juice (page 127)	White Bean and Tomato Salad (page 193)	2 squares of dark chocolate	Beefless Stew (page 189)

WEEK 2 AND 3 – PHASE 2:

Quick Recap of the 'Maintenance Phase'

This week is divided into two parts:
Week 2 with 1 juice a day, 2 optional snacks, and 2 full meals.
Week 3 with 1 juice a day, 2 optional snacks, and 2 full meals.

WEEK 2 – PHASE 2 – SHOPPING LIST

- 85% Chocolate
- Almond Milk, unsweetened
- Apricots, dried
- Asparagus
- Avocado
- Baby Spinach
- Banana
- Bean sprouts
- Bitter greens (arugula, watercress, etc.)
- Black Beans
- Blueberries
- Brown Rice
- Buckwheat
- Buckwheat
- Breadcrumbs
- Buckwheat Flour
- Buckwheat pasta
- Cabbage
- Carrots
- Cauliflower
- Celery
- Chestnuts
- Chickpea flour

- Chickpeas
- Bird's Eye chili
- Coconut Milk
- Coconut Yogurt
- Cucumber
- Dark Chocolate Chips
- Dulse Seaweed
- Eggplant
- Flax Seeds
- Flour
- Garlic
- Ginger
- Green Onions
- Kale
- Kidney Beans
- Lemons
- Lettuce
- Lime
- Mango
- Mint
- Mixed berries, frozen
- Mung sprout
- Mushrooms
- Nutritional Yeast
- Oranges

- Parsley
- Potatoes
- Raisins
- Raspberries, frozen
- Red Bell Peppers
- Red lentils
- Red Onions
- Red Wine
- Rolled Oats
- Scallions
- Seitan
- Self-Raising Flour
- Snow Peas
- Soy Milk
- Spinach
- Strawberries
- Sun-Dried Tomatoes
- Tahini
- Tofu, firm and silken
- Tomato Sauce
- Tomatoes
- Walnuts
- Yams
- Zucchini

<u>Important:</u> The Plan lets you choose your favorite Sirtfood Green Juices Recipes each week. Remember to add the ingredients to this list.

WEEK 2 – PHASE 2 – PLANT-BASED MEAL PLAN

DAY	BREAKFAST	SNACK	LUNCH	SNACK	DINNER
MON	Fluffy Blueberry Pancakes (page 146)	Sirtfood Green Juice (page 127)	Cajun Tofu Ginger Zucchini (page 200/202)	2 squares of dark chocolate	Jamaican Pea Soup (page 205)
TUE	Banana Flax Smoothie (page 198)	Sirtfood Green Juice (page 127)	Armenian Soup (page 197)	Banana Strawberry Smoothie (page 142)	Zucchini Boats (page 210)
WED	Vanilla Coconut Parfait with Berries (page 209)	Sirtfood Green Juice (page 127)	Bitter Greens, Mung Sprouts, Avocado, and Orange Salad (page 200)	2 squares of dark chocolate	Baked Cabbage with Buckwheat and Walnuts (page 198)
THU	Mango Banana Smoothie (page 206)	Sirtfood Green Juice (page 127)	Tofu Patties with Mushrooms and Peas (page 209)	Blueberry Smoothie (page 143)	Golden Chickpea Soup (page 203)
FRI	Overnight Oats with Blueberries and Chocolate (page 206)	Sirtfood Green Juice (page 127)	Hot Garbanzo Beans with Sun Dried Tomatoes (page 203)	2 squares of dark chocolate	Asparagus Seitan with Black Bean Sauce (page 197)
SAT	Raspberry Greens Smoothie (page 208)	Sirtfood Green Juice (page 127)	Scalloped Eggplant Creamy Sea Salad (page 208/201)	Dark Chocolate Mousse (page 202)	Mushroom and Potato Pie (page 207)
SUN	Raspberry Greens Smoothie (page 208)	Sirtfood Green Juice (page 127)	Coconut Spinach Soup (page 201)	2 squares of dark chocolate	Indian Vegetarian Meatballs (page 178)

WEEK 3 – PHASE 2 – SHOPPING LIST

- 85% chocolate
- Almond Milk, unsweetened
- Apples, Red and Green
- Arugula
- Avocado
- Baby Corn
- Baby Spinach
- Bananas
- Basil
- Beets
- Blueberries
- Breadcrumbs
- Broccoli
- Brown Rice
- Buckwheat
- Breadcrumbs
- Buckwheat Flour
- Buckwheat Macaroni
- Buckwheat Noodles
- Buckwheat, puffed
- Capers
- Carrots
- Cauliflower

- Celery
- Chickpea flour
- Chickpeas
- Chilies
- Coconut Milk
- Coconut Yogurt
- Coconut, shredded
- Dark Chocolate Chips
- Dates
- Eggplants
- Garlic
- Ginger
- Green Onions
- Hummus
- Kale
- Leeks
- Lemons
- Lentils, Brown and Red
- Liquid Smoke
- Mango
- Mint
- Mixed Berries, frozen
- Morels

- Mushrooms
- Olives, Black and Green
- Parsley
- Potatoes
- Pumpkin Seeds
- Red Bell Pepper
- Red Onions
- Red Wine
- Rolled Oats
- Scallions
- Seitan
- Self-Raising Flour
- Snow Peas
- Soy Milk
- Strawberries
- Thyme
- Tofu, firm and silken
- Tomato Paste
- Tomato Sauce
- Tomatoes, Cherries and Roma
- Walnuts
- Zucchini

<u>Important:</u> The Plan lets you choose your favorite Sirtfood Green Juices Recipes each week. Remember to add the ingredients to this list.

DAY	BREAKFAST	SNACK	LUNCH	SNACK	DINNER
MON	Strawberry and Walnut Bake (page 222)	Sirtfood Green Juice (page 127)	Potato, Morel and Onion Fricassee (page 219)	Buckwheat Granola (page 158)	Veggie Fajitas (page 222)
TUE	Banana Berry Kale Smoothie (page 214)	Sirtfood Green Juice (page 127)	Baked Eggplant with Turmeric and Garlic with Simple Arugula Salad (page 213/165)	2 squares of dark chocolate	Eggplant, Tomato and Onion Gratin (page 215)
WED	Banana, Vanilla, and Choc Chip Pancake (page 299)	Sirtfood Green Juice (page 127)	Indian Vegetarian Meatballs (page 148)	Blueberry Smoothie (page 158)	Curry Chickpeas Beets with Leek and Parsley (page 214/5)
THU	Overnight Oats and Blueberries and Chocolate (page 206)	Sirtfood Green Juice (page 127)	Lentils and Chickpeas Stew (page 218)	2 squares of dark chocolate	Greek-style Macaroni Casserole (page 217)
FRI	Fluffy Blueberry Pancakes (page 144)	Sirtfood Green Juice (page 127)	White Bean and Tomato Salad (page 193)	Dark Chocolate Mousse (page 202)	Smoky Tofu Stir (page 221)
SAT	Apple and Avocado Smoothie (page 213)	Sirtfood Green Juice (page 127)	Roasted Butternut and Chickpeas Salad (page 162)	2 squares of dark chocolate	Eggplant Creamy Pizza Towers (page 216)
SUN	Vanilla Coconut Parfait with Berries (page 231)	Sirtfood Green Juice (page 127)	Lentil and Onion Soup (page 218)	Mango Coconut Mousse (page 219)	Mushroom and Tomato Risotto (page 220)

WEEK 4 – PHASE 3

Quick Recap of the 'Transition Phase'

After completing successfully Phase 1 and 2, Phase 3 helps you transition to a normal healthy eating plan that continues to include a variety of sirtfoods in daily meals.

Week 4: 1 juice a day, 2 snacks, and 3 full meals.

WEEK 4 – TRANSITION – SHOPPING LIST

- Almond Milk, unsweetened
- Almond Flour
- Arugula
- Avocado
- Baby potatoes
- Baby Spinach
- Banana
- Blueberries
- Broccoli
- Brussels Sprouts

- Buns, whole-wheat
- Butternut Squash
- Buckwheat
- Chickpeas, canned
- Endive
- Coconut, shredded
- Dates
- Lettuce
- Lentils, canned
- Mushrooms
- Oats

- Parsley
- Peanut Butter
- Potatoes
- Red Onions
- Red Peppers
- Red Wine
- Spinach
- Strawberries
- Sweet potatoes
- Tomatoes

Important: The Plan lets you choose your favorite Sirtfood Green Juices Recipes each week. Remember to add the ingredients to this list.

DAY	BREAKFAST	SNACK	LUNCH	SNACK	DINNER
MON	Peanut Butter Cup Smoothie (page 230)	Dark Chocolate Mousse (page 202)	Tomato Bisque (page 232)	Sirtfood Green Juice (page 127)	Spicy Indian Dahl with Basmati Rice (page 173)
TUE	Vanilla Coconut Parfait with Berries (page 231)	Sirtfood Green Juice (page 127)	Romaine Hearts with Tofu and Candied Pecans (page 193)	Walnut Energy Bar (page 232)	Creole Tofu Baked Sweet Potato (page 227/169)
WED	Strawberry and Walnut Bake (page 222)	Mango Coconut Mousse (page 219)	Creamy Potato Leek Soup (page 226)	Sirtfood Green Juice (page 127)	Chickpea Pita Pockets (page 226)
THU	Kale Berry Delight Smoothie (page 227)	Sirtfood Green Juice (page 127)	Baked Eggplant with Turmeric and Garlic, Simple Arugula Salad (page 213)	Dark Chocolate Mousse (page 202)	Stir Fried Tofu and Vegetables in Ginger Sauce (page 231)
FRI	Fluffy Blueberry Pancakes (146)	2 squares of dark chocolate	Tofu Patties with Mushrooms and Peas (page 209)	Sirtfood Green Juice (page 127)	Creamy Broccoli and Potato Soup (page 170)
SAT	Overnight Oats with Blueberries and Chocolate (page 206)	Sirtfood Green Juice (page 127)	Noodles with Walnut Sauce (page 230)	Buckwheat Granola (page 158) ½ cup plain yogurt	Louisiana-style Veggie Sausages Carmelized Fennel (page 229)
SUN	Banana, Vanilla, and Choco Chip Pancake (page 199)	Sirtfood Green Juice (page 127)	Eggplant, Tomato. and Onion Gratin (page 215)	Energy Cocoa Balls (page 170)	Fried Rice with Hot Leek Sauce (page 228)

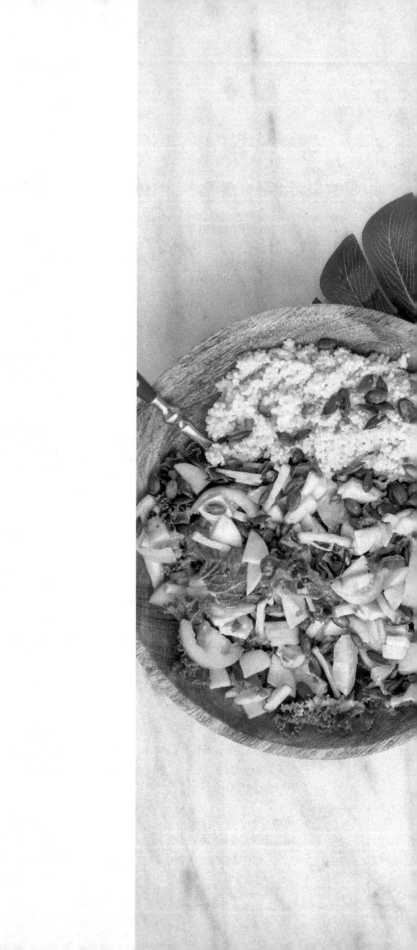

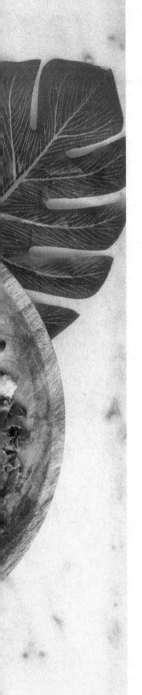

WEEK 1 – PHASE 1 PLANT-BASED RECIPES

AVOCADO WITH RASPBERRY VINEGAR SALAD

 2 25 mins

Ingredients:

4 oz. fresh or frozen raspberries

3 oz, red wine vinegar

1 tsp. extra-virgin olive oil

2 firm-ripe avocados

1 red endive

Directions:

Place half the raspberries in a bowl. Heat the vinegar in a saucepan until it starts to bubble, then pour it over the raspberries and leave too steep for 5 minutes.

Strain the raspberries, pressing the fruit gently to extract all the juices but not the pulp.

Whisk the strained raspberry vinegar together with the oils and seasonings. Set aside.

Carefully halve each avocado and twist out the stone.

Peel away the skin and cut the flesh straight into the dressing.

Stir gently until the avocados are entirely covered in the dressing.

Cover tightly and chill in the fridge for about 2 hours.

Meanwhile, separate the radicchio leaves, rinse and drain them, then dry them on kitchen paper. Store in the fridge in a polythene bag.

To serve, place a few endive leaves on individual plates.

Spoon on the avocado, stir and trim with the remaining raspberries.

NUTRITION FACTS: CALORIES 163KCAL FAT 4 G CARBOHYDRATE 15 G PROTEIN 14 G

BEEFLESS STEW

 4   45 mins

Ingredients:

1 cup dry soy "beef" protein chunks
1 tsp. lemon juice
1 red onion, chopped
1 garlic clove, diced
1 tbsp. extra-virgin olive oil
4 cups water
14 oz. tomatoes
1 tsp. vegan Worcestershire sauce
1 bay leaf
10 oz. peas
6 carrots, chopped
1 stalk celery
3 potatoes, chopped into bite-sized pieces
2 tbsp. cornstarch

Directions:

Put the soy chunks in boiling water and lemon juice. Set aside for 15 minutes, then squeeze out all the water using the hands.

Heat a pan with the oil and sautè the onion and garlic. Add the soy chunks and cook for 5 minutes.

Add 4 cups of water, tomatoes, celery, Worcestershire sauce, bay leaf, salt, pepper, and simmer for 5 minutes.

Add the peas, potatoes, and carrots, and cook for 30 minutes.

Dissolve the cornstarch in a few drops of water and thicken the stew to the desired consistency..

NUTRITION FACTS: CALORIES 199KCAL FAT 5 G CARBOHYDRATE 20 G PROTEIN 18 G

COLORFUL QUINOA SALAD

 4   40 mins

Ingredients:

1 cup dried red quinoa
2 cups of water
2 scallions, chopped
2 carrots, grated
1 stalk celery
1 beet, grated
1/3 cup fresh parsley, chopped
1/3 cup cranberries
1/3 cup walnuts, chopped
2 tbsp. olive oil
1 tsp. toasted sesame oil
2 tsp. lemon juice

Directions:

Cook the quinoa in salted water (1 cup quinoa and 2 cups of water) for about 25 minutes until the water is absorbed. Make it fluffy by mixing it gently with a fork.

Add scallions, carrots, beet, parsley, cranberries, and walnuts, tossing to mix.

In a separate bowl, prepare the dressing. Whisk the olive oil, sesame oil, lemon juice, and salt and pepper to taste. Pour over quinoa and toss to distribute it evenly.

Serve immediately, or refrigerate for a couple of hours.

NUTRITION FACTS: CALORIES 230KCAL FAT 3 G CARBOHYDRATE 24 G PROTEIN 13 G

CRISPY TOFU CUBES

  4   35 mins

Ingredients:

1 lb. firm tofu
2 tbsp. nutritional yeast
2 tbsp. flour
1 tbsp. garlic powder
1 tsp. pepper
2 tbsp. extra-virgin olive oil

Directions:

Cut the tofu into 1/4-inch cubes. Do not pat dry. Put the flour in a bowl, add the nutritional yeast, garlic, pepper, mix with a fork, add the tofu, and coat it well on all sides.

Heat the oil in a saucepan. Cook the tofu over medium heat, turning it after 2-3 minutes until crispy.

NUTRITION FACTS: CALORIES 192KCAL FAT 5 G CARBOHYDRATE 20 G PROTEIN 18 G

GRILLED ASPARAGUS WITH TAPENADE TOAST

 2   *45 mins*

Ingredients:

1 shallot
2 blood oranges
1 ½ tsp. balsamic vinegar
½ tsp. red wine vinegar
4 tsp. extra-virgin olive oil
1 ½ lbs. asparagus (25 –30 spears)
4 slices bread
2 cups black olives
1 garlic clove

Directions:

Blend olives, garlic, olive oil together to prepare the tapenade.

Peel and cut the shallot fine and macerate for 30 minutes in the juice of ½ orange and the balsamic and red wine vinegar. Add the olive oil with salt and pepper to taste and whisk to make a vinaigrette.

Grate the zest of 1 orange and add it to the vinaigrette.

Peel the oranges and slice them. Cut the bottom ends of the asparagus spears, brush them with olive oil and grill them for 5 minutes, until evenly brown.

Toast bread, cut it diagonally, and put the tapenade on top. Arrange asparagus on a platter with the orange cuts on top and the tapenade toasts on the side.

Drizzle vinaigrette over and serve.

NUTRITION FACTS: CALORIES 1990KCAL FAT 5 G CARBOHYDRATE 20 G PROTEIN 18 G

IRISH CABBAGE SOUP

 6   🕐 55 mins

Ingredients:
3 red onions
8 oz. raisins
1/2 cup brown rice, raw
15 oz tomatoes, canned
1 can tomato paste
1 splash of vinegar
2 cups cabbage, shredded

Directions:
Put cabbage, onions, raisins, and rice in a pot. Add water to cover generously.

Cook for 50 minutes until the cabbage is faded and the water is bright purple. Add tomatoes and vinegar. Season with salt and pepper to taste. Cook for another 10 minutes, then blend and serve.

NUTRITION FACTS: CALORIES 210KCAL FAT 4 G CARBOHYDRATE 20 G PROTEIN 6 G

MUSHROOM AND BUCKWHEAT SOUP

🥘 6   🕐 35 mins

Ingredients:
3 tbsp. extra-virgin olive oil
1 onion, chopped
1 leek, chopped
8 cups vegetable broth
1 lb. white potatoes, peeled and diced
1 carrot, chopped
2 cups buckwheat, cooked
3 bay leaves

Directions:
Separate mushroom stems from caps. Cut caps and set aside. Cut stems.

Heat extra-virgin olive oil in a saucepan over medium-high heat. Add mushroom stems, onion, and leek and sauté until tender, about 8 minutes. Stir in vegetable broth, potatoes, carrot, barley, and bay leaves.

Cover, stir, and simmer 10 minutes. Uncover soup, add sliced mushroom caps and buckwheat. Cook for 10 minutes, season with salt and pepper and serve.

NUTRITION FACTS: CALORIES 139KCAL FAT 3 G CARBOHYDRATE 18 G PROTEIN 16 G

ROMAINE HEARTS WITH TOFU AND CANDIED PECANS

 4   20 mins

Ingredients:

2 tsp. agave syrup
1 tsp. extra-virgin olive oil
1/2 cup pecans
3/4 tbsp. balsamic vinegar
1 tsp. Dijon mustard
1 tsp. each chopped fresh parsley and basil
3 tbsp. olive oil
2 romaine hearts, chopped
3½ oz. tofu

Directions:

Mix the agave syrup and 1 tbsp. oil with pecans and place them in a preheated 375°F oven for 10 minutes until lightly toasted. Let cool to room temperature.

Place the vinegar, mustard, salt, pepper, and parsley in a salad bowl and whisk. Slowly whisk in the olive oil. Add the romaine and toss to coat.

Top with the pecans and the tofu, crumbled. Serve immediately..

NUTRITION FACTS: CALORIES 210KCAL FAT 7 G CARBOHYDRATE 21G PROTEIN 13 G

WHITE BEAN AND TOMATO SALAD

4   20 mins

Ingredients:

2 cups cherry tomatoes, halved
4 scallions thinly chopped
2 tbsp. olive oil
14 oz. cannellini beans, cooked
1 tbsp. fresh lemon juice
1 handful parsley

Directions:

Mix cannellini, cherry tomatoes, and scallions in a bowl. Dress with olive oil, lemon juice, salt, and pepper to taste.

Finely chop the parsley. Add it to the beans, mix and serve.

NUTRITION FACTS: CALORIES 209KCAL FAT 4 G CARBOHYDRATE 29 G PROTEIN 11 G

SQUASH AND PEPPERS SOUP

 6 40 mins

Ingredients:
1/2 cup buckwheat, cooked
1/2 lb. chickpeas, cooked
2 cups mushrooms, chopped
2 cups butternut squash, chopped
1/2 cup of chopped green peppers
1/2 cup of chopped red peppers
1 red onion, chopped
2 Roma tomatoes, diced
1/2 gallon water
1 tsp. dill
1 tsp. red cayenne pepper
1 tbsp. extra-virgin olive oil
1 tsp. oregano
1 tsp. basil

Directions:

Bring the water to a boil. Add mushrooms, peppers, onion, tomatoes, butternut squash, salt and pepper, and simmer for 30 minutes.

Add chickpeas, buckwheat, cayenne, oregano, and basil and heat through.

Add the olive oil on top and serve.

NUTRITION FACTS: CALORIES 44KCAL FAT 30 G CARBOHYDRATE 2 G PROTEIN 8 G

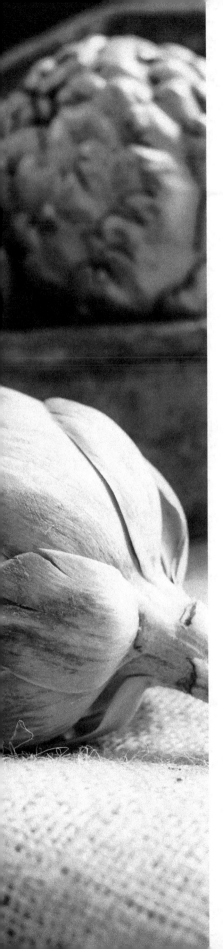

WEEK 2 – PHASE 2 PLANT-BASED RECIPES

ARMENIAN SOUP

 6   🕐 45 mins

Ingredients:
2 oz. red lentils, washed
2 oz. dried apricots
1 potato
4 cups vegetable stock
juice of 1/2 lemon
1 tsp. ground cumin
3 tbsp. parsley, chopped

Directions:
Place lentils in a saucepan. Roughly cut the potato and add it to the pan with the apricots, cumin, and stock. Bring to a boil, and simmer for 30 minutes.

Add lemon juice and blend until smooth.

Top with parsley and serve.

NUTRITION FACTS: CALORIES 219KCAL FAT 4 G CARBOHYDRATE 22 G PROTEIN 16 G

ASPARAGUS SEITAN WITH BLACK BEAN SAUCE

 5   🕐 35 mins

Ingredients:
1/2 cup veggie broth
1 tbsp. soy sauce
1 tbsp. cornstarch
1/2 tsp. sugar
2 cups seitan, sliced
2 tsp. red wine
1 tsp. water
1 tsp. cornstarch
1 tsp. soy sauce
1 tbsp. extra-virgin oil
2 cloves garlic, diced or crushed
2 tsp. black beans, mashed
1 lb. asparagus, into 1-inch pieces

Directions:
Mix the seitan slices with the red wine, 1 tsp. water, 1 tsp. cornstarch and 1 tsp. soy sauce in a bowl. Heat a skillet with oil and, when hot, add the onion, garlic, and mashed black beans.

Sauté for 1 minute over high heat. Add the seitan and cook for another 4 minutes until golden on all sides. Add the asparagus to the pan and stir-fry for 5 minutes.

Lower the heat, add 4 tbsps. of water and let the sauce thicken thanks to cornstarch, about 2 to 3 minutes. Serve hot.

NUTRITION FACTS: CALORIES 340KCAL FAT 5 G CARBOHYDRATE 20 G PROTEIN 18 G

BAKED CABBAGE WITH BUCKWHEAT AND WALNUTS

 4   32 mins

Ingredients:

1 lb. white or green cabbage, finely chopped
1 onion, finely chopped
2 cups buckwheat, cooked
1 cup vegetable stock
1 cup boiling water
2 oz. walnuts
2 tbsp. extra-virgin olive oil
2 oz. raisins

Directions:

Cook the finely chopped onion in some olive oil until it is transparent. Add the cabbage, then add the stock season with salt and pepper to taste.

Simmer for 20 minutes on low heat until the cabbage is still crunchy.

Move the cabbage to an ovenproof dish. While the cabbage is cooking, boil buckwheat in salted water, drain, and stir in the walnuts and raisins.

Spread the buckwheat over the cabbage, and cook for 20 minutes in the oven at 350°F.

NUTRITION FACTS: CALORIES 199KCAL FAT 5 G CARBOHYDRATE 20 G PROTEIN 18 G

BANANA FLAX SMOOTHIE

 2   5 mins

Ingredients:

2 cups kale
½ cup blueberries
1 frozen banana
1 tbsp. flax seeds
1 cup water

Directions:

Add all ingredients to a high-power blender and pulse until smooth.

Pour the smoothie into two glasses and serve immediately.

It can be stored in the refrigerator in an airtight container for up to 3 days.

NUTRITION FACTS: CALORIES 138KCAL FAT 4 G CARBOHYDRATE 18 G PROTEIN 4 G

BANANA, VANILLA, AND CHOC CHIP PANCAKE

 2 25 mins

Ingredients:
1 banana
2 tsp. agave syrup
1 cup rolled oats
¼ tsp. baking powder
A pinch of salt
1 tsp. vanilla extract
½ cup almond milk, unsweetened
1 tbsp. dark chocolate chips

Directions:
Put half of the banana, eggs, oats, vanilla, baking powder, salt, and almond milk in a blender and blend until smooth.

Heat a skillet, and when hot, pour the batter in to form pancakes.

Top with honey and the other half banana

NUTRITION FACTS: CALORIES 232KCAL FAT 5.3 G CARBOHYDRATE 22.8 G PROTEIN 18.6 G

BLUEBERRY PANCAKES

 2 20 mins

Ingredients:
2 oz. self-raising flour
1 oz. buckwheat flour
1/3 cup almond milk, unsweetened
1 cup blueberries
2 tsp. agave syrup

Directions:
Mix the flours in a bowl, add the yolk, and mix in a very thick batter. Keep adding the milk bit by bit to avoid lumps.

In another bowl, beat the egg white until stiff and then mix it carefully to the batter.

Pour enough batter on the skillet to make a 5-inch round pancake to cook 2 minutes per side until done. Repeat until all the pancakes are ready.

Put 1 tsp. honey and ½ cup blueberries on top of each serving.

NUTRITION FACTS: CALORIES 272KCAL FAT 4.3 G CARBOHYDRATE 26.8 G PROTEIN 23.6 G

BITTER GREENS, MUNG SPROUTS, AVOCADO, AND ORANGE SALAD

 4   ⏱ I min

Ingredients:
I cup baby spinach leaves
I cup bitter greens (arugula, dandelion, watercress, etc.)
I cup Mung sprouts
I orange, into wedges
1/2 cup diced avocado
¼ cup walnuts, soaked
2 tbsp. extra-virgin olive oil
I tbsp. lemon juice
I tsp. lemon zest
Fresh cracked black pepper to taste
I Tbsp. tahini
1/2 tsp. diced fresh ginger

Directions:
Mix spinach leaves, bitter greens, and Mung sprouts in a bowl. Add the orange and avocado. In another bowl, whisk the lemon juice, olive oil, lemon zest, salt, pepper, ginger, and tahini.

Pour the dressing over the salad and toss to coat. Trim with the chopped walnuts and serve immediately.

NUTRITION FACTS: CALORIES 173KCAL FAT 4 G CARBOHYDRATE 15 G PROTEIN 9 G

CAJUN TOFU

 4   ⏱ 35 mins

Ingredients:
2 stalks celery, thinly chopped
I red onion, thinly chopped
2 green bell peppers, thinly chopped
2 lbs. firm tofu, diced
2 tomatoes, diced
3 tsp. paprika
3/4 tsp. thyme
1/4 tsp. cayenne
1/2 cup parsley, chopped
3 tbsp. extra-virgin olive oil
1/3 cup water

Directions:
Sauté the onion, bell pepper, and celery in a saucepan with oil for 5 minutes. Add the tofu and sauté until it begins to brown on all sides.

Add tomatoes, paprika, thyme, cayenne, and water and simmer on low heat for 25 minutes. Top with parsley.

It can be served alone, with rice or buckwheat.

NUTRITION FACTS: CALORIES 199KCAL FAT 5 G CARBOHYDRATE 20 G PROTEIN 18 G

COCONUT SPINACH SOUP

 2   20 mins

Ingredients:
1 cup coconut milk
3 cups spinach
1 tsp. curry paste
½ tsp. turmeric
1 1/2-inch fresh ginger, grated
1 tbsp. soy sauce

Directions:
Put spinach, coconut milk, curry, turmeric, ginger, and soy sauce in a pan and simmer until the spinach is cooked, around 15 minutes.

NUTRITION FACTS: CALORIES 234KCAL FAT 5 G CARBOHYDRATE 9 G PROTEIN 8 G

CREAMY SEA SALAD

 4   10 mins

Ingredients:
1 head of lettuce
1 ripe avocado
3 Roma tomatoes
½ cucumber
A handful of dulse seaweed, soaked
2 tbsp. sesame seeds
1 tbsp. extra-virgin olive oil
Juice of ¼ lemon
A handful parsley, chopped

Directions:
Finely shred the lettuce into thin strips using a sharp knife and place it in a bowl. Dice the avocado, tomatoes, and cucumber into medium-sized pieces.

Tear the dulse into small pieces. Add the veggies to the lettuce bowl. Mix oil, sesame seeds, lemon, parsley, salt, and pepper to taste.

Pour the dressing over the salad, stir everything together, and serve.

NUTRITION FACTS: CALORIES 220KCAL FAT 8 G CARBOHYDRATE 15 G PROTEIN 15 G

DARK CHOCOLATE MOUSSE

 4   10mins, 2+h

Ingredients:

1 (16 oz.) package silken tofu, drained
½ cup pure agave syrup
1 tsp. pure vanilla extract
¼ cup of soy milk
½ cup unsweetened cocoa powder
Mint leaves

Directions:

Blend the tofu, agave syrup, and vanilla in a food processor. Add soy milk and cocoa and blend again until smooth.

Pour the mousse into small cups and chill for at least 2 hours. Garnish with fresh mint leaves just before serving.

NUTRITION FACTS: CALORIES 175KCAL FAT 24 G CARBOHYDRATE 18 G PROTEIN 5 G

GINGER ZUCCHINI

 4   15 mins

Ingredients:

1 tbsp. olive oil
1 lb. zucchini chopped into 1/4-inch cuts
1/2 cup vegetarian broth
2 tsp. light soy sauce
1 tbsp. red wine
1 tsp. sesame oil

Directions:

Heat a skillet with oil and when it is hot, add the zucchini and ginger. Stir-fry for 1 minute, then add soy sauce, red wine, and broth.

Cook over high heat until the broth reduces and the zucchini is tender. Drizzle sesame oil and serve.

NUTRITION FACTS: CALORIES 160KCAL FAT 4 G CARBOHYDRATE 12 G PROTEIN 2 G

GOLDEN CHICKPEA SOUP

  6   🕐 40 mins

Ingredients:

6 cloves fresh garlic, crushed
6 cups vegetable broth
1 lb. chickpeas, cooked
1 red onion, chopped
2 carrots, peeled and diced
2 tbsp. parsley
2 bay leaves
1 tbsp. extra-virgin olive oil
1/4 tsp. ground black pepper
4 oz. buckwheat pasta

Directions:

Heat a pot with olive oil and, when hot, add the garlic and sauté for 2 minutes. Add chickpeas, red onion, carrots, bay leaf, and broth, bring to a boil, and simmer for 30 minutes. Remove the bay leaves from the soup.

Blend 2 cups of the soup until smooth, and put them back in the pot.

Add the pasta and simmer for 8 minutes. Serve hot.

NUTRITION FACTS: CALORIES 224KCAL FAT 5 G CARBOHYDRATE 25 G PROTEIN 8 G

HOT GARBANZO BEANS
WITH SUN-DRIED TOMATOES

🗚 2   🕐 40 mins

Ingredients:

2 tbsp. olive oil
4 sun-dried tomatoes, thinly chopped
2 garlic cloves, thinly chopped
½ red onion, thinly chopped
1 tsp. chili flakes
16 oz. garbanzo beans, cooked

Directions:

Sautè the onion, garlic, chili flakes, and sun-dried tomatoes in a hot pan with oil.

Add the garbanzo beans and cook for 5 minutes. Add 1 cup of water and simmer for 10 minutes, until the liquid is almost gone.

Add salt and black pepper to taste and serve immediately.

NUTRITION FACTS: CALORIES 268KCAL FAT 5 G CARBOHYDRATE 29 G PROTEIN 12 G

INDIAN PLANT-BASED MEATBALLS

 2   🕐 35 mins

Ingredients:

1 cup cauliflower
1 cup brown rice
¼ cup breadcrumbs
2 tbsp. chickpea flour
½ tsp. turmeric
1 tsp. smoked paprika
1 tsp. of extra-virgin olive oil
2 cloves garlic, crushed
1 cup tomato sauce
Broth (if needed)
Cooking spray
1 tbsp. extra-virgin olive oil
1 ½ tbsp. garam masala
1 tsp ginger
1 tbsp. parsley, chopped
1 red onion-diced
6 oz. full-fat coconut milk

Directions:

Whisk chickpea flour with 4 tbsp. water and let sit 5 minutes. Steam cauliflower for 5 minutes, then blend it with rice. Use pulse to get a result similar to mince. Add chickpea batter, breadcrumbs, 1 garlic clove, salt, pepper, turmeric, paprika, and finely chopped parsley.

Mix well until you can form meatballs. Note: if it's too dry, add 1 tbsp. egg white and mix. If it's too runny, add 1 tbsp. breadcrumbs and mix. Spray a pan with cooking spray, heat it, and gently cook the meatballs for 5 minutes until golden. Be careful when you turn them so that they don't break. Put them aside

In a different pan, put oil, onion, ginger, garlic, salt, and pepper and cook on low heat until the onion is done. Add tomato sauce and coconut milk and let it simmer around 15 minutes until thickened. Put the meatballs in the sauce and cook another 5 minutes before serving.

NUTRITION FACTS: CALORIES 412KCAL   FAT 7.8 G   CARBOHYDRATE 39.1 G   PROTEIN 18.3 G

JAMAICAN PEA SOUP

 4   🕐 40 mins

Ingredients:

8 oz. red kidney beans, soaked overnight
4 cups water
2 cups coconut milk
2 bay leaves
6 pimento grains
1 Bird's Eye chili
1 red onion, chopped
1 garlic clove
2 carrots, chopped
1 potato, cubed
1/2 lb. yellow yams, cubed
1 sweet potato, cubed
2 scallions, crushed
1 garlic clove, chopped
1/2 tsp. thyme

Directions:

Add beans, 4 cups of water, coconut milk, pimento, and bay leaves to a pot and bring to a boil.

Cook for 2 hours until the beans are almost tender. Add the onion, garlic, carrots, potato, yams, sweet potato, garlic, scallions, and chili. Cook another 20 minutes

Season with salt, pepper, and thyme. Puree half the soup to thicken, put it back in the pot with the other half, stir and serve hot.

NUTRITION FACTS: CALORIES 219KCAL FAT 5 G CARBOHYDRATE 30 G PROTEIN 15 G

MANGO BANANA SMOOTHIE

 2   5 mins

Ingredients:
1 mango
1/2 banana
2 cups greens, including kale
1 cup water

Directions:
Add all ingredients to a high-power blender and pulse until smooth.

Pour the smoothie into two glasses and serve immediately.

It can be stored in the refrigerator in an airtight container for up to 3 days.

NUTRITION FACTS: CALORIES 126KCAL FAT 1 G CARBOHYDRATE 23 G PROTEIN 1 G

OVERNIGHT OATS WITH BLUEBERRIES AND CHOCOLATE

 2   5 mins + 8h

Ingredients:
2 oz. rolled oats
4 oz. almond milk, unsweetened
2 tbsp. coconut yogurt
1 cup blueberries
1 tsp agave syrup
1 square 85% chocolate

Directions:
Mix the oats and the milk in a jar and leave overnight. In the morning, top the jar with yogurt, honey, blueberries, and chocolate cut into small pieces.

It can be prepared in advance and left for up to 3 days in the fridge.

NUTRITION FACTS: CALORIES 258KCAL FAT 3.3 G CARBOHYDRATE 29.8 G PROTEIN 13.6 G

MUSHROOM AND POTATO PIE

  6 🕐 *60 mins*

Ingredients:
2 lbs potatoes
2 cups soy milk
4 celery sticks, grated
1 red onion, chopped
1 lb. mushrooms, chopped
3 tbsp. extra-virgin olive oil
2 garlic cloves, crushed
1 1/2 tbsp. arrowroot
1 handful parsley, chopped
1 tsp. thyme

Directions:
Wash the potatoes to remove any dirt. Cook them in boiling water for 25 to 30 minutes until tender (always check with a stick before draining).

Remove the skin and mash the potatoes. Add 1 tbsp. olive oil, ¼ cup soy milk, salt and pepper, and stir well to make it fluffy.

Sautè onion, garlic, mushrooms, and celery in a saucepan with oil over medium heat for 5 minutes.

Dissolve the arrowroot in a little soymilk, add to the mushrooms, then add the remaining milk and mix well. Add the parsley, thyme, and season with salt and pepper to taste. Simmer gently for 5 minutes.

Move the stir into an ovenproof dish creating two layers. Mushrooms spread on the bottom and mashed potato on top.

Cook at 375°F for about 15 minutes and broil the last 5 minutes to make the top golden and crispy.

NUTRITION FACTS: CALORIES 397KCAL FAT 6 G CARBOHYDRATE 33 G PROTEIN 7 G

RASPBERRY GREENS SMOOTHIE

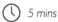 2   5 mins

Ingredients:
1 handful leafy greens
1 cup raspberries (frozen)
2 tbsp. lime juice
1 cup coconut milk

Directions:
Add all ingredients to a high-power blender and pulse until smooth.

Pour the smoothie into two glasses and serve immediately.

It can be stored in the refrigerator in an airtight container for up to 3 days.

NUTRITION FACTS: CALORIES 110KCAL FAT 0.7 G CARBOHYDRATE 16 G PROTEIN 1 G

SCALLOPED EGGPLANT

 4   40 mins

Ingredients:
1 eggplant, diced
2 cups mushrooms, thinly chopped
1 red onion, thinly chopped
1 bell pepper, thinly chopped
3 tbsp. olive oil
1/2 cup soymilk
2 cups buckwheat breadcrumbs
1/2 tsp. paprika
1 tsp. turmeric
1/4 tsp. cayenne

Directions:
Preheat oven to 350°F. In a skillet, sauté the eggplant, mushrooms, onion, and bell pepper in the oil until the eggplant becomes golden, about 10 minutes

Mix the milk, paprika, turmeric, cayenne, salt, and pepper with breadcrumbs. Put the veggie mix on a tray, cover with the breadcrumb mixture and bake for 25 minutes.

NUTRITION FACTS: CALORIES 360KCAL FAT 9 G CARBOHYDRATE 26 G PROTEIN 4 G

TOFU PATTIES WITH MUSHROOMS AND PEAS

 6   55 mins

Ingredients:
1 cup snow peas
1 cup chopped fresh mushrooms
8 green onions, chopped
1 1/2-inch ginger
8 oz. chestnuts, chopped
2 tbsp. oil
2 cups fresh bean sprouts
1 3/4 lbs. tofu, mashed
2 tsp. baking powder
1 cup flour
3 tbsp. nutritional yeast
2 tbsp. soy sauce

Directions:
Heat a skillet with oil and sauté the onions, mushrooms, snow peas, and chestnuts for 5 to 6 minutes. Add the bean sprouts, mix, and set aside. Remove from heat and set aside. Preheat the oven to 375°F.

Blend the tofu and the soy sauce until smooth and creamy. Add flour, nutritional yeast, and baking powder and mix. Add onion, mushrooms, snow peas, and chestnuts.

On lined baking tray, form 6 1/2-inch-thick patties.

Bake for 30 minutes, flip over and bake for 15 more minutes.

NUTRITION FACTS: CALORIES 199KCAL FAT 5 G CARBOHYDRATE 20 G PROTEIN 18 G

VANILLA COCONUT PARFAIT WITH BERRIES

1   5 mins

Ingredients:
4 oz. coconut yogurt
1 tsp agave syrup
1 cup mixed berries, frozen is perfect
1 tbsp. buckwheat granola
½ tsp vanilla extract

Directions:
Mix yogurt, vanilla extract, and honey. Alternate yogurt and berries in a jar and top with granola.

Frozen berries are perfect if the parfait is made in advance because they release their juices in the yogurt.

As far as granola, you can use a tablespoon of the one on page 146.

NUTRITION FACTS: CALORIES 318KCAL FAT 5.4 G CARBOHYDRATE 22.8 G PROTEIN 21.9 G

ZUCCHINI BOATS

 2   🕐 35 mins

Ingredients:

3 zucchini
1 red onion, chopped
1 tbsp. olive oil
1/2 lb. tofu, crumbled
3 tbsp. nutritional yeast flakes
1 garlic clove, crushed
1/2 tsp. oregano
16 oz. tomato sauce

Directions:

Cut the zucchini lengthwise and scoop the pulp out. Heat a pan with oil, sauté the onion for 5 minutes, add the tofu, zucchini pulp, garlic salt, and oregano and cook for 10 more minutes. Let cool for 5 minutes, then add nutritional yeast.

Pour the tomato sauce into a 9x11-inch pan, place the zucchini 'boats' in the sauce and fill the boats with the tofu mixture.

Cook for 30 minutes at 400°F, then broil for 5 minutes until the top becomes golden brown.

NUTRITION FACTS: CALORIES 340KCAL FAT 7 G CARBOHYDRATE 20 G PROTEIN 18 G

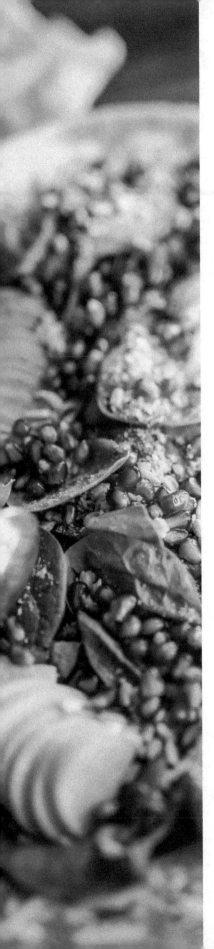

WEEK 3 – PHASE 2 PLANT-BASED RECIPES

APPLE AND AVOCADO SMOOTHIE

 2   🕐 5 mins

Ingredients:
1 apple, cored
1/2 avocado
2 cups raw baby spinach
8 oz. water
1 date

Directions:
Add all ingredients to a high-power blender and pulse until smooth.

Pour the smoothie into two glasses and serve immediately.

It can be stored in the refrigerator in an airtight container for up to 3 days.

NUTRITION FACTS: CALORIES 108KCAL FAT 0.4 G CARBOHYDRATE 18.5 G PROTEIN 1.6 G

BAKED EGGPLANT WITH TURMERIC AND GARLIC

 2   🕐 21 mins

Ingredients:
1 eggplant
2 tbsp. extra-virgin olive oil
2 chilies
1 1/2 tbsp. garlic, diced
1 tsp. green chili
1/4 tsp. turmeric
1/4 cup water
2 tbsp. white poppy seeds made into a paste
1/2 tsp. salt
1/2 tsp. sugar

Directions:
Crush the poppy seeds with a drop of olive oil to form a paste. Preheat oven to 450°F. Cut eggplant lengthwise and place it on a baking sheet with the cut side down.

Bake for 30 to 34 minutes or until the eggplant wrinkles and feels soft to the touch when pressed. Cut. Set aside. Heat a skillet with oil over medium heat.

Fry red chilies until they are soft. Add garlic and green chili. Stir until garlic turns light brown. Add water and turmeric and bring to a boil. Lower the heat and stir in the eggplant cuts.

Add poppy seed paste, salt, and sugar and mix well. Simmer covered for 20 minutes, occasionally stirring. Trim with green onions and serve.

NUTRITION FACTS: CALORIES 160KCAL FAT 7 G CARBOHYDRATE 25 G PROTEIN 3 G

BANANA BERRY KALE SMOOTHIE

  mins

Ingredients:
1 banana
1 cup strawberries (fresh or frozen)
1 cup kale (chopped)
1 cup ice

Directions:
Add all ingredients to a high-power blender and pulse until smooth.

Pour the smoothie into two glasses and serve immediately.

It can be stored in the refrigerator in an airtight container for up to 3 days.

NUTRITION FACTS: CALORIES 98KCAL FAT 0.5 G CARBOHYDRATE 15 G PROTEIN 2 G

BEETS WITH LEEK AND PARSLEY

 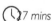 7 mins

Ingredients:
2 lbs. beets, chopped
1 lb. trimmed leeks, thickly chopped
1 tsp. ground cumin
1 tbsp. parsley, chopped
1/2 cups red wine

Directions:
Put the leeks with beets and spices in a pan. Add the wine, bring to a boil and simmer for 30 minutes until the beets are tender.

Season to taste with salt and pepper and serve, either hot or cold.

NUTRITION FACTS: CALORIES 178KCAL FAT 5 G CARBOHYDRATE 16 G PROTEIN 3 G

CURRY CHICKPEAS

 2   25 mins

Ingredients:

1 (15-oz.) can chickpeas, drained and washed
2 tbsp. red wine vinegar
2 tbsp. olive oil
2 tbsp. curry powder
1/2 tbsp. ground turmeric
1/4 tbsp. ground cumin
1/8 tsp. ground cinnamon
1/4 tbsp. salt
1/2 tbsp. pepper
1 handful parsley, chopped

Directions:

Gently crush chickpeas with hands in a bowl, removing skins.

Add oil and vinegar, and toss to coat. Add turmeric, curry powder, and cinnamon; mix gently to blend.

Put chickpeas in a single layer in the oven, and cook at 400°F until crisp, around 15 minutes, shaking them halfway through baking.

Move chickpeas to a bowl. Sprinkle with salt, pepper, and parsley, and toss to cover.

NUTRITION FACTS: CALORIES 173KCAL FAT 8 G CARBOHYDRATE 18 G PROTEIN 7 G

EGGPLANT, TOMATO, AND ONION GRATIN

 6   50 mins

Ingredients:

3 red onions, chopped
3 cloves garlic, crushed
3 tbsp. extra-virgin olive oil
3 sprigs thyme
3 eggplants, sliced
3 ripe tomatoes, sliced

Directions:

Fry onion and garlic in 1 tbsp. oil over medium heat for about 5 minutes until soft, then add thyme, salt, and pepper to taste.

Preheat oven to 400°F. Use 1 tbsp. oil to grease a gratin dish and spread the onions on it.

Alternate tomato and eggplant slices, overlapping them by 2/3, and season with salt and pepper.

Drizzle the remaining 1 tbsp. olive oil on top, and cook, covered with tin foil, until the eggplant is soft enough to be cut with a fork, about 30 minutes.

Uncover and cook for another 15 minutes or more until the liquid is absorbed. The time depends on the vegetables and on the juices they release.

NUTRITION FACTS: CALORIES 316KCAL FAT 5.2 G CARBOHYDRATE 13.1 G PROTEIN 6.9 G

EGGPLANT CREAMY PIZZA TOWERS

 2 *55 mins*

Ingredients:

1 ½ eggplant
1 tbsp. tomato paste
2 cups tomato sauce
½ red onion
1 garlic clove
1 cup soy milk
1 tbsp. buckwheat flour
4 basil leaves
2 tsp. extra-virgin olive oil
Salt and pepper

Directions:

Cut the eggplants into thick slices, add some salt and let them rest so that they let their bitter water out. In the meantime, prepare the salsa. Heat a pan with 1 tsp. oil added, when hot add onion and garlic and cook 5 minutes.

Add tomato sauce, tomato paste, salt, and pepper and cook on low heat for about 15-18 minutes. Add a few leaves of basil. Pat the eggplants with kitchen paper and grill them.

Whisk the flour with little soy milk to avoid lumps. Add the remaining milk. Dress with salt and pepper and cook on medium heat until dense.

Heat the oven to 350°F.

Prepare the towers: put a slice of eggplant, red sauce, white sauce, basil and again eggplant, red sauce, white sauce, basil. Three layers per tower are best. Add 1 tsp. oil on top.

When done, put the tray in the oven for about 10 minutes.

NUTRITION FACTS: CALORIES 353KCAL FAT 4.8 G CARBOHYDRATE 28.1 G PROTEIN 28.3 G

GREEK-STYLE MACARONI CASSEROLE

 8   🕐 50 mins

Ingredients:

1 lb. seitan
16 oz. buckwheat macaroni
3 tbsp. olive oil
1 ½ tsp. soy sauce
1 cup buckwheat breadcrumbs
1 ½ tbsp. arrowroot
1 – 1 ½ cups water
1 ½ cups plain soymilk
1 tbsp. tahini
2 tbsp. capers
2 tbsp. black olives, pitted and chopped

Directions:

Pulse the seitan in a blender to crumble it.
Preheat oven to 400°F.

Cook the pasta al dente in salted boiling water for 8 minutes, then drain it and put it in a bowl.

Heat a skillet with oil, then add the seitan and fry it for 3 to 4 minutes, then add the soy sauce. Add the seitan to the pasta bowl, mix well, and set aside.

Dissolve the arrowroot in a few spoons of water. In a saucepan, heat the soymilk, 1/2 cup water, tahini, olives, capers, salt, and pepper to taste.

Add the arrowroot dissolved in a few spoons of water and cook 2 to 3 minutes until the sauce thickens.

Grease a baking dish with 1 tsp. oil and assemble the casserole by creating 2 layers.

First, spread half the pasta-seitan mix on the dish. Then pour half the sauce on top. Cover with the pasta and spread the remaining sauce. Spread breadcrumbs on top.

Bake for 35 to 40 minutes until the crust is brown and crispy. Serve hot.

NUTRITION FACTS: CALORIES 199KCAL FAT 5 G CARBOHYDRATE 20 G PROTEIN 18 G

LENTILS AND CHICKPEAS STEW

 4   🕐 50 mins

Ingredients:

4 tbsp. extra-virgin olive oil
2 red onions, chopped
4 cloves garlic, finely chopped
1/2 cup parsley, finely chopped
1 cup lentils, soaked overnight
3 cups chickpeas, cooked
4 tomatoes, chopped
1 tsp. cumin
1/2 tsp. thyme
1/8 tsp. cayenne
3 cups water
1/4 cup green olives, chopped
2 tbsp. lemon juice

Directions:

Heat oil in a saucepan and sauté onion, garlic for 6 minutes. Add lentils, chickpeas, tomatoes, cumin, thyme, cayenne, and water. Bring to a boil and simmer for 35 minutes.

Add olives, lemon juice, and parsley, stir and serve.

NUTRITION FACTS: CALORIES 199KCAL FAT 5 G CARBOHYDRATE 20 G PROTEIN 18 G

LENTIL AND ONION SOUP

 2   40 mins

Ingredients:

1 red onion, chopped
2 tbsp. extra-virgin olive oil
1 bay leaf
1 cup red lentils
2 garlic cloves, chopped
1-1/2 cups of water

Directions:

Sauté onions and garlic until soft. Add lentils, bay leaf, salt and pepper to taste, and water.

Cook for 30 minutes until the lentils are soft. Serve hot.

NUTRITION FACTS: CALORIES 149KCAL FAT 5 G CARBOHYDRATE 20 G PROTEIN 7 G

MANGO COCONUT MOUSSE

🍽 1   🕐 5 mins

Ingredients:
1 cup mango
½ cup coconut yogurt
1 tbsp. coconut, shredded
2 squares dark chocolate, chopped

Directions:
Blend mango and yogurt together. Mix coconut, sprinkle chocolate on top, and serve immediately.

NUTRITION FACTS: CALORIES 87KCAL FAT 1.1 G CARBOHYDRATE 11.8 G PROTEIN 1.6 G

POTATO, MOREL, AND ONION FRICASSEE

🍽 6   🕐 30 mins

Ingredients:
1 ½ lbs. potatoes, chopped
1 red onion, chopped
½ lbs. morels
3 tbsp. extra-virgin olive oil
¼ cup chopped parsley

Directions:
Boil the potatoes in salted water until soft, and the edges have started to break down. Drain and set aside. Cut the morels in half and wash them quickly in water. Sauté both morels in the extra-virgin olive oil over high heat. Let the juices evaporate in about 5 to 6 minutes. Fry the potatoes in a skillet

When the potatoes have started to turn golden brown, add the onions until potatoes are crispy and the onions start caramelizing. Add the morels, season with salt and pepper, and add parsley.

Toss and serve.

NUTRITION FACTS: CALORIES 350KCAL FAT 7 G CARBOHYDRATE 21 G PROTEIN 3 G

MUSHROOM AND TOMATO RISOTTO

 4   🕐 1h

Ingredients:
1 red onion, chopped
4 tsp. extra-virgin olive oil
4 cups mushrooms, chopped
2 1/2 cups long-grain brown rice
7 cups boiling broth
2 cloves garlic, crushed
1 lb. tomatoes, peeled and chopped
1 tsp. thyme
1 tsp. oregano

Directions:

Warm a saucepan with 2 tsp. oil and sautè half the onion for 5 minutes. Add the rice and toast it for 2 to 3 minutes on high heat. Add the mushrooms, and cook for 5 minutes.

Add half boiling broth and simmer for around 50 minutes (time will depend on the variety of the brown rice). Keep adding 1 ladle of broth when the previous one has been absorbed. In this way, the rice will not overcook and will not be runny.

In another pan, sauté the remaining onion and garlic. Add the tomatoes, season with salt and pepper to taste, and simmer on low heat for at least 25 minutes, until the sauce thickens.

Add thyme and oregano right before removing the sauce from the heat, then add it to the rice.

Mix well and allow the flavors to combine for a few minutes, then serve.

NUTRITION FACTS: CALORIES 304KCAL FAT 5 G CARBOHYDRATE 30 G PROTEIN 14 G

SMOKY TOFU STIR FRY

 4   🕐 28 mins

Ingredients:

3.75 oz. buckwheat noodles
2 broccoli, chopped
2 green onions
2 tbsp. extra-virgin olive oil
2 chilies
6 garlic cloves, chopped
1-inch ginger, peeled and diced
4 carrots peeled and chopped
3 celery stalks, chopped
1 lb. extra-firm tofu, cubed
1 zucchini, chopped
1 cup snow peas, trimmed
15 oz. baby corn
1 red bell pepper, chopped
1 dash liquid smoke

Directions:

Bring a pot of water to a boil. Add the bean threads, stir, remove from heat, and set aside to soak; they should be ready when the stir-fry is done.

Cut the white and light green sections of the green onions into 3/4-inch-thick cuts. Thinly cut the green sections.

Heat several tbsps. of oil in a skillet.

Put the chilies, garlic, and ginger into a wok. Stir-fry for 1 minute. Add the carrots and cook for 3 minutes. Add the celery and green onions and stir-fry for 2 minutes.

Place the tofu in a hot saucepan with oil and liquid smoke and cook until it begins to brown, 6 to 8 minutes.

Add the zucchini, snow peas, baby corn, and bell pepper to the sauté pan or wok. Stir in the broccoli, then stir-fry until the florets start to turn green, about 2 minutes.

Boil noodles for 5 minutes in salted water. Drain, mix with the stir fry, and serve immediately.

NUTRITION FACTS: CALORIES 472KCAL FAT 8 G CARBOHYDRATE 30 G PROTEIN 26 G

STRAWBERRY AND WALNUT BAKE

 4   35 mins

Ingredients:
4 oz. rolled oats
12 oz. almond milk, unsweetened
1 banana, ripe and mashed
½ tsp. vanilla extract
1 oz. walnuts, chopped
1 cup strawberries
To serve: ½ cup coconut yogurt

Directions:
Heat the oven to 400°F.

Mix the oats, milk, vanilla, banana, strawberries, and walnuts in a bowl. Put on a baking tray lined with parchment paper and cook around 30 minutes.

It can be eaten alone or served with ½ cup of plain yogurt.

NUTRITION FACTS: CALORIES 308KCAL FAT 5.3 G CARBOHYDRATE 35.8 G PROTEIN 15.6 G

VEGGIE FAJITAS

2   25 mins

Ingredients:
6 tbsp. hummus
½ cup cherry tomatoes, halved
1 red onion
5 oz tofu, sliced
1 carrot, grated
1 handful parsley, chopped
2 tbsp. black olives, finely chopped
1 tsp extra-virgin olive oil
2 whole-wheat tortillas

Directions:
Sauté the onion with olive oil on medium heat for 5 minutes, add the tofu and heat for 4 to 5 minutes..

Quick heat the tortillas on a pan (keep them soft), spread the hummus and add the tofu with onions. Add cherry tomatoes, carrots, parsley and olives on top, and serve immediately.

NUTRITION FACTS: CALORIES 353KCAL FAT 4.8 G CARBOHYDRATE 28.1 G PROTEIN 28.3 G

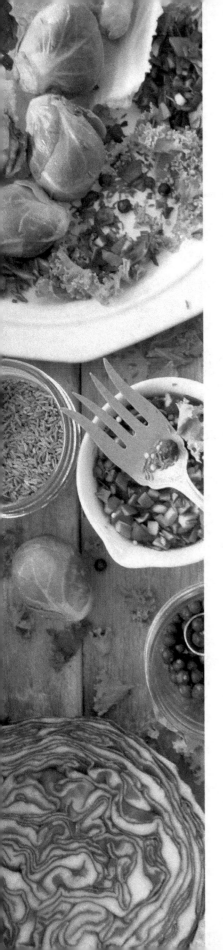

WEEK 4 – PLANT-BASED TRANSITION RECIPES

BAKED SWEET POTATO

 1 55 mins

Ingredients:
1 medium sweet potato
1 tsp. extra-virgin olive oil

Directions:
Heat the oven to 425°F.

Clean the potato very well under running water to get rid of the dirt.

Prick it several times and put it in the oven for 50 minutes. Always remember to test if it's done using a stick.

Cut the upper part and pour the oil over the sweet potato

NUTRITION FACTS: CALORIES 353KCAL FAT 4.8 G CARBOHYDRATE 28.1 G PROTEIN 28.3 G

CARAMELIZED FENNEL

 4 15 mins

Ingredients:
2 fennel bulbs
2 tbsp. extra-virgin olive oil
salt and pepper

Directions:
Trim the fennel bulbs, removing the outer layers. Cut bulbs in half vertically and then into 1/8-inch-thick cuts.

Heat a sauté pan with olive oil over medium heat. Add fennel.

Cook, occasionally stirring, for 8 to 10 minutes until fennel is caramelized and tender. Season with salt and pepper.

NUTRITION FACTS: CALORIES 104KCAL FAT 5 G CARBOHYDRATE 16 G PROTEIN 1 G

CHICKPEA PITA POCKETS

 4   20 mins

Ingredients:

1 16 oz. can chickpeas, cooked
1/3 cup celery, chopped
1 tbsp. red onion, chopped
2 tbsp. pickle relish
2 tbsp. vegan mayonnaise
1 tsp. mustard
Dash of garlic powder
4 whole-wheat pitas
4 leaves lettuce
1 tomato, sliced
1 carrot, grated

Directions:

Mash the chickpeas with a potato masher or quickly blend them in a blender without making them too smooth.

Add the mash to a bowl and add celery, onion, relish, mayonnaise, mustard, and garlic powder. Stir well, then season with salt and pepper to taste.

Cut the pitas in half and fill them with 1/4 of the chickpea spread, top with lettuce, tomato, and carrot and serve immediately.

NUTRITION FACTS: CALORIES 199KCAL FAT 5 G CARBOHYDRATE 20 G PROTEIN 18 G

CREAMY POTATO LEEK SOUP

 4   30 mins

Ingredients:

4 cups potatoes, diced
8 cups water
2-3 leeks, diced
1/4 lb. mushrooms, chopped
½ stalk celery, finely chopped
2 tbsp. extra-virgin olive oil
1 (12oz.) firm tofu

Directions:

Boil the potatoes in salted water until cooked, about 14 minutes.

Heat a pan and sauté the mushrooms and leeks in oil for 5 minutes, then add 1/4 cup water and cook until soft, about 6 to 8 minutes. Add them to the potatoes and blend until smooth and creamy.

Crumble the tofu into the pot, return it over medium heat for 3 minutes. Season with salt and pepper to taste.

NUTRITION FACTS: CALORIES 197KCAL FAT 5 G CARBOHYDRATE 20 G PROTEIN 18 G

CREOLE TOFU

 8   🕐 30 mins

Ingredients:
2 lbs. tofu, chopped 1/4 inch thick
2 tbsp. extra-virgin olive oil
1 red onion diced
3 cloves garlic, crushed
1 red bell pepper diced
2 stalks celery, diced
1/4 tsp. cayenne
1/4 tbsp. chili powder
1/4 cup garlic powder
6 tomatoes, diced
1/2 lemon, thinly chopped
1/4 cup parsley, chopped

Directions:
Heat a saucepan with 1 tbsp. oil and sauté the tofu until golden. Set aside. Add garlic, onion, celery, bell pepper, cayenne, chili, garlic powder in the remaining oil and sauté for 5 minutes. Add the tomatoes with a splash of water and cook for 15 minutes. Add the tofu, lemon, parsley, heat through.

Very good when served over hot rice or steamed buckwheat.

NUTRITION FACTS: CALORIES 199KCAL FAT 5 G CARBOHYDRATE 20 G PROTEIN 18 G

KALE BERRY DELIGHT SMOOTHIE

 2   🕐 5 mins

Ingredients:
1 cup blueberries
1 apple
2 cups kale
1 cup strawberries
1 cup coconut milk

Directions:
Add all ingredients to a high-power blender and pulse until smooth.

Pour the smoothie into two glasses and serve immediately.

It can be stored in the refrigerator in an airtight container for up to 3 days.

NUTRITION FACTS: CALORIES 109KCAL FAT 0.9 G CARBOHYDRATE 17 G PROTEIN 2 G

FRIED RICE WITH HOT LEEK SAUCE

4   55 mins

Ingredients:

1 tbsp. cornstarch
2 tsp. extra-virgin olive oil
1 leek diced
1/2-inch cube fresh ginger, peeled and diced
1 Bird's Eye chili, chopped
1 tbsp. garlic, chopped
1/4 cup teriyaki sauce
2 tbsp. extra-virgin olive oil
1-inch cube fresh ginger, peeled and diced
6 scallions, diced
2 tbsp. garlic, chopped
16 oz. firm tofu, cubed
1/2 cup cashews
½ cup walnuts
2 carrots, shredded
2 celery stalks, thinly chopped
1 cup mushrooms, chopped
15 oz. baby corn
2 broccoli, cut into florets
1/4 cup teriyaki sauce
3 cups rice, cooked

Directions:

Heat oil in a saucepan over medium heat. Add the leek, ginger, and chili and sauté for 5 to 7 minutes, or until the leek is golden brown. Add the teriyaki sauce and cornstarch dissolved in a little water and cook for 2 to 3 minutes until the sauce thickens. Set aside.

Heat 2 tbsp. oil in another pan. Add the ginger, scallions, and garlic and sauté for 3 minutes. Add the tofu and cook for 8 to 10 minutes, until brown on all sides.

Add the cashews, walnuts, celery, mushrooms, broccoli, baby corn, and carrots and sauté for 10 minutes over high heat. Stir well and sauté for 7 to 10 minutes or until the veggies are cooked and crispy.

Serve fried rice with the sauce on the side.

NUTRITION FACTS: CALORIES 109KCAL FAT 0.9 G CARBOHYDRATE 17 G PROTEIN 2 G

LOUISIANA-STYLE VEGGIE SAUSAGES

🍲 4   🕐 1h + 15 mins

Ingredients:

3 cups chickpeas, soaked overnight
2 cups flour
2 garlic cloves, crushed
1 cup rolled oats
1 cup nutritional yeast flakes
3/4 cups extra-virgin olive oil
1 cup soymilk
1/2 tsp. salt
2 tsp. garlic powder
2 tsp. oregano
1 tsp. fennel seeds
1/4 cup soy sauce

Directions:

Drain the chickpeas, wash them in running water, and then grind them in a food processor until very fine.

In a bowl, mix flour, rolled oats, nutritional yeast, salt, garlic powder, oregano, fennel seed. In a separate bowl, mix soy milk, soy sauce, and chickpeas. Mix and add to the flour. Stir well to create a dough.

Cut 4 pieces of aluminum foil 14 x 12 inches. Divide the mixture into 4 parts, and roll it up in a sausage shape. Close the foil packages by rolling the ends. Steam for 55 minutes and let cool before opening.

It can be served like this, with some arugula salad as a side, or they can be chopped and sautéed in 1 tsp oil until brown.

NUTRITION FACTS: CALORIES 368KCAL   FAT 5 G   CARBOHYDRATE 29 G   PROTEIN 15 G

NOODLES WITH WALNUT SAUCE

 4   🕐 25 mins

Ingredients:
1/2 lb. cooked buckwheat spaghetti
1/2 cup walnuts
4 tbsp. soy sauce
2 tbsp. rice vinegar
1 tsp. chili powder
1 dash cayenne
1-inch ginger, grated

Directions:
Bring a pot of salted water to a boil and cook the spaghetti al dente (around 8 minutes).

Put the walnuts in a blender with 1/2 cup lukewarm water and blend until smooth. Add the soy sauce, ginger, rice vinegar, chili powder, and cayenne pepper and mix again.

When the spaghetti is done, drain and place them in a bowl. Add the walnut sauce and toss well until the spaghetti is coated with the sauce.

NUTRITION FACTS: CALORIES 316KCAL FAT 5.2 G CARBOHYDRATE 13.1 G PROTEIN 6.9 G

PEANUT BUTTER CUP SMOOTHIE

🍵 2   🕐 5 mins

Ingredients:
1 pear, cored
1 tbsp. all-natural peanut butter
1/2 tbsp. cacao powder
2 cups baby spinach
8 oz. unsweetened almond milk

Directions:
Add all ingredients to a high-power blender and pulse until smooth.

Pour the smoothie into two glasses and serve immediately.

It can be stored in the refrigerator in an airtight container for up to 3 days.

NUTRITION FACTS: CALORIES 202KCAL FAT 4 G CARBOHYDRATE 21 G PROTEIN 9 G

STIR-FRIED TOFU AND VEGETABLES IN GINGER SAUCE

 4   75 mins

Ingredients:
3/4 cup soy sauce
3/4 cup lemon juice
1-2 tsp. grated fresh ginger
1 lb. extra firm tofu
2 tbsp. olive oil
1 cup broccoli florets
1 cup cauliflower florets
3 carrots chopped into 2-inch strips
1 red onion, chopped
1 green pepper, chopped
1 cup snow peas
1 cup chopped mushrooms
2 green onions, chopped
2 cups cooked rice

Directions:
Whisk the lemon juice, soy sauce, and ginger and add the marinade to the tofu.

Let marinate for 45 minutes. Drain the tofu saving the marinade. Heat the oil in a pan, and add the cauliflower, broccoli, carrots, onion, green pepper, and tofu.

Stir frequently, cooking evenly. Add the snow peas, mushrooms, and green onions.

Continue to stir frequently until the vegetables are cooked but still crunchy.

Serve over rice, topped with the marinade.

NUTRITION FACTS: CALORIES 358KCAL FAT 7 G CARBOHYDRATE 20 G PROTEIN 28 G

VANILLA COCONUT PARFAIT WITH BERRIES

 1   5 mins

Ingredients:
4 oz. coconut yogurt
1 tsp agave syrup
1 cup mixed berries, frozen is perfect
1 tbsp. buckwheat granola
½ tsp vanilla extract

Directions:
Mix yogurt, vanilla extract, and honey. Alternate yogurt and berries in a jar and top with granola.

Frozen berries are perfect if the parfait is made in advance because they release their juices in the yogurt.

As far as granola, you can use a recipe from the ones on this book.

NUTRITION FACTS: CALORIES 318KCAL FAT 5.4 G CARBOHYDRATE 22.8 G PROTEIN 21.9 G

TOMATO BISQUE

🍲 4   🕐 20 mins

Ingredients:
1 1/2 cups tofu
1 cup water
1 (14oz.) can diced tomatoes
2 tbsp. tomato paste
1/2 red onion, chopped
1 cup vegetable broth
½ tsp. turmeric

Directions:
Blend the tofu and water until smooth. Add the tomatoes, tomato paste, red onion, turmeric, and broth and let simmer for 40 minutes.
Serve hot.

NUTRITION FACTS: CALORIES 190KCAL FAT 6 G CARBOHYDRATE 20 G PROTEIN 11 G

WALNUT ENERGY BAR

🍲 4   🕐 35 mins

Ingredients:
4 oz. rolled oats
1 oz. shredded coconut
8 walnuts, chopped
½ cup almond milk, unsweetened
3 tbsp. agave syrup
1 pinch salt
½ tsp vanilla extract
1 tbsp. peanut butter

Directions:
Mix all the ingredients, put them on a baking tin lined with parchment paper, and cook 20-25 minutes at 325°F until golden and crisp.

NUTRITION FACTS: CALORIES 192KCAL FAT 4.3 G CARBOHYDRATE 32.8 G PROTEIN 6.6 G

THE SIRTFOOD DIET AND WORKOUTS

The Sirtfood Diet is intended as a lifestyle; it is certainly not a one-time diet plan. For this reason, it's very important to talk, not only about what you eat but also about exercise. Exercise can act to prevent many kinds of diseases as we age.

So let's answer a common question when it comes to working out, "It possible to combine exercising during the phases of a Sirtfood Diet, or do we need to keep workout routines out of the way?"

The answer is, actually, that it depends.

Especially during Phase 1, when caloric intake is drastically reduced, reducing physical activity seems to be the best option for most people while the body adapts to the changes. It's essential to be kind to yourself and support your body, especially the first three days.

After the first three days, though, if you are already in the habit of exercising moderately, you can start back. It will depend on you and how far you can push yourself. Manage your fitness regime according to your diet regime and to listen to your body. In case you are feeling low-energy or fatigued, stop working out for a few days. Dedicate that time to focusing on the Sirtfood Diet principles for a healthy life.

If you have never exercised before, or you have but never established a routine, it's probably better if you wait until the end of Phase 2 when caloric intake is higher. Then, it will be easier for your body to support proper training.

It is essential to find a healthy and sustainable exercise routine. It should be something that won't keep you from enjoying your life and won't need you to exercise all the time.

IMPORTANCE OF EXERCISING

Proper exercise should involve all parts of the body, allowing your body to burn calories and make your muscles work. You can opt for various physical exercises such as running, walking, jogging, swimming, dancing, etc. As you start increasing your physical activity, you will experience multiple benefits in both your mental and physical. Coupling moderate exercise with a Sirtfood Diet can help you shed extra pounds.

EXERCISE SUPPORTS METABOLISM

The main aim of the Sirtfood Diet is to erase the extra pounds from your body. Staying inactive can result in obesity and weight gain. To understand the overall effect exercise has on weight reduction, you need a clear understanding of the relationship between energy expenditure and exercise.

The human body expends energy in three ways: exercise, digestion, and the maintenance of body functions, such as breathing and heart rate. The diet begins with calorie reduction, and which can lower the metabolism. This might result in slowed weight loss. On the other hand, exercising along with your diet plan can improve the metabolic rate, helping you burn more calories. Thus, you will be able to lose more weight without affecting your muscle mass.

It has been found that the combination of aerobic exercise and resistance training can improve fat loss and can also help in the maintenance of muscle mass. So, make sure that you opt for moderate exercise as soon as you can, preferably before the end of Phase 2.

EXERCISE CAN SUPPORT YOUR MOOD

Exercise can help uplift your mood. It can also help you deal with depression, stress, and anxiety. As you begin the Sirtfood Diet, your body will enter a state of shock during the first few days due to the sudden calorie restriction. Moderate exercise can help you deal with this kind of stress. Exercising causes specific changes in the brain that can regulate anxiety and stress. It can also improve the brain's sensitivity to hormones such as norepinephrine and serotonin, which help relieve depression.

Also, exercising can improve endorphins production, which promotes positive feelings, helping people who suffer from anxiety. With moderate exercise, you will become more aware of your mental state. It does not matter how intensively you exercise; you will benefit even from moderate exercise. As you cut down calories during the first phase of the diet, you will most likely experience mood swings. If you feel strong enough, exercise can play a profound role in regulating your mood, especially during this phase.

EXERCISE IMPROVES ENERGY LEVELS

Exercise has the incredible power of boosting your energy levels. If you suffer from a medical condition, it can help improve your energy as well. While on the Sirtfood Diet, energy is provided by the body by burning body fat. When you couple it with proper exercise, you can improve the benefits. Exercise can boost the energy levels also of CFS, or chronic fatigue syndrome, sufferers.

EXERCISE CAN REDUCE CHRONIC DISEASES

A chronic lack of physical activity can lead to chronic diseases. Regular exercise can improve sensitivity to insulin, body composition, and also cardiovascular fitness. It can also help maintain blood pressure and body fat levels.

Lack of physical exercise, even for a short period, can result in the development of body fat and can also increase the overall risk of developing type II diabetes. Physical exercise must be combined with a proper diet to reduce belly fat.

EXERCISING IS BENEFICIAL FOR BONES AND MUSCLES

Exercise can play a beneficial role in maintaining and building strong bones and muscles. Different types of physical activity, such as weight lifting, can help build muscles when coupled with proper protein intake. This is mainly because exercise helps release certain hormones that can promote the muscles' capability to absorb amino acids. This ultimately helps grow muscles and reduce their breakdown. As our bodies age, we tend to lose muscle mass along with muscle function. This can result in disabilities and injuries. It is essential to opt for daily physical activity to retain muscle mass while following a diet. It can help maintain your strength with age.

Exercising can improve bone density and help prevent osteoporosis later in life. Studies show that high impact exercise, such as running and gymnastics, or sports such as basketball and soccer, improve bone density at higher rates than non-impact activities, such as cycling and swimming.

IMPROVES SKIN HEALTH

Skin quality is affected by high amounts of oxidative stress on the body. Oxidative stress occurs when the body's antioxidant defenses cannot mend the damage caused to cells. Exhausting and intense physical activity can also result in oxidative damage; moderate daily exercise, on the other hand, can improve the production of antioxidants naturally. This can help protect skin cells. Similarly, exercise can help stimulate blood flow and induce adaptations of the skin cells that delay skin aging.

IMPROVES MEMORY AND HEALTH

It has been found that brain function can be improved with the help of regular exercise. Exercise can also help protect your memory and cognition since it improves blood circulation to the brain. Regular exercise with a proper diet is even more critical for older adults as increased rates of inflammation and oxidative stress linked to aging can also lead to changes in brain structure and function.

EXERCISE CAN IMPROVE SLEEP QUALITY

Regular exercise with a balanced diet can help you relax and sleep well because they help release stress and increase body temperature directly related to sleep quality. Exercising can help with sleep disorders, as well. You can be completely flexible regarding the type of exercise that you want to choose. The best results have been shown with aerobic exercise, coupled with resistance training.

EXERCISE CAN HELP REDUCE PAIN

Chronic pain can be debilitating. But, with the help of exercise, you can deal with it very easily. Exercise helps tone the muscles that remain inactive, which, in turn, results in the reduction of pain. You will be able to improve your level of pain tolerance and decrease pain perception with daily exercise.

MINDSET: A FUNDAMENTAL ASPECT

All diets work. But not all dieters manage to lose weight.

This concept can be applied to all fields of our life. For example, many people graduate with high marks, but few manage to get the job they dream of. Many people play basketball, but very few play in the NBA.

Why do some succeed and others fail? What are they doing differently?

And, returning to the world of diets, why is losing weight so difficult?

The answer is Mindset!

To be able to talk about it, we must first define what mindset is. With this expression, we want to refer, in general, to all the conditionings and beliefs that our mind has assimilated during life. This habitual mental attitude characterizes our ways of reacting and acting in certain circumstances. In a sense, we can define mindset as our usual behavior in the face of the situations that arise.

For example, a person convinced that he cannot speak publicly will tend to avoid occasions when it is necessary to speak in front of others. This creates general insecurity, which, if not addressed, will take root more and more deeply in the mind, causing them to give up and surrender for fear of making mistakes.

This is precisely one of the reasons why it is essential to know ourselves deeply. Knowing our limits, our fears, and our difficulties, and being able to admit them is a crucial step towards the possibility of overcoming them. Although they are often theoretical limits that we place on ourselves, when, in reality, our fears speak and make us believe that there are obstacles that cannot be overcome.

We said that mindset is a mental setting that has taken root in each of us year after year. So how is it possible to change what seems to be so intrinsic to ourselves?

It is possible by practicing new behaviors until our mind accepts them as a new mindset.

This step may not be easy and immediate, and you may not be able to put the correct strategy into practice immediately. Different tactics correspond to different activities and situations.

This means that the transition to practice requires adjustments along the way. There is no definitive or right mindset for all situations, but you have to model ad hoc strategies for every occasion. Mindset is not a point of arrival but a process in progress, a continuous evolution of your personal way of approaching things.

MINDSET FOR A SUCCESSFUL DIET

Now that we have explained what mindset is and how it influences our way of thinking, we can explain what interests us most: how to use it to follow a diet successfully.

Let's start by saying that food, from a psychological point of view, represents a fundamental need for people: pleasure.

Now, if food is related to pleasure, and if pleasure is a fundamental emotion (one of the four fundamental emotions for survival - the others are fear, anger, and pain), in your opinion, can we withstand being deprived of food? Of course, the answer is no.

What typically happens in all diets is this: you follow them for a while and then stop. In the worst case, you follow them for some days and then explode in a binge that makes you recover all the weight lost, and perhaps, even more.

In short, the more you deprive yourself of something, the more you desire it.

THE SOLUTION

The solution is changing our behavior and, in particular, changing our habits to make dieting feel less restrictive and unpleasant, and instead, make it as pleasurable as possible. The Sirtfood Diet, with its massive list of allowed foods, including chocolate and wine, surely helps to make our weight loss journey less deprived of the things we love.

But there's more. For example, let's talk about where we eat and how good it looks to the eye. For sure, it is more lovely to eat with a nice setting, than to do it with a plastic plate or a sandwich wrapped in paper. It's great to find a bench, a corner of greenery, or any other pleasant space when eating outside. Listening to some music or in the pleasant sound of silence when eating is better than eating with the TV on or, worse, while continuing to work. The environment should help us appreciate our food; we shouldn't pass it mindlessly from mouth to stomach.

As long as you finish following the 4-week Meal plan, which includes many satisfying recipes and even some healthy chocolate snacks, consider that a happy, healthy life cannot be achieved when you are continuously depriving yourself.

You made an effort to change your eating habits and are now able to put together a weekly menu to maintain your results. Just know that sometimes it's ok to give in to temptation.

From time to time, there should be the option to enjoy something you may crave, even if it's not "healthy." An afternoon chocolate, a plate of pasta now and then, a less restrictive Sunday, without exaggerating, of course, but ensure that no food is permanently denied. This will be your secret weapon to maintaining long-lasting results for life.

CONCLUSION

Congratulations, you have now finished all the stages of the Sirtfood Diet!

Let's take a look at what you have achieved. You've entered the hyper-success phase 1, probably achieving a remarkable weight loss of around 7 pounds and an increase in muscle mass.

You also maintained your weight loss throughout the fourteen-day maintenance phase 2 and further improved your body composition. You have marked the beginning of your lifetime transformation thanks to phase 3, where you had a sample of how your new way of eating could be.

You took a stand against diseases that often strike as we get older and enhanced your strength, productivity, and health.

By now, you are familiar with the top twenty sirtfoods, and you've gained a sense of how powerful they are. Not only that, you probably have become quite good at including them in your diet and loving them. These items must stay a prominent feature in your everyday diet to continue to see the sustained weight loss and health benefits they offer.

Good luck to you as you move towards this new chapter of your healthy, happy life!

APPENDIX A - FREQUENTLY ASKED QUESTIONS

Below is included a list of the most frequently asked questions and their answers.

DO I EXERCISE DURING PHASE 1?

Regular exercise is one of the best things you can do for your health. Doing some moderate exercise can improve your weight loss and well-being. As a general rule, during the Sirtfood Diet's first seven days, we advise you to maintain your average exercise and physical activity level. We suggest staying in your usual comfort zone, as prolonged or overly intense training can simply put too much stress on the body during this time. Check your body. There's no need to force yourself to do more exercise during Phase 1; instead, let the sirtfoods do the hard work.

I AM SLIM — CAN I FOLLOW THE DIET?

For anyone underweight, we do not recommend Phase 1 of the Sirtfood Diet as you don't need to lose any more weight. Calculating your body mass index or BMI is a safe way to understand if you are underweight. You can easily calculate this by using one of the numerous online BMI calculators, as long as you know your height and weight. If your BMI is 18.5 or less, we do not suggest embarking on phase 1 of the diet. We would also advise caution if your BMI is between 18.5 and 20 because following the diet could mean that your BMI falls below 18.5. While many people strive to be super-skinny, the fact is that being underweight may have a detrimental effect on your health, leading to a weakened immune system, an increased risk of osteoporosis (weakened bones), and fertility issues. What you could do is follow Phase 3 – Transition and use the recipes in the book to create your Meal Plan. You should follow the guidelines of Phase 3, as it does not include caloric restriction but helps you set up a diet rich in sirtfoods.

I AM OBESE — IS THE SIRTFOOD DIET RIGHT FOR ME?

Of course! Join the thousands of people who already tried the diet and lost weight. You will reap considerable improvements in your well-being, thanks to sirtuin activation. Being obese increases the risk of many chronic health problems, yet these are the very illnesses that sirtfoods will help you avoid.

I REACHED MY TARGET WEIGHT, AND DON'T WANT TO LOSE ANY MORE — DO I STOP EATING SIRTFOODS?

First of all, congratulations on your success! With sirtfoods, even if you have seen great success, it doesn't stop when you reach your goal. While we do not recommend further calorie restriction, your diet should still provide ample sirtfoods. The great thing about sirtfoods is that they are a lifestyle. In terms of weight control, the best way to think of them as a way to help get the body into the weight and shape it was meant to be and stay there. They will continue to work to maintain your weight and keep you looking fantastic and feeling great.

I TAKE MEDICATION — IS IT OK TO FOLLOW THE DIET?

The Sirtfood Diet is ideal for most people. Still, due to its powerful effects on fat burning and well-being, it can alter the processes of certain diseases and the medication plan recommended by your doctor.

If you suffer from a significant health condition, take prescription medications, or have any reasons to think about going on a diet, we recommend that you speak to your doctor about it. Likely, you could profoundly benefit from the Sirtfood Diet, but you should check with your physician first.

I AM PREGNANT – CAN I FOLLOW THE DIET?

If you are trying to conceive, are pregnant, or breastfeeding, we do not suggest embarking on the Sirtfood Diet. It is a powerful diet for weight loss, which makes it inappropriate for women in these conditions. However, don't be put off eating plenty of sirtfoods, as these are incredibly nutritious foods that can be consumed as part of a balanced and varied pregnancy diet. Because of its alcohol content, you will want to avoid red wine and limit caffeinated items such as coffee, green tea, and cocoa, as it is not recommended to exceed 200 milligrams of caffeine per day during pregnancy (one mug of instant coffee typically contains about 100 milligrams of caffeine). It is also recommended to drink less than four cups of green tea a day and avoid matcha altogether. Other than that, the benefits of having sirtfoods in your diet are free to reap.

ARE SIRTFOODS SUITABLE FOR CHILDREN?

The Sirtfood Diet is an intense diet for weight loss and not intended for kids. However, that doesn't mean that kids can't partake in the excellent health benefits provided by adding more sirtfoods to their overall diet. Of course, not all sirtfoods are suitable for children, like red wine and coffee, but it's just common sense.

WILL I GET A HEADACHE OR TIRED FEEL DURING PHASE 1?

This diet can include mild headaches or tiredness, but these effects are slight and short-lived. Of course, if the symptoms are severe or give you cause for concern, seek medical advice promptly. Occasional mild symptoms will quickly resolve, and within a few days, most people have a renewed sense of energy, vigor, and well-being.

SHOULD I REPEAT PHASES 1, 2, AND 3?

You can repeat Phase 1 if you feel you need to lose more weight or need a health boost. To ensure no long-term adverse effects of calorie restriction appear, you should wait at least a month before repeating it. Most people need to repeat it no more than once every three months and to see excellent results. Instead, if you have gone off course, need some fine-tuning, or want a little more sirtfood pressure, we suggest that you repeat Phase 2 and 3 as often as you want, as these are about developing lifelong eating habits. Remember, the Sirtfood Diet's beauty is that it doesn't require you to feel like you're endlessly on a diet. Instead, it's the foundation for developing positive lifelong dietary changes that will create a lighter, leaner, healthier you.

DOES THE SIRTFOOD DIET HAVE ENOUGH FIBER?

Many sirtfoods are naturally rich in fiber. Onions, endives, and walnuts are notable sources, with buckwheat and Medjool dates standing out too, meaning The Sirtfood Diet is not short in the fiber department. Even during Phase 1, when food consumption is reduced, most dieters will still consume an acceptable fiber quantity, particularly if recipes are selected from the menu containing buckwheat, beans, and lentils. However, for others known to be susceptible to intestinal problems such as constipation without high fiber intake, a suitable fiber supplement may be considered during Phase 1, especially days 1 to 3, which should be discussed with your health care professional.

CAN I EAT WHAT I WANT ONCE I EAT PLENTY OF SIRTFOODS AND STILL SEE RESULTS?

One of the main reasons why the Sirtfood Diet works so well in the long term is that it encourages good food rather than demonizing mediocre food. Exclusion diets just aren't effective long-term. Processed foods high in sugars and fats decrease sirtuin activity in the body, thus reducing the benefits of sirtfood consumption. However, if you stay focused on eating a diet rich in sirtfoods, you will end up consuming much less garbage than the average person, and, as a result, you will feel happy and fulfilled and have less appetite for certain refined foods. If you sometimes indulge in these refined foods, don't worry about it — the strength of sirtfoods, the rest of the time, will ensure that you are still reaping the benefits.

SIRTFOOD DIET COOKBOOK

200 TASTY IDEAS FOR HEALTHY, QUICK, AND EASY MEALS

Enjoy the Anti Inflammatory Power of Sirtuine Foods Combined in Delicious Recipes to Lose Weight and Feel Great in Your Body

KATE HAMILTON

First published in the United States of America in 2020

Copyright © 2020 Kate Hamilton

Typeset by Leah Jespersen

Images from Unsplash

ISBN 979-8668852222

SIRTFOOD DIET COOKBOOK

INTRODUCTION

It would probably surprise you, but people knew about healthy foods long before recent studies. In ancient times, they discovered the effects of different plants and adopted some of them in their regular diet. Of course, back then, food was natural, so they weren't dealing with the same problem we are dealing with today. Thousands of years ago, people were dying from many causes; but most were not related to bad nutrition. They didn't have the knowledge and technology to process food. Nowadays, medicine has evolved, but bad nutrition, unfortunately, causes plenty of deaths.

You are probably wondering how the Sirtfood Diet was discovered. The founders of this meal plan, Dr. Aidan Goggins and Dr. Glen Matten, have targeted foods with a higher concentration of sirtuin-activating nutrients. They had a hunch about what these foods can do to your body. Their research analyzed the eating habits and lifestyles of different people worldwide who have a diet rich in sirtuin-activating nutrients. Therefore, if the Mediterranean diet was inspired by the eating habits and lifestyle of the people living on the Mediterranean shores, the Sirtfood Diet tried the same approach, but the analyzed population was spread all over the world.

There are regions worldwide called the blue zones, where people normally eat plenty of sirtfoods. These people have much lower rates of Alzheimer's disease, diabetes, heart disease, osteoporosis, and even cancer. Don't be surprised if you see people in their 90s walking, working, and dancing. This probably sounds like a fairy tale, a legend, or a myth, but people in the blue zones are less affected by the typical "western world" lifestyle. They have less stress, and they are enjoying life to the fullest.

Suppose you have the privilege of visiting the San Blas Islands of Panama. In that case, you will meet the Kuna American Indians, an indigenous population with incredibly low rates of high blood pressure, diabetes, obesity, cancer, and early deaths. Do you know what their secret is? It is the consumption of cocoa, which happens to have a high concentration of sirtuin-activating nutrients. Cocoa can increase memory performance and enhance brain functionality. It works miracles when it comes to preventing diabetes and even cancer, plus it can be used for better oral hygiene, as it can protect teeth from cavities and plaque.

Let's move on to India, which used to be the jewel in the British Empire's crown. India can be easily considered a micro-continent, as its vast territory is home to some of the most amazing veggies, fruits, plants, and spices. Speaking of spices, do you know which spice is called the "Indian solid gold"? The answer is turmeric, and India is responsible for more than 80 percent of the global supply. This is a frequently used condiment in Indian cuisine and an excellent curcumin source, a potent sirtuin-activating nutrient. As it turns out, the consumption of turmeric can have anti-inflammatory and healing effects. Curcumin even has anticancer effects, so turmeric should be included in your diet.

China is considered the home ground for green tea, one of the drinks with the most health benefits. People in China have been drinking green tea for more than 4,700 years, and now this beverage has become extremely popular worldwide. The consumption of green tea is associated with a lower risk of different forms of cancer (breast, prostate, and lung) and lower rates of coronary heart disease. Green tea works wonders on metabolism, and it is the perfect drink to have when you want to burn fat while keeping your existing muscle mass intact.

If you have the pleasure of traveling to the Mediterranean region, you will notice how common extra-virgin olive oil is in their daily diet. People living in this area like to consume healthy fats, like nuts (and especially walnuts), which are a good source of lipids. Their diet is designed to burn fats in the body and keep blood sugar and insulin levels to a minimum, avoiding diabetes, obesity, heart diseases, and even some cancers. No wonder there are so many people from this region who are aging slowly and feeling fabulous.

If you look at the top 20 sirtfoods, you can easily see that some of the ingredients come from specific regions of the world. The Sirtfood Diet practically brings the whole world to your plate so that you can reap the weight loss and health benefits of the best ingredients from all over the world.

QUICK RECAP OF THE SIRTFOOD DIET

SIRTFOOD DIET PHASES

As a newbie, you must understand that the Sirtfood Diet does not start with a single list of ingredients in your hands. Its implementation and adaptation are more than a mere selective grocery shopping list. Every diet can only work effectively when we allow our body to embrace the sudden shift and change in food intake. Similarly, the Sirtfood Diet comes with two phases of adaptation. Going through these phases leads to following the Sirtfood Diet efficiently and successfully. After the two weight loss phases, there is a third one, which is a maintenance phase that aims to consolidate your weight loss results in the long run.

PHASE ONE

The first seven days of this diet plan are known as Phase One. In this phase, a dieter must focus on calorie restriction and the intake of green juices. These seven days are crucial to initiate your weight loss and usually lead to seven pounds of weight loss if the diet is followed correctly. Suppose you find yourself achieving this target that means that you are on the right track.

In the first three days of Phase One, caloric intake is set around 1,000 calories. While doing so, the dieter must also drink green juice three times per day. The recipes given in the book provide a great variety of juices to chose from.

After the first three days, the caloric intake is increased to 1,500 calories per day for the next four days. In these four days, the green juices are reduced to two per day, paired with Sirtuin-rich food in every meal.

PHASE TWO

Phase Two starts right after the first week of the Sirtfood Diet, or Phase One. Pase 2 is about continuing with the diet, and it begins to feel easier thanks to your body's adaptation to the new regimen. According to the diet, the first week enables the body to embrace the change and start working towards the weight loss goal, while the second phase allows the body to keep losing weight slowly and steadily. Therefore, the duration of this phase is almost two weeks.

So how is this phase different from Phase One? In this phase, there is no restriction on caloric intake, as long as the food is rich in sirtuins, and you are having three meals per day. As far as green juices, the intake is decreased to one per day, which will be more than enough to guarantee weight loss. You can drink the juice any time during the day, even after any meal, in the morning or the evening.

AFTER THE DIET

With the end of Phase 2 comes the most crucial time, and that is the after-diet phase. If you haven't achieved your weight loss target by the end of phase two, then you can restart the phases all over again. Or even when you have reached the goals but still want to lose more weight.

In any case, continue eating good quality sirtfoods to keep your everyday diet rich in sirtuins. It is also good to continue the habit of drinking green juice each day. The recipes in this book will help you arrange a colorful, tasty meal plan which everyone in your household will enjoy.

20 SUPERFOOD LIST

MAIN CHARACTERISTICS AND BENEFITS	CALORIES
RED WINE is considered the first original sirtfood discovered. It contains a compound called Resveratrol, which protects the body against conditions like heart attacks and cancer. When consumed in moderate quantities, it is also responsible for weight loss in a sirtuin rich diet.	Calories: 153kcal Carbohydrate: 4.7g Protein: 0.1g Fat: 0g
COFFEE is one of the most common sirtfoods known. Coffee contains a nervous system stimulant. The nervous system comprises the brain and the spinal cord. Stimulation of the nervous system signals the body to break down fat cells.	Calories: 1 kcal Carbohydrate: 0g Protein: 0.3g Fat: 0g
KALE is an essential component of many effective green juices. Kale helps the body by enhancing fast and easy absorption of nutrients, making skin and hair glow, hardening nails, and alkalizing the whole body.	Calories: 49 kcal Carbohydrate: 9g Protein: 4.3 g Fat: 0.9 g
ONIONS contain a large fraction of antioxidants and help reduce cell inflammation. They are also a significant source of sirtuin activators that prevent and control oxidation of fatty acids in the cells.	Calories: 40 kcal Carbohydrate: 9g Protein: 1.1g Fat: 0.1g
SOY is a highly nutritious ingredient, rich in proteins, vitamins, and minerals. Regular consumption of soy in the Sirtfood diet helps prevent tumors and prostate and breast cancers. Soy has no cholesterol and is low in saturated fatty acids	Calories: 173 kcal Carbohydrate: 9.9g Protein: 16.6g Fat: 9g
STRAWBERRIES. Fresh, juicy, and sweet, they are very low in calories thanks to their high water content. They are useful in the Sirtfood diet because they are an excellent source of Vitamin C. They contain Elleagic Acid, very useful in fighting cancer and heart diseases.	Calories: 53 kcal Carbohydrate: 12.75 g Protein: 1.11g Fat: 0.50 g

CAPERS are the flower buds of a small bush very common in the Mediterranean region. Rich in quercetin, they are used in many meat, fish, and salad recipes. They contain sodium, calcium, magnesium, and potassium and are very low in calories. They are also rich in antioxidants	Calories: 23 kcal Carbohydrate: 4.9 g Protein: 2.4 g Fat: 0.9 g Potassium: 40 mg
BLUEBERRIES are a significant source of minerals such as iron, phosphorous, and calcium; thus, they help maintain healthy bones. These minerals are also important for mental health, digestion, and weight loss.	Calories: 57 kcal Carbohydrate: 21.45 g Protein: 1.1 g Fat: 0.49 g
RED CHICORY. Rich in water and fibers, its consumption helps promote healthy digestion, improve blood sugar control, and support weight loss by regulating appetite. It contains a fair amount of Vitamin C, Vitamin B, Vitamin K, and potassium.	Calories: 20 kcal Carbohydrate 4 g Protein: 1.2 g Fat: 0 g
MEDJOOL DATES. This is an edible sweet fruit coming from the date palm tree with plenty of vitamins, minerals like potassium and phosphorus, and fiber. They help in preventing constipation and decreasing cholesterol due to soluble fiber intake.	Calories: 133 kcal Carbohydrate: 36 g. Protein: 0.8 g Fat: 0g
PARSLEY is a flowering plant rich in vitamin B, vitamin C, potassium, and calcium. It is essential in reducing the risk of heart disease and strengthening bones and the immune system. Used in many recipes, it's better to add it raw to keep its health benefits intact.	Calories: 36 kcal Carbohydrates: 6 g Protein: 3 g Fat: 0.3g
EXTRA VIRGIN OLIVE OIL is a rich source of antioxidants and healthy fats, which protect from cardiovascular diseases. Additionally, it is important in lowering the risk of type 2 diabetes and protects against stroke.	Calories: 119 kcal Carbohydrate: 0g Protein: 0g Fat: 13.5g.
DARK CHOCOLATE is a very important source of antioxidants. Flavonoids, polyphenols, and tryptophan reduce the probability of heart disease, improve brain function, and improve mood, protecting against depression.	Calories: 604 kcal Carbohydrate: 46.36 g Protein: 7.87 g Fat: 43.06 g
MATCHA GREEN TEA is a variety of tea that is easy to prepare. It boosts brain and liver function. Catechins have a strong antibiotic effect on the body, while potassium, Vitamin A, and Vitamin C are potent antioxidants that help burn fat and lead to weight loss.	Calories: 2.5 kcal Carbohydrate:0g Protein: 0.5g Fat:0 g
TURMERIC is a yellow-orange spice frequently used in sauces or curries for its anti-inflammatory and antioxidant properties. Rich in curcumin, it improves the immune system, protects the liver, and helps digestion, among many other positive benefits.	Calories: 29 kcal Carbohydrate: 6.31 g Protein: 0.91 g Fat: 0.31 g

BUCKWHEAT is a seed high in fiber, essential amino acids, and minerals like phosphorus, calcium, iron, copper, magnesium, and potassium. It has a very low glycemic index, which helps keep blood sugar under control. It's very rich in Vitamin A and Vitamins B that help improve heart health by reducing inflammation and cholesterol levels.	Calories: 343 kcal Carbohydrate: 33 g Protein: 5.50g Fat: 1 g
WALNUTS are a significant source of fiber, healthy fats, minerals, and vitamins. They are rich in antioxidants and a better source of Omega-3 fats than any other nut. They help keep blood pressure and cholesterol low. Since they are very caloric, it's suggested to have 3-4 walnuts per day to appreciate their benefits while keeping calorie intake under control.	Calories: 650 kcal Carbohydrate: 3.89 g Protein: 5 g Fat: 20 g
ARUGULA is rich in fibers and minerals like potassium that are very important for heart and nerve system function. It's also rich in calcium and can be considered one of this mineral's best vegetal sources. Its vitamin content includes Vitamin A, B, C, and E, which support liver function.	Calories: 2.5 kcal Carbohydrate: 0.4g. Protein: 0.3g. Fat: 0.1g.
CHILIS contain high amounts of capsaicin, which has a powerful anti-inflammatory effect that can impact inflammation disorders such as arthritis. It's very high in vitamin C, which is also an antioxidant.	Calories: 6 kcal Carbohydrate: 1.3 g Protein: 0.3 g Fat: 0.1 g
LOVAGE Thanks to the resins, tannins, sugars, vitamin C, essential oils, it is used for phytotherapeutic use (especially the roots, but also the leaves and seeds) for its potential diuretic, antispasmodic and disinfectant action.	Calories: 5 kcal Carbohydrate: 1 g Protein: 0.2 g Fat: 0.1 g

PREP YOUR KITCHEN, FRIDGE, AND PANTRY

You want this change to happen, and you want to lose weight and finally reach your goal. So, first things first. Let's start with cleaning out the old to make room for the new.

Do a quick inventory of what is currently in your fridge and pantry: you may find several items that are not compatible with the Sirtfood Diet.

The best thing to do would be tossing them out or giving them away, even if you just bought them. It's better not to have items around that won't help you reach your goal of better health and a better-looking you.

If this is too extreme for you, or if you live with others who aren't following the diet, just set these items aside, at least for the very first part of the diet.

If there are others in the household, it is a great idea to get them on board and excited about what you are planning to accomplish so that they can either follow the same diet or at least cheer you on every day as you work towards your goal.

ESSENTIAL KITCHEN TOOLS

Some tools will make life easier in the kitchen; these are listed below. If you don't have these items already, our suggestion is to check out garage sales and thrift shops before going to the department store. You can probably get most of them for a quarter of the price of a department store.

COOKING TOOLS

○ Saucepans with lids – 1.5 qt. and 3 qt.

○ Stockpot with lid – 6 qt.

○ Nonstick skillet – 9.5" and 12"

○ Cast iron skillet – at least 12"

○ Set of stainless steel mixing bowls (s, m, l)

○ Pyrex bakeware – 9x13 pan, large pie dish

○ Stainless bakeware – 9x9, 9x13, 9" pie pan

○ Vegetable knife (12" wedge shape blade)

○ Paring knife (3" blade)

○ Ladle

○ Meat fork (sturdier than a regular fork)

○ Spatulas (variety of metal and rubber)

○ Measuring spoons

○ Measuring cups (1 c. and 2c.)

○ Whisk

○ Zester (tiny grater)

○ Peppermill

○ Food processor

○ Microwave oven

COOKING TERMS & TECHNIQUES

Poaching – Protein cooked in liquid.

Blanching – Process to trap nutrients in vegetables, kill bacteria, and lock in color. It is also a method of popping skins off of nuts.

Sweating – Cooking vegetables (usually onions and garlic) over low heat with the lid on until translucent and limp.

Caramelizing – Cooking vegetables at low heat in a little fat for a long time so that the natural sugars in the vegetables brown as they cook.

Sauté – A quick fry in very little fat.

Simmer – Liquid that stays just below the boiling point.

Braising – A technique that uses quick hot, dry heat followed by long low heat and liquid. Pot roast is made using braising. The roast is first seared on all sides over high heat with oil only. The heat is then reduced, and liquid is added as the roast cooks slowly to break down connective fibers (collagen) that make the meat tough.

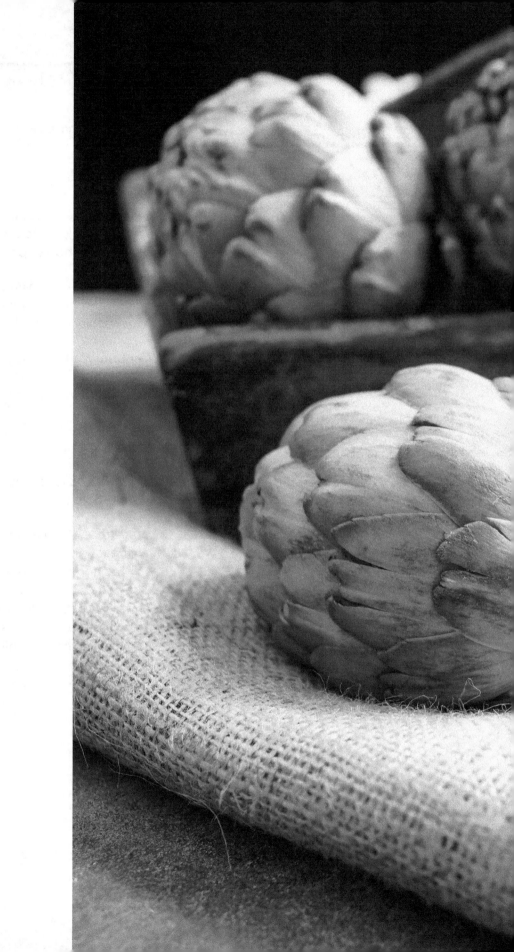

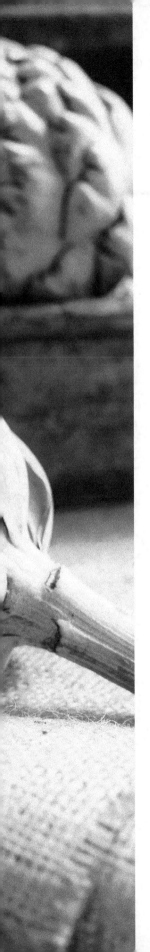

RECIPES

Nutritional Facts are intended per serving.

JUICES AND SMOOTHIES

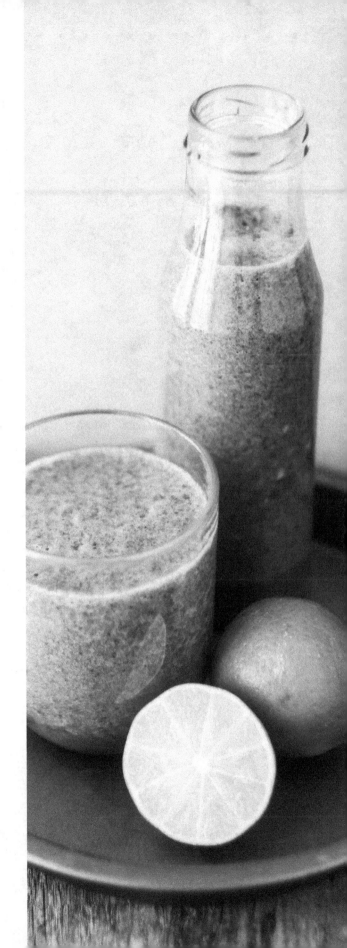

APPLE & CELERY JUICE

 2   🕐 10 mins

Ingredients:
4 large green apples, cored and sliced
4 large celery stalks
1 lemon, peeled

Directions:
Add all ingredients into a juicer and extract the juice according to the manufacturer's method.

In case you don't have one, add all the ingredients in a blender and pulse until well combined.

Filter the juice through a fine-mesh strainer and transfer it into two glasses.

Serve immediately.

NUTRITION FACTS: CALORIES 62KCAL FAT 0.6 G CARBOHYDRATE 6.7 G PROTEIN 1.8 G

APPLE, CUCUMBER & CELERY JUICE

 2   🕐 10 mins

Ingredients:
3 apples, cored and sliced
2 cucumbers, sliced
4 celery stalks
1 1-inch piece fresh ginger, peeled
1 lemon, peeled

Add all ingredients into a juicer and extract the juice according to the manufacturer's method.

In case you don't have one, add all the ingredients in a blender and pulse until well combined.

Filter the juice through a fine-mesh strainer and transfer it into two glasses.

Serve immediately.

Directions:

NUTRITION FACTS: CALORIES 71KCAL FAT 0.7 G CARBOHYDRATE 9.2 G PROTEIN 1.3 G

APPLE, GRAPEFRUIT & CARROT JUICE

 2   10 mins

Ingredients:

3 cups fresh kale
2 large apples, cored and sliced
2 medium carrots, peeled and chopped
2 medium grapefruit, peeled and sectioned
1 tsp fresh lemon juice
½ cup filtered water

Directions:

Add all ingredients into a juicer and extract the juice according to the manufacturer's method.

In case you don't have one, add all the ingredients in a blender and pulse until well combined.

Filter the juice through a fine-mesh strainer and transfer it into two glasses.

Serve immediately.

NUTRITION FACTS: CALORIES 67KCAL FAT 0.2 G CARBOHYDRATE 8 G PROTEIN 0.8 G

APPLE & CARROT JUICE

2   10 mins

Ingredients:

5 carrots, peeled and chopped
1 large apple, cored and chopped
1 ½-inch piece fresh ginger, peeled and chopped
½ of lemon
½ cup filtered water

Directions:

Add all ingredients into a juicer and extract the juice according to the manufacturer's method.

In case you don't have one, add all the ingredients in a blender and pulse until well combined.

Filter the juice through a fine-mesh strainer and transfer it into two glasses.

Serve immediately.

NUTRITION FACTS: CALORIES 125KCAL FAT 0.3 G CARBOHYDRATE 21.4 G PROTEIN 1.7 G

CELERY JUICE

 2　　 10 mins

Ingredients:
8 celery stalks with leaves
2 tbsp. fresh ginger, peeled
1 lemon, peeled
½ cup filtered water
Pinch of salt

Directions:
Add all ingredients into a juicer and extract the juice according to the manufacturer's method.

In case you don't have one, add all the ingredients in a blender and pulse until well combined.

Filter the juice through a fine-mesh strainer and transfer it into two glasses.

Serve immediately.

NUTRITION FACTS: CALORIES 32KCAL FAT 0.5 G CARBOHYDRATE 6.5 G PROTEIN 1 G

GREEN FRUIT JUICE

 2　　 10 mins

Ingredients:
3 kiwis, peeled and chopped
3 green apples, cored and sliced
2 cups seedless green grapes
2 tsp fresh lime juice
½ cup filtered water

Directions:
Add all ingredients into a juicer and extract the juice according to the manufacturer's method.

In case you don't have one, add all the ingredients in a blender and pulse until well combined.

Filter the juice through a fine-mesh strainer and transfer it into two glasses.

Serve immediately.

NUTRITION FACTS: CALORIES 105KCAL FAT 0.5 G CARBOHYDRATE 12.5 G PROTEIN 1 G

FRUITY KALE JUICE

 1   55 mins

Ingredients:

2 green apples, cored and sliced
2 pears, cored and sliced
3 cups fresh kale leaves
3 celery stalks
1 lemon, peeled
½ cup filtered water

Directions:

Add all ingredients into a juicer and extract the juice according to the manufacturer's method.

In case you don't have one, add all the ingredients in a blender and pulse until well combined.

Filter the juice through a fine-mesh strainer and transfer it into two glasses.

Serve immediately.

NUTRITION FACTS: CALORIES 65KCAL FAT 0.3 G CARBOHYDRATE 5.9 G PROTEIN 2.5 G

LEMONY APPLE & KALE JUICE

 2   10 mins

Ingredients:

2 green apples, cored and sliced
4 cups fresh kale leaves
4 tbsp. fresh parsley leaves
1 tbsp. fresh ginger, peeled
1 lemon, peeled
½ cup filtered water
Pinch of salt

Directions:

Add all ingredients into a juicer and extract the juice according to the manufacturer's method.

In case you don't have one, add all the ingredients in a blender and pulse until well combined.

Filter the juice through a fine-mesh strainer and transfer it into two glasses.

Serve immediately.

NUTRITION FACTS: CALORIES 55KCAL FAT 0.3 G CARBOHYDRATE 6.9 G PROTEIN 1.2 G

ORANGE & KALE JUICE

 2   10 mins

Ingredients:
5 oranges, peeled
2 cups fresh kale

Directions:
　　Add all ingredients into a juicer and extract the juice according to the manufacturer's method.
　　In case you don't have one, add all the ingredients in a blender and pulse until well combined.
　　Filter the juice through a fine-mesh strainer and transfer it into two glasses.
　　Serve immediately.

NUTRITION FACTS: CALORIES 52KCAL FAT 0.7 G CARBOHYDRATE 8.5 G PROTEIN 1.5 G

APPLE, ORANGE & BROCCOLI JUICE

  2   10 mins

Ingredients:
2 broccoli, chopped
2 green apples, cored and sliced
3 oranges, peeled
4 tbsp. fresh parsley

Directions:
　　Add all ingredients into a juicer and extract the juice according to the manufacturer's method.
　　In case you don't have one, add all the ingredients in a blender and pulse until well combined.
　　Filter the juice through a fine-mesh strainer and transfer it into two glasses.
　　Serve immediately.

NUTRITION FACTS: CALORIES 82KCAL FAT 0.3 G CARBOHYDRATE 8.5 G PROTEIN 2 G

STRAWBERRY JUICE

 2   10 mins

Ingredients:

2½ cups fresh ripe strawberries, hulled
1 apple, cored and chopped
1 lime, peeled

Directions:

Add all ingredients into a juicer and extract the juice according to the manufacturer's method.

In case you don't have one, add all the ingredients in a blender and pulse until well combined.

Filter the juice through a fine-mesh strainer and transfer it into two glasses.

Serve immediately. It can be stored in the fridge in a proper container for up to 3 days.

NUTRITION FACTS: CALORIES 108KCAL FAT 0.8 G CARBOHYDRATE 18.5 G PROTEIN 1.6 G

APPLE & CINNAMON SMOOTHIE

 2   5 mins

Ingredients:

2 apples, peeled, cored, sliced
4 tbsp. pecans
4 Medjool dates, pitted
½ tsp. vanilla extract, unsweetened
2 cups almond milk, unsweetened
1 ½ tbsp. ground cinnamon

Directions:

Add all ingredients to a high-power blender and pulse until smooth.

Pour the smoothie into two glasses and serve immediately.

It can be stored in the fridge in a proper container for up to 3 days.

NUTRITION FACTS: CALORIES 183KCAL FAT 5.5 G CARBOHYDRATE 12.8 G PROTEIN 4.5 G

AVOCADO SMOOTHIE

 1　　 5 mins

Ingredients:
½ avocado
1 banana
1 cup spinach
1 tbsp. linseed
¼ cup almond milk, unsweetened
½ cup filtered water

Directions:
Add all ingredients to a high-power blender and pulse until smooth.

Pour the smoothie into two glasses and serve immediately

NUTRITION FACTS: CALORIES 161KCAL FAT 5.5 G CARBOHYDRATE 29.5 G PROTEIN 1 G

BANANA STRAWBERRY SMOOTHIE

 1　　 5 mins

Ingredients:
1 cup strawberries
½ banana
½ cup almond milk, unsweetened
½ tsp cocoa powder
3 cubes ice (optional)

Directions:
Blend all ingredients and serve immediately.

NUTRITION FACTS: CALORIES 92KCAL FAT 1.3 G CARBOHYDRATE 12.8 G PROTEIN 3.6 G

BERRIES VANILLA PROTEIN SMOOTHIE

🥤 2   🕐 5 mins

Ingredients:
2 oz. blackberries
2 oz. strawberries
2 oz. raspberries
2 scoops of vanilla protein powder
1 ½ cup almond milk, unsweetened

Directions:
Add all ingredients to a high-power blender and pulse until smooth.

Pour the smoothie into two glasses and serve immediately.

It can be stored in the refrigerator in a proper container for up to 3 days.

NUTRITION FACTS: CALORIES 151KCAL FAT 2.8 G CARBOHYDRATE 10.9 G PROTEIN 20.3 G

BLUEBERRY SMOOTHIE

 🥤 1   🕐 5 mins

Ingredients:
1 cup blueberries
½ banana
½ cup orange juice
3 cubes ice (optional)

Directions:
Blend all ingredients and serve immediately.

NUTRITION FACTS: CALORIES 87KCAL FAT 1.1 G CARBOHYDRATE 11.8 G PROTEIN 1.6 G

BLUEBERRY & KALE SMOOTHIE

 2   10 mins

Ingredients:

2 cups frozen blueberries

2 cups fresh kale leaves

2 Medjool dates, pitted

1 tbsp. chia seeds

1 ½-inch piece fresh ginger, peeled and chopped

1 ½ cups almond milk, unsweetened

Directions:

Add all ingredients to a high-power blender and pulse until smooth.

Pour the smoothie into two glasses and serve immediately.

It can be stored in the refrigerator in a proper container for up to 3 days.

NUTRITION FACTS: CALORIES 230KCAL FAT 4.5 G CARBOHYDRATE 28.8 G PROTEIN 5.6 G

CHOCOLATE & DATE SMOOTHIE

  2   10 mins

Ingredients:

4 Medjool dates, pitted

2 tbsp. cacao powder

2 tbsp. flaxseed

1 tbsp. almond butter

1 tsp. vanilla extract

¼ tsp. ground cinnamon

1 ½ cups almond milk, unsweetened

4 ice cubes

Directions:

Add all ingredients to a high-power blender and pulse until smooth.

Pour into two glasses and serve immediately.

It can be stored in the refrigerator in a proper container for up to 3 days.

NUTRITION FACTS: CALORIES 234KCAL FAT 5 G CARBOHYDRATE 25.5 G PROTEIN 6 G

GREEN PINEAPPLE SMOOTHIE

 I 5 mins

Ingredients:
1 cup spinach
1 apple
1 cup pineapple
1 tsp. of flax seeds
½ cup filtered water

Directions:
Add all ingredients to a high-power blender and pulse until smooth.

Pour the smoothie into two glasses and serve immediately.

NUTRITION FACTS: CALORIES 102KCAL FAT 0.3 G CARBOHYDRATE 18.5 G PROTEIN 1 G

KALE SMOOTHIE

 I 5 mins

Ingredients:
1 cup kale
½ mango
½ banana
1 tbsp. chia seeds
¼ cup coconut milk, unsweetened
½ cup filtered water

Directions:
Add all ingredients to a high-power blender and pulse until smooth.

Pour the smoothie into two glasses and serve immediately

NUTRITION FACTS: CALORIES 156KCAL FAT 4.5 G CARBOHYDRATE 20.5 G PROTEIN 3.2 G

LETTUCE SMOOTHIE

 1   mins

Ingredients:
½ head of lettuce
3 fresh plums, seeded
½ banana
1 tbsp. linseed
½ cucumber
½ cup almond milk, unsweetened

Directions:
Add all ingredients to a high-power blender and pulse until smooth.

Pour the smoothie into two glasses and serve immediately.

NUTRITION FACTS: CALORIES 138KCAL FAT 2.5 G CARBOHYDRATE 19.8 G PROTEIN 3 G

SPINACH SMOOTHIE

 1   mins

Ingredients:
1 cup spinach
1 pear
½ bananas
¼ zucchini
½ cup almond milk, unsweetened

Directions:
Add all ingredients to a high-power blender and pulse until smooth.

Pour the smoothie into two glasses and serve immediately.

NUTRITION FACTS: CALORIES 123KCAL FAT 0.9 G CARBOHYDRATE 18.5 G PROTEIN 2.4 G

STRAWBERRY & BEET SMOOTHIE

 2   10 mins

Ingredients:
2 cups frozen strawberries, pitted and chopped
2/3 cup frozen beets, chopped
1 ½-inch piece ginger, chopped
1 ½-inch piece fresh turmeric, chopped (or 1 tsp turmeric powder)
½ cup fresh orange juice
1 cup almond milk, unsweetened

Directions:
Add all ingredients to a high-power blender and pulse until smooth.

Pour the smoothie into two glasses and serve immediately.

It can be stored in the fridge in a proper container for up to 3 days.

NUTRITION FACTS: CALORIES 130KCAL FAT 0.2 G CARBOHYDRATE 22.5 G PROTEIN 2 G

STRAWBERRY, MANGO, & YOGURT SMOOTHIE

 2   5 mins

Ingredients:
1 mango, diced
4 oz. strawberries
1.3 oz. yogurt
2 cups almond milk, unsweetened

Directions:
Add all ingredients to a high-power blender and pulse until smooth.

Pour the smoothie into two glasses and serve immediately.

It can be stored in the fridge in a proper container for up to 3 days.

NUTRITION FACTS: CALORIES 166KCAL FAT 3.7 G CARBOHYDRATE 27 G PROTEIN 3.5 G

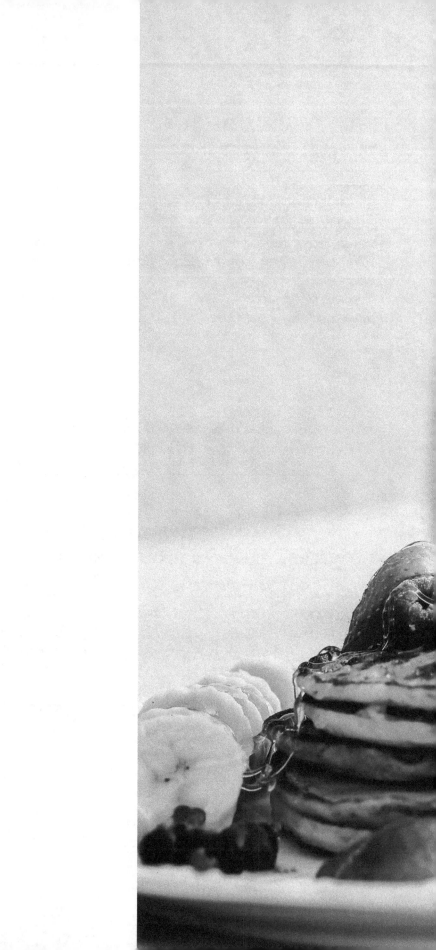

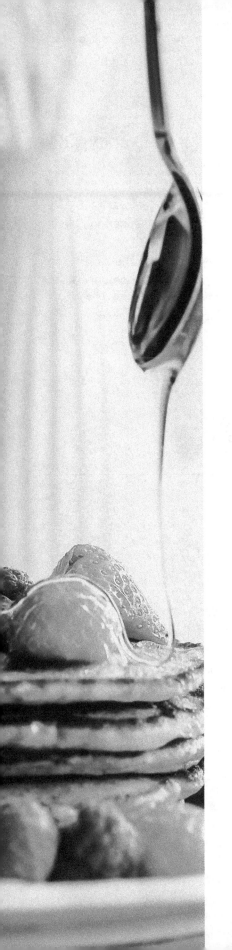

BREAKFAST

BANANA VANILLA PANCAKE

 2   25 mins

Ingredients:

1 egg
1 egg white
1 banana
2 tsp. honey
1 cup rolled oats
¼ tsp. baking powder
A pinch of salt
1 tsp. vanilla extract
½ cup almond milk, unsweetened

Directions:

Put half of the banana, eggs, oats, vanilla, baking powder, salt, and almond milk in a blender and blend until smooth.

Heat a skillet, and when hot, pour the batter in to form pancakes. Cook 2 minutes per side until done. Repeat until all the pancakes are ready.

Top with honey and the other half banana.

NUTRITION FACTS: CALORIES 232KCAL   FAT 5.3 G   CARBOHYDRATE 22.8 G   PROTEIN 18.6 G

BLUEBERRY AND WALNUT BAKE

  4   35 mins

Ingredients:

4 oz. rolled oats
12 oz. almond milk, unsweetened
1 banana, ripe and mashed
½ tsp. vanilla extract
1 oz. walnuts, chopped
1 cup blueberries
To serve: ½ cup plain yogurt

Directions:

Heat the oven to 400°F.

Mix the oats, milk, vanilla, banana, blueberries, and walnuts in a bowl. Put on a baking tray lined with parchment paper and cook around 30 minutes.

It can be eaten alone or served with ½ cup of plain yogurt.

NUTRITION FACTS: CALORIES 308KCAL   FAT 5.3 G   CARBOHYDRATE 35.8 G   PROTEIN 15.6 G

BLUEBERRIES PANCAKE

 2   🕐 15 mins

Ingredients:

1 banana, peeled
4 tbsp. peanut butter
¼ cup whole-wheat flour
2 oz. blueberries
1 tbsp. agave syrup
A pinch of ground cinnamon
½ cup almond milk, unsweetened
Cooking spray

Directions:

Add all the ingredients to a blender and then pulse for 2 minutes until smooth. Spray a skillet pan with cooking spray, place it over medium heat until it gets hot.

Pour some batter into the pan, shape batter to form a pancake, and cook for 2 to 3 minutes per side until golden brown.

Transfer cooked pancakes to a plate and then repeat with the remaining batter. Serve straight away.

Pancakes can be stored up to 3 days in the fridge using a proper container with a lid. When ready to eat, reheat in the microwave oven for 1 to 2 minutes until hot and then serve.

NUTRITION FACTS: CALORIES 408KCAL FAT 14 G CARBOHYDRATE 53 G PROTEIN 10.2 G

BRUSSELS SPROUTS EGG SKILLET

 2   🕐 35 mins

Ingredients:

½lb Brussels sprouts, halved
1 red onion, chopped
10 cherry tomatoes, halved
4 eggs
1 tsp. extra-virgin olive oil

Directions:

In an 8 inch cast iron skillet, heat olive oil over medium heat.

Add in onion and sauté for 1-2 minutes.

Add in Brussels sprouts and tomatoes and season with salt and pepper to taste.

Cook for 3-4 minutes, then crack the eggs, cover, and cook until egg whites have set, and egg yolk is desired consistency.

NUTRITION FACTS: CALORIES 194KCAL FAT 18.2 G CARBOHYDRATE 11.4 G PROTEIN 7.1 G

BUCKWHEAT PORRIDGE

 2   25 mins

Ingredients:

1 cup buckwheat, rinsed
1 cup almond milk, unsweetened
1 cup water
½ tsp ground cinnamon
½ tsp. vanilla extract
¼ cup fresh blueberries
1 tbsp. honey (optional)

Directions:

In a pan, add all the ingredients (except honey and blueberries) over medium-high heat and bring to a boil.

Now, reduce the heat to low and simmer, covered for about 10 minutes. Stir in the honey and remove from the heat.

Set aside, covered, for about 5 minutes. With a fork, fluff the mixture, and transfer into serving bowls.

Top with blueberries and serve.

NUTRITION FACTS: CALORIES 358KCAL FAT 4.7 G CARBOHYDRATE 3.7 G PROTEIN 12 G

CHERRY AND VANILLA PROTEIN SHAKE

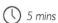 1   5 mins

Ingredients:

2 oz. cherries, destemmed
1 scoop vanilla protein powder
1 cup almond milk, unsweetened

Directions:

Place all the ingredients in the order into a food processor or blender, then pulse for 1 to 2 minutes until smooth.

Serve immediately.

NUTRITION FACTS: CALORIES 193KCAL FAT 5.2 G CARBOHYDRATE 38 G PROTEIN 5.2 G

CASHEW BISCUITS

 8   39 mins

Ingredients:

1 ¼ cups whole-wheat flour
1/3 cup toasted whole cashews, unsalted
½ tsp fine sea salt
1 ½ teaspoons baking powder
1 tbsp. coconut oil
3 tbsp. natural smooth cashew butter
½ cup soft silken tofu or unsweetened plain yogurt

Directions:

Preheat the oven to 425°F. Line a baking sheet with parchment paper. Place the flour and nuts in a food processor.

Pulse until almost all the nuts are chopped: a few larger pieces are okay and add texture to the cookies. Add salt and baking powder and pulse a couple of times.

Add oil and nut butter and pulse to combine. Add tofu or yogurt, and pulse until a crumbly (but not dry) dough forms.

Gather the dough on a piece of parchment and pat it together to shape into a 6-inch square.

Cut into nine 2-inch square biscuits. Transfer the cookies to the baking sheet. Bake for 12 to 14 minutes or until golden brown at the edges. Cool on a wire rack and serve.

NUTRITION FACTS: CALORIES 166KCAL FAT 3.7 G
CARBOHYDRATE 27 G PROTEIN 3.5 G

CHERRY PARFAIT

 1   5 mins

Ingredients:

3 oz. cherries, destemmed
3 tbsp. chia seeds
2 ½ tbsp. shredded coconut
3 tbsp. agave syrup
8 oz. almond milk, unsweetened
½ tsp. vanilla extract, unsweetened

Directions:

Take a bowl, place chia and coconut in it; add agave syrup and vanilla, pour in the milk, and whisk until well combined.

Let the mixture rest for 30 minutes, then stir it and refrigerate for a minimum of 3 hours or overnight.

Assemble the parfait: divide half of the chia mixture into the bottom of the serving glass, and then top evenly with three-fourths of cherries.

Cover cherries with remaining chia seed mixture and then place remaining cherries on top. Serve straight away.

NUTRITION FACTS: CALORIES 236KCAL FAT 9.2 G CARBOHYDRATE 34.7 G PROTEIN 3.5 G

FLAX WAFFLES

 2   10 mins

Ingredients:

½ cup whole-wheat flour
½ tbsp. flaxseed meal
½ tsp. baking powder
1 tbsp. olive oil
½ cup almond milk, unsweetened
¼ tsp. vanilla extract, unsweetened
2 tbsp. honey, or a few stevia drops (optional)

Directions:

Switch on a mini waffle maker and let it preheat for 5 minutes. Meanwhile, take a bowl, place all the ingredients in it, and then mix by using an immersion blender until smooth.

Pour the batter evenly into the waffle maker, shut with lid, and let it cook for 3 to 4 minutes until firm and golden brown.

Serve straight away. Cool the waffles, divide them between two meal prep containers, evenly add berries into the container, and then add agave syrup in mini-meal prep cups.

Cover each container with a lid and store in the refrigerator for up to 5 days.

When ready to eat, enjoy them cold or reheat them in the microwave for 40 to 60 seconds or more until hot.

NUTRITION FACTS: CALORIES 220KCAL   FAT 3.7 G   CARBOHYDRATE 7 G   PROTEIN 21.5 G

GREEN OMELET

 I 20 mins

Ingredients:

I tsp. of olive oil
I scallion peeled and finely chopped
2 eggs
Salt and freshly ground black pepper
A handful of parsley, finely chopped
A handful of arugula leaves

Directions:

Heat the oil in a frying pan over medium-low heat. Add the scallion and gently fry for about 5 minutes. Increase the heat and cook for two more minutes.

In a cup or bowl, whisk the eggs, distribute the scallion in the pan then add in the eggs. Evenly distribute the eggs by tipping the pan on all sides.

Cook for about a minute before lifting the sides and allowing the runny eggs to move to the pan's base.

Sprinkle arugula leaves and parsley on top and season with pepper and salt to taste.

When the base is just starting to brown, tip it onto a plate and serve right away.

NUTRITION FACTS: CALORIES 221KCAL FAT 28 G CARBOHYDRATE 10.6 G PROTEIN 9.5 G

KALE AND MUSHROOM FRITTATA

 4 45 mins

Ingredients:

8 eggs
½ cup unsweetened almond milk
Salt and ground black pepper, to taste
I tbsp. extra-virgin olive oil
I red onion, chopped
I garlic clove, minced
I cup fresh mushrooms, chopped
I ½ cups fresh kale, chopped

Directions:

Preheat oven to 350°F. In a bowl, place the eggs, almond milk, salt, and black pepper and beat well. Set aside. In a ovenproof pan, heat the oil over medium heat and sauté the onion and garlic for about 3–4 minutes. Add the kale salt and black pepper, and cook for about 8–10 minutes.

Stir in the mushrooms and cook for about 3–4 minutes. Place the egg mixture on top evenly and cook for about 4 minutes without stirring. Transfer the pan to the oven and bake for about 12–15 minutes or until desired doneness.

Remove from the oven and let rest for about 3–5 minutes before serving.

NUTRITION FACTS: CALORIES 151KCAL FAT 10.2 G CARBOHYDRATE 5.6 G PROTEIN 10.3 G

KALE SCRAMBLE

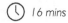 2   16 mins

Ingredients:
4 eggs
1/8 tsp ground turmeric
Salt and ground black pepper, to taste
1 tbsp. water
2 teaspoons olive oil
1 cup fresh kale, chopped

Directions:
In a bowl, add the eggs, turmeric, salt, black pepper, and water, and with a whisk, beat until foamy. In a skillet, heat the oil over medium heat.

Add the egg mixture and stir to combine.

Reduce the heat to medium-low and cook for about 1 to 2 minutes, stirring frequently.

Stir in the kale and cook for about 3 to 4 minutes, stirring frequently.

Remove from the heat and serve immediately.

NUTRITION FACTS: CALORIES 183KCAL FAT 13.4 G CARBOHYDRATE 4.3 G PROTEIN 12.1 G

OVERNIGHT OATS WITH STRAWBERRIES AND CHOCOLATE

 2   5 mins + 8h

Ingredients:
2 oz. rolled oats
4 oz. almond milk, unsweetened
2 tbsp. plain yogurt
1 cup strawberries
1 tsp honey
1 square 85% chocolate

Directions:
Mix the oats and the milk in a jar and leave overnight. In the morning, top the jar with yogurt, honey, strawberries, and chocolate cut into small pieces.

It can be prepared in advance and left for up to 3 days in the fridge.

NUTRITION FACTS: CALORIES 258KCAL FAT 3.3 G CARBOHYDRATE 29.8 G PROTEIN 13.6 G

PANCAKES WITH APPLES AND BLACKCURRANTS

 4 30 mins

Ingredients:

2 apples cut into small chunks
2 cups of quick-cooking oats
1 cup flour
2 egg whites
1 ¼ cups almond milk, unsweetened
Cooking spray
1 cup blackcurrants, stalks removed
3 tbsp. water may use less
2 tbsp. honey, or a few stevia drops (optional)

Directions:

Place the ingredients for the topping in a small pot. Simmer. Stir frequently for about 10 minutes until it cooks down, and the juices are released. Take the dry ingredients and mix them in a bowl.

After, add the apples and the milk a bit at a time (you may not use it all) until it is a batter. Whisk the egg whites until they are firm and gently mix them into the pancake batter.

Set aside in the refrigerator. Spray a pan with cooking spray, and when hot, pour some of the batter into it in a pancake shape. When the pancakes start to have golden brown edges and form air bubbles, they are ready to be flipped. Repeat for the next pancakes. Top each pancake with the berry topping.

NUTRITION FACTS: CALORIES 370KCAL   FAT 10.8 G   CARBOHYDRATE 79 G   PROTEIN 11.7 G

PANCAKES WITH BLACKCURRANT COMPOTE

 4  40 mins

Ingredients:

1 cup plain flour
½ cup porridge oats
2 apples peeled and cut into tiny pieces
1 tsp. of baking powder
2 egg whites
1 cup almond milk, unsweetened
Cooking spray
Pinch of salt
4 oz. blackcurrants, stalks removed
3 tbsp. of water
2 tbsp. honey of a few drops of stevia

Directions:

Make the compote first. Place the blackcurrants, water, and sugar in a pan. Bring it to a simmer and let it cook for 10 to 15 minutes. Place oats, baking powder, flour, and salt in a bowl and stir well. Add in the apple then the milk while you whisk until you have a smooth batter.

Whisk the egg whites into stiff peaks and fold into the pancake batter. Transfer the ready batter to a jug. Spray a pan with cooking spray, place it on medium-high heat, and add approximately a quarter of the batter. Let it cook on both sides until it turns golden brown.

Remove when ready, then repeat to make four pancakes. Drizzle the blackcurrant compote over the pancakes and serve.

NUTRITION FACTS: CALORIES 210KCAL FAT 7 G CARBOHYDRATE 40 G PROTEIN 5.8 G

PEANUT BUTTER CUP PROTEIN SHAKE

 1   🕐 5 mins

Ingredients:
1 banana, peeled
1 scoop of chocolate protein powder
1 tbsp. nutritional yeast
2 tbsp. peanut butter
½ cup almond milk, unsweetened
½ tsp. turmeric powder

Directions:
Place all the ingredients in the order into a food processor or blender, then pulse for 1 to 2 minutes until smooth.

Distribute smoothie between two glasses and then serve.

Divide smoothie between two jars or bottles, cover with a lid and store the containers in the refrigerator for up to 3 days.

NUTRITION FACTS: CALORIES 233KCAL FAT 11 G CARBOHYDRATE 17 G PROTEIN 14 G

RASPBERRIES PARFAIT

 2   5 mins

Ingredients:
4 oz. raspberries
3 tbsp. chia seeds
2 ½ tbsp. shredded coconut
3 tbsp. agave syrup
8 oz. almond milk, unsweetened
½ tsp. vanilla extract, unsweetened

Directions:
Take a medium bowl, place chia and coconut in it; add agave syrup and vanilla, pour in the milk, and whisk until well combined. Let the mixture rest for 30 minutes, then stir it and refrigerate for a minimum of 3 hours or overnight.

Assemble the parfait: divide half of the chia mixture into the bottom of the serving glass, and then top evenly with three-fourth of raspberries.

Cover berries with remaining chia seed mixture and then place remaining berries on top. Serve straight away.

Use wide-mouth pint jars to layer parfait, cover tightly with lids, and store jars in the refrigerator for up to 7 days. When ready to eat, enjoy it cold.

NUTRITION FACTS: CALORIES 239KCAL FAT 9.5 G
CARBOHYDRATE 9.9 G PROTEIN 34 G

RASPBERRY WAFFLES

 2   20 mins

Ingredients:

½ cup whole-wheat flour

1 ½ tbsp. chopped raspberry

½ tsp. baking powder

1 tbsp. olive oil

½ cup almond milk, unsweetened

¼ tsp vanilla extract, unsweetened

2 tbsp. coconut sugar or a few drops of stevia (optional)

Directions:

Switch on the waffle maker and let it preheat for 5 minutes. Meanwhile, take a medium bowl, place all the ingredients in it, and then mix by using an immersion blender until smooth.

Pour the batter evenly into the waffle maker, shut the lid, and let it cook for 3 to 4 minutes until firm and golden brown.

Serve straight away. Cool the waffles, divide them between two meal prep containers, evenly add berries into the container, and then add agave syrup in mini-meal prep cups.

Cover each container with a lid and store in the refrigerator for up to 5 days.

When ready to eat, enjoy them cold or reheat them in the microwave for 40 to 60 seconds or more until hot.

NUTRITION FACTS: CALORIES 229KCAL FAT 3.7 G CARBOHYDRATE 35.4 G PROTEIN 3.5 G

SAUTÉED MUSHROOMS AND POACHED EGGS

 2   25 mins

Ingredients:
2 eggs
1 white onion, sliced
1 tsp. extra-virgin olive oil
10 oz. mushrooms, sliced
10 oz. tomatoes, chopped
1 tsp. marjoram

Directions:
Sauté the onions in a frying pan with the oil for 5 minutes. Add mushrooms, tomatoes, marjoram, and season with salt and pepper to taste.

While the mushrooms are cooking, bring some water to a boil, crack one egg at a time and poach it. Put the poached egg on top of mushrooms and serve.

NUTRITION FACTS: CALORIES 270KCAL FAT 4.3 G CARBOHYDRATE 19.8 G PROTEIN 22.8 G

SUPER EASY SCRAMBLED EGGS AND CHERRY TOMATOES

 1   4 mins

Ingredients:
2 eggs
1 tbsp. parmesan or other shredded cheese
Salt and pepper
½ cup cherry tomatoes

Directions:
Put eggs and cheese with a pinch of salt and pepper in a jar. Microwave for 30 seconds, then quickly stir with a spoon.

Put back in the microwave for 60 seconds, and they are ready to eat with cherry tomatoes.

In case you don't own a microwave, cook the scrambled eggs in a skillet for 2 minutes, stirring continuously until done.

NUTRITION FACTS: CALORIES 278KCAL FAT 5.4 G CARBOHYDRATE 12.8 G PROTEIN 18.9 G

STRAWBERRY BUCKWHEAT PANCAKES

 4   30 mins

Ingredients:
3½ oz. strawberries, chopped
3½ oz. buckwheat flour
1 egg
8 fl. oz. milk
1 tsp olive oil
1 tsp olive oil for frying
1 orange, juiced

Directions:
Pour the milk into a bowl and mix in the egg and a tsp of olive oil. Sift in the flour to the liquid mixture until smooth and creamy.

Allow it to rest for 15 minutes. Heat a little oil in a pan and pour in a quarter of the mixture or the size you prefer.

Sprinkle in a quarter of the strawberries into the batter. Cook for around 2 minutes on each side.

Serve hot with a drizzle of orange juice.

Try this recipe with other berries such as blueberries and blackberries.

NUTRITION FACTS: CALORIES 180KCAL FAT 7.5 G CARBOHYDRATE 22.5 G PROTEIN 7.4 G

TOMATO FRITTATA

2   30 mins

Ingredients:
¼ cup cheddar cheese, grated
¼ cup kalamata olives halved
8 cherry tomatoes, halved
4 eggs
1 tbsp. fresh parsley, chopped
1 tbsp. fresh basil, chopped
1 tbsp. olive oil
1 tbsp. tomato paste

Directions:
Whisk eggs together in a mixing bowl.

Toss in the parsley, basil, olives, tomatoes, and cheese, stirring thoroughly. In a skillet, heat the olive oil over high heat.

Pour in the frittata mixture and cook until firm (around 10 minutes).

Remove the skillet from the hob and place it under the grill for 5 minutes until golden brown.

Divide into portions and serve immediately.

NUTRITION FACTS: CALORIES 269KCAL FAT 23.7 G CARBOHYDRATE 5.5 G PROTEIN 9.2 G

VANILLA PARFAIT WITH BERRIES

 | 5 mins

Ingredients:

4 oz. Greek yogurt

1 tsp honey or agave syrup

1 cup mixed berries, frozen is perfect

1 tbsp. buckwheat granola

½ tsp vanilla extract

Directions:

Mix yogurt, vanilla extract, and honey. Alternate yogurt and berries in a jar and top with granola.

Frozen berries are perfect if the parfait is made in advance because they release their juices in the yogurt.

As far as granola, you can usea one of the recipes on this book..

NUTRITION FACTS: CALORIES 318KCAL FAT 5.4 G CARBOHYDRATE 22.8 G PROTEIN 21.9 G

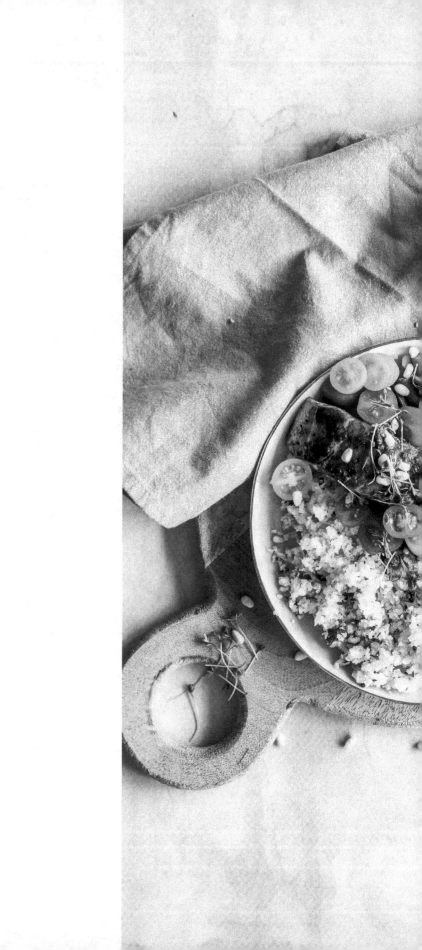

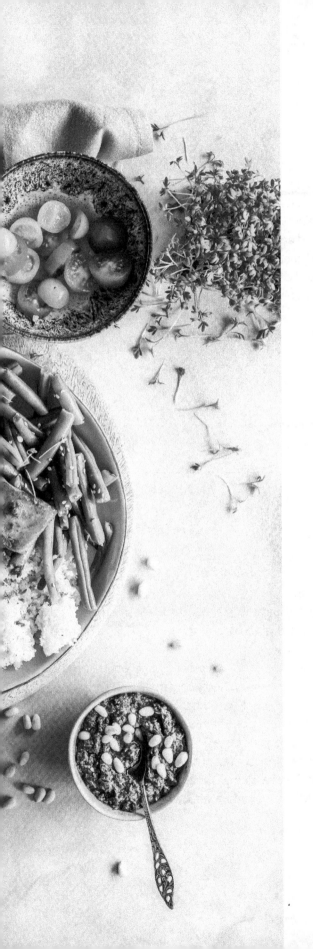

MAIN DISHES

ARTICHOKES AND KALE WITH WALNUTS

 2    40 mins

Ingredients:

1 cup of artichoke hearts
1 tbsp. parsley, chopped
½ cup of walnuts
1 cup of kale, torn
1 cup of Cheddar cheese, crumbled
½ tbsp. balsamic vinegar
1 tbsp. olive oil
Salt and black pepper, to taste

Directions:

Preheat the oven to 250°-270°F and roast the walnuts in the oven for 10 minutes until lightly browned and crispy and then set aside.

Add artichoke hearts, kale, oil, salt, and pepper to a pot and cook for 20 to 25 minutes until done.

Add cheese and balsamic vinegar and stir well. Divide the vegetables onto two plates and garnish with roasted walnuts and parsley.

NUTRITION FACTS: CALORIES 152KCAL FAT 32 G CARBOHYDRATE 59 G PROTEIN 23 G

ASIAN BEEF SALAD

 2   23 mins

Ingredients:

3 tsp. extra-virgin olive oil
8 oz. sirloin steak
½ red onion, finely sliced
½ cucumber, sliced
½ cup cherry tomatoes, halved
2 cups lettuce
1 handful parsley
1 tbsp. soy sauce
½ bird's eye chili
3 tbsp. lemon juice

Directions:

Crush the garlic, mix it with finely sliced chili and parsley, 2 tsp olive oil, and soy sauce. This will be the dressing.

Prepare the salad in a bowl placing lettuce on the bottom, then onion, cherry tomatoes, and cucumber. Heat a skillet until very hot. Brush the steaks with remaining oil, season them with salt and pepper and cook them to your taste.

Transfer the steaks onto a cutting board for 5 minutes before slicing. Drizzle the dressing on the salad and mix well. Place steak slices on top and serve.

NUTRITION FACTS: CALORIES 262KCAL FAT 12 G CARBOHYDRATE 15.2 G PROTEIN 25.2 G

AUTUMN STUFFED ENCHILADAS

🍽 4   🕐 1h

Ingredients:

1 lemon, juiced
1 cup cashews
½ oz. parsley
1 oz. roasted pumpkin seeds
8 corn tortillas
2 cups Butternut squash
1 cup salsa
1 can black beans
2 tbsp. olive oil
¼ tbsp. cayenne pepper
1 tsp. chili flakes
1 tsp. cumin
3 cloves garlic
1 jalapeno
1 red onion
1 cup Brussels sprouts

Directions:

Soak the cashews in boiling water and set aside.

Cut the squash in half, and after scooping out the seeds, lightly rub olive oil. Sprinkle with a little salt and pepper before putting on a baking sheet face down. Cook for about forty-five minutes at 400°F until it is cooked.

Heat one tbsp. olive oil in a pan on medium heat and put chopped onion in, stirring until soft. Finely dice the jalapeno and garlic and finely slice the Brussel sprouts. Add these three things to the frypan and cook until the Brussels begin to wilt through.

Strain and rinse the black beans, then add them to the frypan and mix well.

When the squash is cooked and cool enough to handle, scrape out the soft insides away from the skin and put in a big bowl along with the Brussels mixture. Mix well again with salt and pepper to taste.

Put the tortillas in the oven to soften up (don't let them get crispy)

Spoon the squash mixture into the middle of the soft tortillas. Carefully roll them up to make little open-ended wraps, and then put in on a baking tray with the open ends down to stop them from unrolling.

Do this for all twelve tortillas, then pour the rest of the salsa on top and spread to coat evenly.

Change the temperature of the oven to 350°F and bake for 30 minutes.

While these cooks put the drained, soaked cashews into a blender with one and a half cups cold water, lemon juice, and a quarter tsp. salt.

Blend until smooth, adding water if it becomes too thick; this is your sour cream.

When enchiladas are done, leave to cool while you chop parsley.

Then drizzle the sour cream generously over the dish and top with parsley and pumpkin seeds.

NUTRITION FACTS: CALORIES 333KCAL   FAT 11 G   CARBOHYDRATE 36 G   PROTEIN 14 G

BAKED POTATOES WITH SPICY CHICKPEA STEW

 4　　　🕐 70 mins

Ingredients:

4 baking potatoes, pricked around
2 tbsp. olive oil
2 red onions, finely chopped
4 tsp. garlic, crushed or grated
1-inch ginger, grated
1/2 tsp. chili flakes
2 tbsp. cumin seeds
2 tbsp. turmeric
2 tins chopped tomatoes
2 tbsp. cocoa powder, unsweetened
2 tins chickpeas – do not drain
2 yellow peppers, chopped

Directions:

Preheat the oven to 400°F, and start preparing all ingredients. When the oven is ready, put in baking potatoes and cook for 50 minutes to 1 hour until they are done.

While potatoes are cooking, put olive oil and sliced red onion into a wide saucepan and cook lightly, using the lid, for 5 minutes until the onions are tender but not brown.

Remove the lid and add ginger, garlic, cumin, and cook for another minute on very low heat. Then add the turmeric and a tiny dab of water and cook for a few more minutes until it becomes thicker, and the consistency is ok.

Then add tomatoes, cocoa powder, peppers, chickpeas with their water and salt. Bring to the boil, and then simmer on a very low heat for 45 to 50 minutes until it's thick. Finally, stir in the 2 tbsp. of parsley, some pepper and salt if you desire, and serve the stew with the potatoes.

NUTRITION FACTS: CALORIES 520KCAL FAT 8 G CARBOHYDRATE 91 G PROTEIN 32 G

BAKED ROOT VEGGIES WITH CHILI

🍲 6   🕐 70 mins

Ingredients:

3 Potatoes
3 Sweet potatoes
3 Yam
2 cups vegetable broth
1 can Red kidney beans
1 can white kidney beans
2 cans diced tomatoes
1 can black beans
1 tbsp. oregano
2 tbsp. paprika
1 tsp. cumin
2 tsp. chili powder
2 stalks celery
2 carrots
1 bell pepper
2 red onions
3 tbsp. Olive oil
½ oz. Parsley
2 avocados
1 bay leaf
1 can sweet corn
2 tomatoes
2 limes, juiced
1 head romaine

Directions:

Scrub and fork the potatoes and yams. Drizzle them with oil. Sprinkle with salt and put on a baking tray for 45 minutes or until you can pierce easily with a knife.

Heat the oil in a frying pan on medium heat and add the diced onion with the chopped bell pepper, diced carrots, celery, and a quarter tsp. of salt.

Cook until the carrot is tender, then add the paprika, oregano, cumin, and chili powder.

Put in tomato, the bay leaf, and the vegetable broth. Rinse the beans and drain well before adding to the pot.

Stir well and leave to simmer for a further 30 minutes. After this time has passed, get a potato masher and mash the chili a few times to crush part of the beans and thicken the mixture.

Add the juice of one lime and salt and pepper to taste.

In a bowl, finely dice the avocado and lightly mash with salt, pepper, and the juice of another lime.

In another bowl, drain and rinse the corn and toss in parsley, finely chopped, shredded romaine lettuce, a pinch of salt, and a tbsp. olive oil.

Serve potatoes, chili, avocado, and salad so that everyone can assemble his/her masterpiece. Enjoy!

NUTRITION FACTS: CALORIES 493KCAL FAT 14 G CARBOHYDRATE 96 G PROTEIN 14 G

BAKED SALMON SALAD WITH CREAMY MINT DRESSING

 1   45 mins

Ingredients:

1 salmon fillet
1 cup mixed salad leaves
1 cup lettuce leaves
Two radishes, thinly sliced
½ cucumber, sliced
2 spring onions, trimmed and chopped
½ oz. parsley, roughly sliced
1 tsp. low-carb mayonnaise
1 tbsp. natural yogurt
1 tbsp. rice vinegar
2 stalks mint, finely chopped

Directions:

Put the salmon fillet onto a baking tray and bake for 16 to 18 minutes until cooked

In a bowl, blend the mayonnaise, yogurt, rice vinegar, mint leaves, and salt. Set aside 5 minutes for the flavors to mix well.

Arrange the salad leaves and lettuce onto a serving plate and top with all the radishes, cucumber, lettuce, celery, spring onions, and parsley.

Drizzle the dressing.

NUTRITION FACTS: CALORIES 433KCAL FAT 9 G CARBOHYDRATE 32 G PROTEIN 18 G

BAKED SALMON WITH STIR-FRIED VEGETABLES

 2   50 mins

Ingredients:

Zest and juice of 1 lemon
1 tsp. sesame oil
2 tsp. extra-virgin olive oil
2 carrots cut into matchsticks
1 bunch of kale, chopped
2 tsp. of root ginger, grated
8 oz. wild salmon fillets

Mix ginger lemon juice and zest together. Place the salmon in an ovenproof dish and pour over the lemon-ginger mixture. Cover with foil and leave for 30-60 minutes to marinate.

Bake the salmon at 375°F in the oven for 15 minutes. While cooking, heat a wok or frying pan, then add sesame oil and olive oil. Add the vegetables, and cook, constantly stirring for a few minutes.

Once the salmon is cooked, spoon some of the salmon marinades onto the vegetables and cook for a few more minutes. Serve the vegetables onto a plate and top with salmon.

Directions:

NUTRITION FACTS: CALORIES 458KCAL FAT 13.2 G CARBOHYDRATE 15.3 G PROTEIN 21.4 G

BROCCOLI AND PASTA

 2   🕐 30 mins

Ingredients:

5 oz. buckwheat spaghetti
5 oz. broccoli
1 garlic clove, finely chopped
3 tbsp. extra-virgin olive oil
2 scallions sliced
¼ tsp. crushed chilies
12 sage shredded leaves
Grated Parmesan (optional)

Directions:

Put broccoli in boiling water for 5 minutes, then add spaghetti and cook until both pasta and broccoli are done (around 8 to 10 minutes).

In the meantime, heat the oil in a frying pan and add scallions and garlic.

Cook for 5 minutes until it becomes golden.

Mix chilies and sage to the pan and gently cook for 1 minute. Drain pasta and broccoli; mix with the scallion mixture in the pan. Add some Parmesan, if desired, and serve.

NUTRITION FACTS: CALORIES 350KCAL FAT 8 G CARBOHYDRATE 38 G PROTEIN 6 G

BUCKWHEAT WITH MUSHROOMS AND GREEN ONIONS

2   🕐 50 mins

Ingredients:

1 cup buckwheat groats
2 cups vegetable or chicken broth
3 green onions, thinly sliced
1 cup mushrooms, sliced
2 tsp. extra-virgin olive oil

Directions:

Combine all ingredients in a pot and cook on low heat for about 35 to 40min until the broth is completely absorbed.

Divide between two plates and serve immediately.

NUTRITION FACTS: CALORIES 340KCAL FAT 10 G CARBOHYDRATE 51 G PROTEIN 11 G

BUCKWHEAT WITH ONIONS

 4   50 mins

Ingredients:

3 cups of buckwheat, rinsed
4 red onions, chopped
1 white onion, chopped
5 oz. extra-virgin olive oil
3 cups of water
Salt and pepper, to taste

Directions:

Soak the buckwheat in warm water for around 10 minutes. Then add the buckwheat to your pot. Add in the water, salt, and pepper and stir well.

Close the lid and cook for about 30-35 minutes until the buckwheat is ready. In the meantime, in a skillet, heat the extra-virgin olive oil and fry the chopped onions for 15 minutes until transparent and caramelized.

Add some salt and pepper and mix well. Portion the buckwheat into four bowls or mugs. Then dollop each bowl with the onions. Remember that this dish should be served warm.

NUTRITION FACTS: CALORIES 132KCAL FAT 32 G CARBOHYDRATE 64 G PROTEIN 22 G

CAJUN TURKEY RICE

 4   35 mins

Ingredients:

5 quarts chicken broth
2 cups white rice, raw
1 ½ cups celery, chopped
1 ½ cups red onion, chopped
1 tbsp. garlic, minced
16 oz. ground turkey
2 tbsp. Cajun seasoning
1 tbsp. thyme
1 tbsp. parsley
1 tbsp. oregano

Directions:

Place the chicken broth, rice, celery, and 1 cup of chopped onion into a pot. Bring to a boil over high heat. Reduce heat to medium-low, cover, and simmer until the rice is tender, 20 to 25 minutes.

Meanwhile, place the remaining ½ cup of onion into a skillet with the garlic, and turkey.

Cook and stir over medium-high heat until the meat is brown and crumbly. Stir the meat into the cooked rice along with the thyme, parsley, and oregano.

Stir well and serve.

NUTRITION FACTS: CALORIES 134KCAL CARBOHYDRATE 27 G PROTEIN 4 G

BUTTERNUT SQUASH ALFREDO

 4   🕐 40 mins

Ingredients:

9 oz. buckwheat linguine
2 cups vegetable broth
3 cups butternut squash, diced
I tsp. paprika
2 cloves garlic
I white onion
I cup green peas
I zucchini
2 tbsp. olive oil
2 tbsp. sage

Directions:

Heat the oil in a frypan with medium heat. While it heats, ensures the sage leaves are clean and dry, then put in the oil to fry, moving around not to burn.

Pull them out and put them on a paper towel.

Into the frying pan, put the peeled and diced squash along with paprika, diced onion, and black pepper.

Cook until the onion is soft, then add the broth and salt to taste.

Bring to a boil before turning down to low heat and leaving the squash to cook through. In another pot, cook the linguine in water with a little salt.

When the squash is tender, put it in a blender with all the liquid and other ingredients. Blend until creamy and taste to see if more salt, pepper, or spice is needed.

Put it back in the frying pan to keep warm on low heat.

Using a grater, grate the zucchini lengthwise to make long noodles. Make as many long ones as you can to blend in with the linguine.

Add them to the sauce with the green peas and cook in the butternut squash for five minutes.

When the pasta is done, save one cup of liquid before you drain it. Add the linguine to the pasta and stir well to coat the linguine.

If the sauce is too thick, add a little pasta water. Serve the pasta topped with the fried sage leaves and a little blacker pepper.

NUTRITION FACTS: CALORIES 432KCAL FAT 14 G CARBOHYDRATE 36 G PROTEIN 34 G

CAPRESE SKEWERS

 2   🕐 15 mins

Ingredients:

4 oz. cucumber, cut into 8 pieces
8 cherry tomatoes
8 small balls of mozzarella or 4 oz. mozzarella cut into
8 pieces
1 tsp. of extra-virgin olive oil
8 basil leaves
2 tsp. of balsamic vinegar

Directions:

Use 2 medium skewers per person or 4 small ones. Alternate the ingredients in the following order: tomato, mozzarella, basil, yellow pepper, cucumber, and repeat.

Mix oil, vinegar, salt, and pepper and pour the dressing over the skewers.

NUTRITION FACTS: CALORIES 280KCAL FAT 8.6 G CARBOHYDRATE 14.4 G PROTEIN 17.2 G

CASSEROLE WITH SPINACH AND EGGPLANT

  2   🕐 1h

Ingredients:

1 eggplant
2 white onions
3 tbsp. extra-virgin olive oil
3 cups spinach, fresh
4 tomatoes
2 eggs
¼ cup almond milk, unsweetened
2 tsp. lemon juice
4 tbsp. parmesan

Directions:

Preheat the oven to 400°F. Cut the eggplants, onions, and tomatoes into slices and sprinkle salt on the eggplant slices. Brush the eggplants and onions with olive oil and fry them in a grill pan.

Cook spinach in a saucepan over moderate heat and drain in a sieve. Put the vegetables in layers in a greased baking dish: first the eggplant, then the spinach, and then the onion and the tomato.

Repeat this. Whisk eggs with almond milk, lemon juice, salt, and pepper and pour over the vegetables.

Sprinkle parmesan over the dish and bake in the oven for about 30 to 40 minutes.

NUTRITION FACTS: CALORIES 446KCAL FAT 31.8 G CARBOHYDRATE 30.5 G PROTEIN 13.9 G

CHICKPEAS, QUINOA, AND TURMERIC CURRY

🍳 4   🕐 70 mins

Ingredients:

1 lb. potatoes
3 garlic cloves, crushed
3 tsp. ground turmeric
1 tsp. mild curry
1 tsp. ground ginger
2 cups coconut milk, unsweetened
1 tbsp. tomato purée
1 can of tomatoes
6 oz. quinoa
1 can chickpeas, drained
2 cups spinach

Directions:

Put the potatoes in a pan, cover in cold water, bring to boil, and then cook for 25 minutes until they are soft (always check with a stick). Drain them well, remove the skin, and put them aside.

Put garlic, turmeric, bean stew, ginger, coconut milk, tomato purée, and tomatoes in a skillet. Bring to boil, season with salt and pepper; at that point, add the quinoa with an additional cup of water.

Put on low heat, put a lid on and let simmer for 30 minutes, stirring occasionally. Halfway through cooking, add the chickpeas. When there are only 5 minutes left, add in the spinach and potatoes, roughly chopped.

Split into 4 portions and serve immediately.

NUTRITION FACTS: CALORIES 609KCAL FAT 12.1 G CARBOHYDRATE 85.3 G PROTEIN 23 G

CHICKEN AND BROCCOLI CREAMY CASSEROLE

 2   45 mins

Ingredients:

3 cups broccoli
8 oz. chicken breast, cubed
1/2 onion
1 cup mushrooms
½ cup broth
2 tbsp. red wine
1 tbsp. flour
2 tbsp. parmesan

Directions:

Heat the oven to 350°F. Steam the broccoli for 5 minutes, drain and cool in water and ice to set the bright green color.

Cut the chicken breast into medium-sized cubes. Mix chicken and broccoli and put them in a baking tray.

Prepare the creamy sauce. Sauté the onion with olive oil on low heat, then set to high heat. Add in the mushrooms, a pinch of salt and pepper, flour, and mix.

Add the red wine and mix until it has evaporated. Add the broth, cook for 5 minutes, then hand blend until smooth.

Pour the sauce over the chicken and broccoli, spread 2 tbsp. of parmesan and cook in the oven for 30-35 minutes. Turn on the broiler for the last 5 minutes.

NUTRITION FACTS: CALORIES 353KCAL FAT 4.8 G CARBOHYDRATE 28.1 G PROTEIN 28.3 G

CHILI SWEETCORN AND WILD GARLIC FRITTERS

 4   15 mins

Ingredients:

¾ cup self-rising flour
2 cups tinned or frozen sweetcorn
3 eggs
1 Bird's Eye chili, finely chopped
Fry-light extra-virgin olive oil spray
¾ cup wild garlic leaves and bulbs, finely diced
2 cups lettuce, chopped

Directions:

Mix the eggs, flour, chili, diced wild garlic, and sweetcorn in a bowl, season with the pepper and the salt.

Spray a non-stick frypan and put it on medium heat.

Use a spoon to scoop the egg mixture into the frypan batch by batch. The mixture will give you two large fritters per person or four small fritters.

Fry the pancakes for about 4 minutes on one side, and then gently turn it to the other side and fry for another 3 minutes until it is set and golden brown.

Serve immediately with salad.

NUTRITION FACTS: CALORIES 198KCAL FAT 7 G CARBOHYDRATE 30 G PROTEIN 3 G

CHICKEN WITH KALE AND CHILI SALSA

2   45 mins

Ingredients:

3 oz. buckwheat
1 tsp. fresh ginger
½ lemon, juiced
1 tsp. turmeric
2 cups kale, chopped
1 oz. onion, sliced
8 oz. chicken breast
2tsp. extra-virgin olive oil
1 tomato
1 handful parsley
1 bird's eye chili, chopped
1tsp. paprika

Directions:

Finely chop the tomato, mix it with chili, parsley, lemon juice, salt, pepper, and 1 tsp. olive oil.

Heat the oven to 220F.

Marinate the chicken with 1 tsp. oil, turmeric, paprika, and let it rest for 10 minutes.

Heats a pan over medium heat until it is hot, then add marinated chicken and allow it to cook for a minute on both sides until golden. Transfer the chicken to the oven (and bake for 8 to 10 minutes or until it is cooked through.

In a little oil, fry the ginger and red onions until they are soft and then add in the kale and sauté it for 5-10 minutes until it's done.

Cook the buckwheat in 25 to 30 minutes, dress it with the chili tomato sauce, and serve with kale and chicken.

NUTRITION FACTS: CALORIES 290KCAL FAT 3.8 G CARBOHYDRATE 24.3 G PROTEIN 22 G

CREAMY TURKEY AND ASPARAGUS

 2   40 mins

Ingredients:

8 oz. turkey breast

2 cups asparagus

2 cloves garlic

½ red onion

½ Bird's Eye chili

2 tsp. extra-virgin olive oil

½ cup full fat coconut milk

Directions:

Heat a skillet over medium-high heat, add the oil, onion, garlic, chili, and cook for 5 minutes.

Add turkey, cut in strips, and cook it another 5 minutes until golden on all sizes. Add the asparagus, cut into 2-inch pieces, and after 2 minutes, add the coconut milk.

Let it simmer for 25 minutes until the sauce is creamy.

NUTRITION FACTS: CALORIES 353KCAL FAT 4.8 G CARBOHYDRATE 28.1 G PROTEIN 28.3 G

DAHL WITH KALE, RED ONIONS, AND BUCKWHEAT

2   25 mins

Ingredients:

1 tsp. of extra-virgin olive oil

1 tsp. of mustard seeds

1 ½ oz. red onions, finely chopped

1 clove of garlic, very finely chopped

1 tsp. very finely chopped ginger

1 Thai chili, very finely chopped

1 tsp. curry powder

2 tsp. turmeric

10 fl. oz. vegetable broth

1 ½ oz. red lentils

1 ⅝ oz. kale, chopped

1.70 fl. oz. coconut milk

4 oz. buckwheat

Directions:

Heat oil in a pan at medium temperature and add mustard seeds. When they crack, add onion, garlic, ginger, and chili. Heat until everything is soft.

Add the curry powder and turmeric, mix well. Add the vegetable stock, bring to a boil.

Add the lentils and cook them for 25 to 30 minutes until they are ready. Then add the kale and coconut milk and simmer for 5 minutes.

While the lentils are cooking, prepare the buckwheat. Serve buckwheat with the dahl.

NUTRITION FACTS: CALORIES 273KCAL FAT 2.4 G CARBOHYDRATE 24.8 G PROTEIN 7.6 G

CREAMY VEGETABLE CASSEROLE

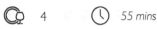 4   55 mins

Ingredients:

2 tbsp. Fresh rosemary
1 tsp. basil
1 tsp. oregano
3 cloves garlic
¼ cup nutritional yeast
2 tbsp. olive oil
2 tbsp. apple cider vinegar
1 cup cashews
2 zucchini
1 stalk broccoli
1 cauliflower
4 russet potatoes

Directions:

Pour boiled water over the cashews and leave to soak. Cut up the cauliflower into florets and cook until soft. When the cauliflower is done, drain it and put it in a blender along with the drained cashews and one and a half cups of cold water.

Add a good half tsp. of salt along with the apple cider vinegar and nutritional yeast. Blend until creamy.

Wash and grate the zucchini, set aside. Cut the broccoli into bite-sized pieces and set aside.

Spread the sides and bottom of a baking tray with olive oil. Cut the potatoes as thin as you can and spread them in the tray, forming an even layer. Pour half of the cauliflower sauce to cover and spread evenly.

Add the grated zucchini and spread out to cover the sauce. Sprinkle the oregano and basil over the zucchini, then push the broccoli pieces into the zucchini to keep the surface as even as possible.

Drizzle a little more cauliflower sauce around the broccoli pieces to fill in the gaps.

Do another layer to use up the rest of the potatoes, then pour the rest of the remaining cauliflower sauce over top of that.

Spread it out as evenly as possible, right to the edges to fill in all the gaps around the sides.

Sprinkle the top with a half tsp. of black pepper and a generous pinch or two of salt. Finely chop the fresh rosemary and sprinkle that on top also.

Put in the oven at 400°F for 45 minutes. It will be done when a knife pierces the potatoes without pulling them up, and the top should be beautifully browned. Let it cool before serving.

NUTRITION FACTS: CALORIES 389KCAL FAT 4 G CARBOHYDRATE 37 G PROTEIN 26 G

EGGPLANT PIZZA TOWERS

 2   55 mins

Ingredients:

1 ½ eggplant
1 tbsp. tomato paste
2 cups tomato sauce
½ red onion
1 garlic clove
½ cup mozzarella
4 basil leaves
1 tsp. extra-virgin olive oil
1 tbsp. parmesan

Directions:

Cut the eggplants into thick slices, add some salt and let them rest so that they let their bitter water out. In the meantime, prepare the salsa. Heat a pan with oil added, when hot add onion and garlic and cook 5 minutes.

Add tomato sauce, tomato paste, salt, and pepper and cook on low heat for about 15-18 minutes. Add a few leaves of basil. Pat the eggplants with kitchen paper and grill them. Heat the oven to 350°F.

Compose the towers: put a slice of eggplant, sauce, a few dices of mozzarella and again eggplant, sauce, mozzarella. Three layers per tower are best. Sprinkle parmesan on top.

When done, put the tray in the oven for about 10 minutes until the mozzarella is melted.

NUTRITION FACTS: CALORIES 353KCAL FAT 4.8 G CARBOHYDRATE 28.1 G PROTEIN 28.3 G

FRAGRANT ASIAN HOT POT

2   25 mins

Ingredients:

1 tsp tomato purée
1 star anise, crushed
½ oz. parsley, finely chopped
Juice of 1/2 lime
2 cups chicken stock
½ carrot, cut into matchsticks
½ cup cauliflower cut into florets
2 oz. bean sprouts
4 oz. raw tiger prawns
2 oz. rice noodles
2 oz. chestnuts, cooked
2 inch. ginger, sliced
1 tbsp. miso paste

Directions:

Set the tomato purée, star anise, parsley stalks, lime juice, and chicken stock in a pan and simmer for about 10 minutes.

Add the beansprouts, cauliflower, carrot, prawns, tofu, noodles, chestnuts, and simmer gently until the prawns are cooked.

Remove from the heat and stir in miso paste. Serve sprinkled with the parsley leaves.

NUTRITION FACTS: CALORIES 397KCAL   FAT 15 G   CARBOHYDRATE 33 G   PROTEIN 19 G

FRIED CAULIFLOWER RICE

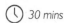 2   🕐 30 mins

Ingredients:

1 cauliflower
2 tbsp. coconut oil
1 red onion
4 cloves garlic
¼ cup vegetable broth
2-inch ginger
1 tsp. chili flakes
1/2 carrot
1/2 red bell pepper
1/2 lemon, juiced
2 tbsp. pumpkin seeds
2 tbsp. fresh parsley

Directions:

Cut the cauliflower into rice grains using a food processor.

Finely chop the onion, garlic, and ginger, cut the carrot into thin strips, dice the bell pepper and finely chop the herbs. Melt 1 tbsp. of coconut oil in a pan, add half of the onion and garlic, and fry briefly until translucent.

Add cauliflower rice and season with salt. Pour in the broth and stir everything until it evaporates and the cauliflower rice is tender.

Take the rice out of the pan and set it aside. Melt the rest of the coconut oil in the pan and add the remaining onions, garlic, ginger, carrots, and peppers.

Fry for a few minutes until the vegetables are tender. Season them with a little salt.

Add the cauliflower rice again, heat the whole dish, and add the lemon juice.

Garnish with pumpkin seeds and parsley before serving.

NUTRITION FACTS: CALORIES 230KCAL   FAT 17.8 G   CARBOHYDRATE 17.2 G   PROTEIN 5.1 G

GARLIC CHICKEN BURGERS

 2   20 mins

Ingredients:

8 oz. chicken mince
¼ red onion, finely chopped
1 garlic clove, crushed
1 handful of parsley, finely chopped
1 cup arugula
½ orange, chopped
1 cup cherry tomatoes
3 tsp extra-virgin olive oil

Directions:

Put chicken mince, onion, garlic, parsley, salt, and pepper to taste in a bowl and mix well. Form 2 patties and let rest 5 minutes.

Heat a pan with olive oil, and when very hot, cook 3 minutes per patty.

They are also delicious when grilled. If you opt for grilling, just brush the patties with a bit of oil right before cooking.

Put the arugula on two plates; add cherry tomatoes and orange on top, dress with salt and the remaining olive oil. Put the patties on top and serve.

NUTRITION FACTS: CALORIES 353KCAL FAT 4.8 G CARBOHYDRATE 28.1 G PROTEIN 28.3 G

GARLIC SALMON WITH BRUSSELS SPROUTS AND RICE

 2   35 mins

Ingredients:

8 oz. salmon fillet slices
1 garlic clove, crushed
2 tbsp. red wine
1 cup Brussels sprouts
1 cup cherry tomatoes
1 tsp. extra-virgin olive oil
3 oz. basmati rice
3 tbsp. stock (or water), if needed

Directions:

Boil the basmati rice until tender and set aside.

Crush the garlic and coat the top of the salmon. Put a skillet on medium-high heat, and when hot, put the salmon fillets skin down. Cook for 5 minutes, then turn them. Cook them until it becomes brown and crispy (around 5-6 more minutes).

Remove the salmon from the pan and add Brussels sprouts, tomatoes, wine, and salt and cook them around 10 minutes. Add stock or water if needed. When done, add the basmati rice and mix to combine the flavors. Add the parmesan and serve, putting the salmon on top.

NUTRITION FACTS: CALORIES 353KCAL FAT 4.8 G CARBOHYDRATE 28.1 G PROTEIN 28.3 G

GOAT CHEESE SALAD WITH CRANBERRIES AND WALNUT

 2   🕐 15 mins

Ingredients:

10 walnuts, chopped
1 cup lettuce
½ cup arugula
½ cup baby spinach
1 tbsp. balsamic vinegar
1 tsp mustard
4 oz. goat cheese
2 tsp extra-virgin olive oil
Salt and pepper to taste

Directions:

Mix lettuce, arugula, and baby spinach in a bowl. Whisk oil, mustard, salt, pepper, and vinegar, put the dressing on the salad, and mix well.

Transfer to a serving plate. Crumble goat cheese over the top.

Add cranberries and walnuts on top and serve.

NUTRITION FACTS: CALORIES 250KCAL FAT 20.9 G CARBOHYDRATE 23.4 G PROTEIN 20.9 G

GREEK FRITTATA WITH GARLIC GRILLED EGGPLANT

 2   🕐 35 mins

Ingredients:

1 ½ cups shredded zucchini
3 eggs
3 oz. feta cheese
2 tbsp. milk
2 leaves mint, finely chopped
1 eggplant
2 tbsp. oil
1 garlic clove, crushed
1 tsp. balsamic vinegar

Directions:

Heat the oven to 350°F. Cut the eggplant into thin slices; mix with a pinch of salt and let rest.

Mix the shredded zucchini with a pinch of salt and let it rest in a colander until some water has drained. After 10 minutes, squeeze the rest of the water out and put zucchini in a bowl.

Add 3 eggs, crushed feta cheese, milk, salt, pepper, mint, whisk well and pour in a silicone baking tray and cook 25-30 minutes in the oven. Pat the eggplant slices dry and grill them.

Mix garlic, oil, salt, pepper, and balsamic vinegar and pour the dressing on the eggplants. Serve the frittata alongside the eggplant.

NUTRITION FACTS: CALORIES 359KCAL FAT 7.8 G CARBOHYDRATE 18.1 G PROTEIN 21.3 G

GREEN BEANS WITH CRISPY CHICKPEAS

 4   🕐 20 mins

Ingredients:

1 can chickpeas, rinsed
1 tsp. parsley
1 lb. green beans, trimmed
2 tbsp. olive oil
1 tsp. cumin seeds
Grilled lemons, for serving

Directions:

Heat grill to medium. Gather chickpeas, parsley, cumin, and 1 tbsp. oil in a medium cast-iron skillet. Put a skillet on the grill and cook chickpeas, occasionally mixing, until golden brown and parsley begin to pop, 5 to 6 minutes. Season with salt and pepper.

Transfer to a bowl. Add green beans and remaining tbsp. olive oil to the skillet. Add salt and pepper. Cook, turning once, until charred and barely tender, 3 to 4 minutes.

Toss green beans with chickpea mixture and serve with grilled lemons alongside.

NUTRITION FACTS: CALORIES 460KCAL FAT 15 G CARBOHYDRATE 57 G PROTEIN 16 G

GREEN VEGGIES CURRY

 2   🕐 40 mins

Ingredients:

3 tbsp. coconut oil
¼ red onion, chopped
1 tsp. garlic, minced
1 tsp. fresh ginger, minced
1 cup broccoli florets
1 tbsp. curry paste or powder
2 cups spinach
½ cup coconut cream
2 tsp. low-sodium soy sauce
½ Bird's Eye chili
1 tsp. fresh parsley, chopped finely

NUTRITION FACTS: CALORIES 324KCAL FAT 24.5 G
CARBOHYDRATE 8 G PROTEIN 17.5 G

Directions:

In a skillet, melt 2 tbsp. of the coconut oil over medium-high heat and sauté the onion for about 3-4 minutes. Add the garlic, chili, and ginger, and sauté for about 1 minute. Add the broccoli and stir to combine well.

Immediately reduce the heat to medium-low and cook for about 1-2 minutes, stirring continuously.

Stir in the curry paste and cook for about 1 minute, stirring continuously. Add in the spinach and cook or about 2 minutes, stirring frequently.

Add the coconut cream and remaining coconut oil and stir until smooth.

Stir in the soy sauce and simmer for about 5-10 minutes, stirring occasionally or until curry reaches the desired thickness.

Remove from the heat and serve hot, topped with parsley.

INDIAN VEGETARIAN MEATBALLS

 2   50 mins

Ingredients:

1 cup cauliflower
1 cup brown rice
¼ cup breadcrumbs
1 egg
½ tsp. turmeric
1 tsp. smoked paprika
1 tsp. of extra-virgin olive oil
1 cloves garlic crushed
1 cup tomato sauce
Broth (if needed)
1 tbsp. extra-virgin olive oil
1 ½ tbsp. garam masala
1 tsp ginger
1 tbsp. parsley, chopped
1 red onion-diced
6 oz. full-fat coconut milk

Directions:

Steam cauliflower for 5 minutes, then blend it with rice. Use pulse to get a result similar to mince. Add egg, breadcrumbs, 1 garlic clove, salt, pepper, turmeric, paprika, and finely chopped parsley.

Mix well until you can form meatballs. Note: if it's too dry, add 1 tbsp. egg white and mix. If it's too runny, add 1 tbsp. breadcrumbs and mix. Spray a pan with cooking spray, heat it, and gently cook the meatballs for 5 minutes until golden. Be careful when you turn them so that they don't break. Put them aside

In a different pan, put oil, onion, ginger, garlic, salt, and pepper and cook on low heat until the onion is done. Add tomato sauce and coconut milk and let it simmer around 15 minutes until thickened. Put the meatballs in the sauce and cook another 5 minutes before serving.

NUTRITION FACTS: CALORIES 412KCAL FAT 7.8 G CARBOHYDRATE 39.1 G PROTEIN 18.3 G

KALE AND RED ONION DHAL WITH BUCKWHEAT

 4　　　🕐 40 mins

Ingredients:

1 tbsp. olive oil

1 red onion, sliced

3 garlic cloves, crushed or grated

2-inch ginger, grated

1 Bird's Eye chili deseeded, chopped

2 tsp. turmeric

2 tsp. garam masala

6 oz. snow peas

2 cups coconut milk, unsweetened

1 cup water

1 cup carrot, thinly sliced

6 oz. buckwheat

Directions:

Place the olive oil into a , deep skillet and then add the chopped onion. Cook on very low heat, with the lid for 5 minutes until softened.

Add the ginger, garlic, and chili and cook 1 minute. Add turmeric and garam masala along with a dash of water, and then cook for 1 minute.

Add the snow peas, coconut milk, and 1 cup of water. Mix everything and cook for 20 minutes on low heat covered. Stir occasionally and add a bit more water if the dhal begins to stick.

After 20 minutes, add the carrot, stir thoroughly and cook for another 5 minutes.

While the dhal is cooking, steam the buckwheat in salted boiling water for 15 minutes, drain it and serve it with the dhal.

NUTRITION FACTS: CALORIES 340KCAL FAT 4 G CARBOHYDRATE 30 G PROTEIN 4 G

KALE, EDAMAME AND TOFU CURRY

 4   75 mins

Ingredients:

1 tbsp. extra-virgin olive oil
1 big onion, chopped
4 cloves garlic, peeled and grated
1 3-inch fresh ginger, peeled and grated
1 Bird's Eye chili, thinly sliced
1/2 tsp. ground turmeric
1/4 tsp. cayenne pepper
1 tsp. paprika
1/2 tsp. ground cumin
1 tsp. salt
8 oz. dried red lentils
2 oz. soya edamame beans
8 oz. firm tofu, cubed
2 tomatoes, roughly chopped
Juice of 1 lime
½ cup parsley, stalks removed

Directions:

Put the oil in a pan on medium heat. When the oil is hot, add the onion and cook for 5 minutes. Add ginger, garlic, and chili and cook for another 2 minutes.

Add turmeric, cayenne, paprika, cumin, and salt. Stir and add red lentils, soya edamame beans, and tomatoes.

Pour in 4 cups boiling water and then bring to a simmer for about 10 minutes, lower the heat and cook for a further 40 minutes until the curry becomes thicker and all flavors are blended.

Add lime juice and parsley, stir and serve.

NUTRITION FACTS: CALORIES 325KCAL FAT 6 G CARBOHYDRATE 77 G PROTEIN 28 G

LAMB, BUTTERNUT SQUASH AND DATE TAGINE

 4   1h + 30 mins

Ingredients:

2 tbsp. extra-virgin olive oil
1 red onion, chopped
1-inch ginger, grated
3 garlic cloves, crushed
1 tsp. chili flakes
2 tsp. cumin seeds
1 cinnamon stick
2 tsp. ground turmeric
16 oz. lamb shoulder, cut into pieces
½ tsp. salt
2 oz. dates, pitted and sliced
2 cups tomatoes
1 cup broth
2 cups butternut squash, cubed
1 can chickpeas, drained
2 tbsp. fresh parsley
1 cup basmati rice

Directions:

Heat the oven to 325°F. Add oil into a tagine pot or an ovenproof saucepan with lid, heat on low heat, and when hot, gently cook the onions until they are soft.

Add the grated ginger and garlic, chili, cumin, cinnamon, and turmeric. Stir well and cook 1 minute. Add a dash of water if it becomes too dry. Add the lamb and stir to coat it with spices and onions. Add dates, tomatoes, and 1 cup broth.

Bring the tagine to the boil, set the lid, and place on your preheated oven for about 1 hour and 15 minutes. Steam the basmati rice and put aside. After 45 minutes, add butternut squash and drained chickpeas to the tagine. Stir everything together, place the lid back on and return to the oven for 30 minutes.

Serve with basmati rice on the side.

NUTRITION FACTS: CALORIES 380KCAL FAT 13.1 G SUGAR 51.6 G PROTEIN 80.6 G

LEMON CHICKEN WITH SPINACH, RED ONION, AND SALSA

   1   ( ) 65 mins

Ingredients:

4 oz. chicken breast, skinless, boneless

1 tomato

1 Bird's Eye chili, finely chopped

1 oz. capers

Juice of 1/2 lemon

2 tbsp. extra-virgin olive oil

2 cups spinach

1/2 red onion, chopped

2 tsp. chopped garlic

3 oz. buckwheat

Directions:

Heat the oven to 400°F. To make the salsa, chop the tomato very finely and put it with its liquid in a bowl. The liquid is very important because it's delicious.

Mix with chili, capers, onion, 1 tbsp oil, and some drops of lemon juice. Marinate the chicken breast with garlic, lemon juice, and ½ tbsp oil for 10 minutes.

Heat an ovenproof skillet until warm, add the chicken and cook for a minute on every side, until light gold, then move to the oven (put on a baking tray if your pan is not ovenproof) for 5 minutes until cooked.

Remove from the oven, and cover with foil. Leave to rest for 5 minutes before serving. Meanwhile, sauté the spinach for 5 minutes with ½ tbsp. oil and 1 tbsp. garlic. Serve alongside chicken with salsa and spinach.

NUTRITION FACTS: CALORIES 342KCAL FAT 8 G CARBOHYDRATE 18 G PROTEIN 33 G

LEMON PAPRIKA CHICKEN WITH VEGETABLES

 2 55 mins

Ingredients:
2 carrots, chopped
2 bay leaves
2 tbsp. red wine
Juice of 1 lemon
½ celeriac, peeled and chopped
3 turnips, peeled and chopped
8 oz. of chicken wings
3 tbsp. extra-virgin olive oil
2 tbsp. paprika
2 cups stock
Sprigs of rosemary and thyme
2 cups kale, chopped

Directions:
Heat the oil with a tight-fitting lid inside a saucepan. Add the carrots, paprika, celeriac, turnips, and chicken wings to the saucepan and cook for a few minutes. Add the wine, mix, and let it evaporate.

Stir in the pan the stock, spices, salt, pepper, and lemon juice and bring to the boil.

Turn the heat down, cover it with a lid, and gently simmer for 40 minutes.

Add the kale and cook until the kale and the chicken are cooked for a few more minutes.

NUTRITION FACTS: CALORIES 154KCAL FAT 2.2 G CARBOHYDRATE 32.1 G PROTEIN 21.4 G

LEMON TUNA STEAKS WITH BABY POTATOES

 2 35 mins

Ingredients:
10 oz. tuna steaks
12 oz. baby potatoes, chopped
1 garlic clove, crushed
1 tbsp. thyme
½ tbsp. oregano
1 tbsp. rosemary
1 lemon
2 tsp. extra-virgin olive oil

Directions:
Heat the oven to 400°F. Marinate the tuna for 20 minutes with 1 tsp. oil, herbs, salt, pepper, and the juice of a half lemon. Chop the baby potatoes and season them with oil, salt, pepper, and rosemary.

Put potatoes in a baking tray, spreading the potatoes so that they are in a single layer. Cook them for 12 minutes. Cut the remaining half lemon in slices and put them on the tuna steaks. Take the tray out of the oven and add tuna steaks. Cook for another 10 minutes and serve immediately.

NUTRITION FACTS: CALORIES 305KCAL FAT 5.5 G CARBOHYDRATE 34.2 G PROTEIN 23.7 G

LEMONY CHICKEN BURGERS

 2   🕐 20 mins

Ingredients:

8 oz. chicken mince
¼ red onion, finely chopped
1 garlic clove, crushed
1 handful of parsley, finely chopped
Juice and zest of ¼ lemon
2 leaves lettuce
½ tomato
2 tsp. extra-virgin olive oil
2 whole-wheat buns

Directions:

Put chicken mince, onion, garlic, parsley, salt pepper, lemon zest, and juice in a bowl and mix well. Form 2 patties and let rest 5 minutes.

Heat a pan with olive oil, and when very hot, cook 3 minutes per part. They are also delicious when grilled. If you opt for grilling, just brush the patties with a bit of oil right before cooking.

Put the patties in the buns with lettuce and tomato and enjoy.

NUTRITION FACTS: CALORIES 353KCAL FAT 4.8 G CARBOHYDRATE 28.1 G PROTEIN 28.3 G

LEMON CHICKEN SKEWERS WITH PEPPERS

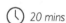 8   🕐 20 mins

Ingredients:

8 oz. chicken breast
2 cups peppers, chopped
1 cup tomatoes, chopped
3 tsp. extra-virgin olive oil
1 garlic clove
½ lemon, juiced
½ tsp. paprika
½ tsp turmeric
1 handful parsley, chopped

Directions:

Cut the breast into small cubes and let it marinate with oil and spices for 30 minutes.

Prepare the skewers and set aside.

Heat a pan with oil. When hot, add garlic and cook 5 minutes, then remove the clove.

Add peppers, tomatoes, salt, and pepper and cook on high heat for 5-10 minutes.

Heat another pan to high heat. When very hot, put the skewers in and cook 10-12 minutes until golden on every side. Serve the skewers alongside the peppers.

NUTRITION FACTS: CALORIES 315KCAL FAT 20.9 G CARBOHYDRATE 5.4 G PROTEIN 15.8 G

LEMONGRASS AND GINGER MACKEREL

 4   🕐 35 mins

Ingredients:

4 mackerel fillets
2 tbsp. extra-virgin olive oil
1 tbsp. ginger, grated
2 lemongrass sticks, chopped
2 red chilies, chopped
Juice of 1 lime
Handful parsley, chopped

Directions:

In a roasting pan, combine the mackerel with the oil, ginger, and the other ingredients, toss and bake at 390° F for 25 minutes. Divide between plates and serve.

NUTRITION FACTS: CALORIES 251KCAL FAT 3.7 G CARBOHYDRATE 14 G PROTEIN 30 G

MEXICAN CHICKEN CASSEROLE

4   🕐 45 mins

Ingredients:

Ingredients:
½ cup buckwheat
½ red onion
8 oz. chicken mince
1 tbsp. paprika
½ Bird's Eye chili
1 garlic clove
4 oz. black beans, rinsed
2 cups spinach
1 cup shredded cheddar

Directions:

Boil buckwheat for 25 minutes, then rinse and put aside.

When hot, add onion, garlic, and chili, heat a pan with oil, and cook for 5 minutes. Add mince and spices and cook for 10 minutes, stirring repeatedly. Add spinach and cook another 3 minutes.

Take a baking dish and put buckwheat as the first layer, then add chicken mince.

Spread the cheese on top and bake for 10 minutes until the cheese is melted.

NUTRITION FACTS: CALORIES 353KCAL FAT 4.8 G CARBOHYDRATE 28.1 G PROTEIN 28.3 G

MINCE STUFFED PEPPERS

 4   🕐 75 mins

Ingredients:
4 oz. lean mince
¼ cup brown rice, cooked
2 yellow bell peppers
2 red bell peppers
1 tbsp. parmesan
2 tbsp. breadcrumbs
3 oz. mozzarella
1 egg
¼ cup walnuts, chopped
2 cups arugula
2 tsp. extra-virgin olive oil
A few drops of lemon juice

Directions:
Preheat oven to 350 degrees F.

In a bowl, mix the mince, parmesan, brown rice, egg, and mozzarella. Mix well and set aside.

Cut peppers lengthwise, remove the seeds, fill them with the mince mix, and put them on a baking tray. Distribute breadcrumbs on top and lightly spray with cooking spray to have a crunchy top without adding calories to the recipe.

Cook for 50-60 minutes until peppers are soft. Let cool for a few minutes.

Serve stuffed peppers with an arugula salad dressed with olive oil, salt, and a few lemon drops.

NUTRITION FACTS: CALORIES 375KCAL FAT 8.2 G CARBOHYDRATE 24.7 G PROTEIN 15.3 G

MOROCCAN SPICED EGGS

 2   🕐 55 mins

Ingredients:
1 tsp. extra-virgin olive oil
1 scallion, finely chopped
1 red bell pepper, finely chopped
1 garlic clove, finely chopped
1 zucchini, finely chopped
1 tbsp. tomato paste
½ tsp. mild curry
¼ tsp. ground cinnamon
¼ tsp. ground cumin
½ tsp. salt
1 can tomatoes
1 can chickpeas, drained
1/3 oz. parsley
4 eggs

Directions:
Heat the oil in a pan; include the scallion and red bell pepper and fry on low heat for 5 minutes. Add garlic and zucchini and cook for 2 minutes. Add tomato paste, spices, and salt and stir well.

Add tomatoes and chickpeas and bring to medium heat. Put a lid on and simmer for 30 minutes until thicker. Remove from heat and add chopped parsley. Preheat the grill to 350°F.

Spread the tomato sauce into a cooking tray and crack the eggs in the middle. Put the tray under the grill for 10 minutes and serve.

NUTRITION FACTS: CALORIES 316KCAL FAT 5.2 G CARBOHYDRATE 13.1 G PROTEIN 7 G

MISO CARAMELIZED TOFU

 2   45 mins

Ingredients:

1 tbsp. mirin
¾ oz. miso paste
10 oz. firm tofu
2 oz. celery, trimmed
2 oz. red onion
4 ¼ oz. zucchini
1 Bird's Eye chili
1 garlic clove, finely chopped
1 tsp. fresh ginger, finely chopped
5 oz. kale, chopped
2 tsp. sesame seeds
1 ¼ oz. buckwheat
1 tsp. ground turmeric
2 tsp. extra-virgin olive oil
1 tsp. tamari (or soy sauce)

Directions:

Preheat your oven to 400°F. Cover a tray with parchment paper. Combine the mirin and miso. Dice the tofu and let it marinate in the mirin-miso mixture. Chop the vegetables (except for the kale) at a diagonal angle to produce long slices.

Using a steamer, cook the kale for 5 minutes and set aside. Disperse the tofu across the lined tray and garnish with sesame seeds. Roast for 20 minutes, or until caramelized. Rinse the buckwheat using running water and a sieve.

Add to a pan of boiling water with turmeric and cook the buckwheat according to the packet instructions.

Heat the oil in a skillet over high heat. Toss in the vegetables, herbs, and spices, then fry for 2 to 3 minutes. Reduce to medium heat and fry for another 5 minutes or until cooked but still crunchy.

NUTRITION FACTS: CALORIES 101KCAL FAT 4.7 G CARBOHYDRATE 12.4 G PROTEIN 4.2 G

MUSHROOM & TOFU SCRAMBLE

 | 25 mins

Ingredients:

3 ½ oz. tofu, extra firm
1 tsp. ground turmeric
1 tsp. mild curry powder
4 oz. kale, roughly chopped
1 tsp. extra-virgin olive oil
¾ oz. red onion, thinly sliced
4 oz. mushrooms, thinly sliced
A few parsley leaves, finely chopped

Directions:

Place 2 sheets of kitchen towel under and on top of the tofu, then rest a considerable weight such as saucepan onto the tofu to ensure it drains off the liquid.

Combine the curry powder, turmeric, and 1-2 tsp. of water to form a paste. Using a steamer, cook kale for 3 to 4 minutes.

In a skillet, warm oil over medium heat. Add the chili, mushrooms, and onion, cooking for several minutes or until brown and tender.

Break the tofu into small pieces and toss in the skillet. Coat with the spice paste and stir, ensuring everything becomes evenly coated.

Cook for up to 5 minutes, or until the tofu has browned. Add the kale and fry for 2 more minutes. Garnish with parsley before serving.

NUTRITION FACTS: CALORIES 333KCAL FAT 22.9 G CARBOHYDRATE 18.8 G PROTEIN 20.9 G

ORANGE CUMIN SIRLOIN

2   15 mins + 8h

Ingredients:
8 oz. sirloin
2 cloves garlic, crushed
2 tbsp. extra-virgin olive oil
Juice of ½ a lime
Juice of ½ an orange
¼ cup parsley
½ tsp cumin
½ Bird's Eye chili
2 tbsp. soy sauce

Directions:
Prepare the marinade combining all the ingredients, reserve 2 tbsp. for later and put the rest on the sirloin in a small tray. Turn the meat several times so that the marinade covers it completely. Cover with aluminum foil and put it in the fridge for 8 hours.

Drain the meat from the marinade; pat it with kitchen paper to dry it.

Heat the grill or a skillet until very hot and cook to your taste. Let the cooked meat sit on a plate for 5 minutes, slice it and dress it with the 2 tablespoons of marinade you kept aside.

NUTRITION FACTS: CALORIES 353KCAL FAT 4.8 G CARBOHYDRATE 28.1 G PROTEIN 28.3 G

PECAN CRUSTED CHICKEN BREAST

4   30 mins

Ingredients:
½ cup whole-wheat breadcrumbs
1/3 cup pecans
2 tbsp. parmesan
1 egg white
4 8oz. chicken breasts, sliced
1 tbsp. grapeseed oil
1 cup mixed greens
1 tbsp. extra-virgin olive oil

Directions:
Preheat oven to 425°F. In a food processor, blitz bread, pecans, and parmesan; season with salt and pepper until you get thin breadcrumbs.

Move to a bowl. In another bowl, beat egg white until foamy. Season chicken with salt and pepper. Coat each chicken breast slice with egg white first, then put it in the breadcrumb bowl and mix until completely covered.

In a nonstick ovenproof skillet, heat grapeseed oil over medium heat. When hot, put in chicken breasts cook until gently seared, 1 to 3 minutes.

Turn chicken over and put the skillet in the oven. Cook until chicken is done (around 8 to 12 minutes). Serve chicken with a plate of mixed greens seasoned with olive oil, lemon, and salt.

NUTRITION FACTS: CALORIES 250KCAL FAT 8 G
CARBOHYDRATE 27 G PROTEIN 17 G

PRAWN ARRABBIATA

 I 40 mins

Ingredients:

5 oz. raw prawns
4 oz. Buckwheat pasta
1 tbsp. extra-virgin olive oil
½ red onion, finely chopped
1 garlic clove, finely chopped
1 oz. celery, thinly sliced
1 Bird's Eye chili, thinly sliced
1 tsp. dried mixed herbs
1 tsp. extra-virgin olive oil
2 tbsp. red wine
½ can tomatoes, chopped
1 tbsp. parsley, chopped

Directions:

Fry the garlic, onion, celery, and herbs in oil on low heat for 1 to 2 minutes. Turn up the heat to medium, add the red wine and cook until evaporated. Add the tomatoes and leave the sauce simmer for 20 to 30 minutes, until it will reduce and get a creamy texture.

While the sauce is cooking, bring some water to the boil and cook the pasta as per the package directions. When cooked, drain it and put it aside.

Put prawns into the sauce and cook for a further 3 to 4 minutes, till they've turned opaque and pink, then add the parsley and the cooked pasta into the sauce, mix, and serve.

NUTRITION FACTS: CALORIES 335KCAL FAT 12 G CARBOHYDRATE 38 G PROTEIN 19 G

PRAWN AND CHILI BOK CHOY

 I 45 mins

Ingredients:

2 ¼ oz. brown rice
1 bok choi
2 fl. oz. chicken stock
1 tbsp. extra-virgin olive oil
1 garlic clove, finely chopped
1 ⅝ oz. red onion, finely chopped
½ Bird's Eye chili, finely chopped
1 tsp. freshly grated ginger
4 ¼ oz. raw king prawns
1 tbsp. soy sauce
1 tbsp. parsley, chopped

Directions:

Bring a saucepan of water to a boil, cook the brown rice for 25 to 30 minutes, or until soft.

Tear the bok choi into pieces. Warm the chicken stock in a skillet over medium heat and toss in the bok choi, cooking until the bok choi has slightly wilted.

In another skillet, warm olive oil over high heat. Toss in the ginger, chili, red onions, and garlic, frying for 2 to 3 minutes.

Put in the prawns, five-spice, and soy sauce and cook for 6 to 8 minutes, or until cooked.

Drain the brown rice and add to the skillet, stirring and cooking for 2 to 3 minutes. Add the bok choi, garnish with parsley and serve.

NUTRITION FACTS: CALORIES 403KCAL FAT 15.3 G CARBOHYDRATE 50.8 G PROTEIN 16.2 G

ROASTED MACKEREL AND SIMPLE VEGGIES

🍽 2   🕐 30 mins

Ingredients:

2 oz. pitted black olives
2 leeks, chopped
7 oz. Cherry tomatoes
2 sweet potatoes, chopped
1 tbsp. extra-virgin olive oil
1 lemon, juiced
11 oz. mackerel fillets
¼ pint vegetable stock

Directions:

Heat your oven to 375° F. Place the chopped leeks and sweet potatoes in a roasting tray. Pour the vegetable stock over them and drizzle with the extra-virgin oil.

Place the tray in the oven to roast for about 15 to 20 minutes.

Take out of the oven, add the black olives, cherry tomatoes, and mackerel fillets, and then squeeze the lemon juice all over. Return to the oven to roast for another 10 minutes.

Serve immediately.

NUTRITION FACTS: CALORIES 374KCAL FAT 12 G CARBOHYDRATE 48 G PROTEIN 17 G

SALMON AND KALE OMELET

 2   🕐 17 mins

Ingredients:

6 eggs
2 tbsp. almond milk, unsweetened
2 tbsp. extra-virgin olive oil
4 oz. smoked salmon, cut into small chunks
2 cup kale leaves
4 scallions, chopped finely

Directions:

In a bowl, put eggs, almond milk, salt, and black pepper, and whisk well. Set aside.

In a non-stick skillet, heat the oil over medium heat.

Place a scoop of egg mixture, distribute it evenly by rotating the skillet and cook for about 1 minute.

Place salmon kale and scallions on top of the egg mixture evenly. Reduce heat to low and cook for about 4 to 5 minutes or until omelet is done completely.

Carefully transfer the omelet onto a serving plate and serve.

NUTRITION FACTS: CALORIES 210KCAL FAT 14.9 G CARBOHYDRATE 5.2 G PROTEIN 14.8 G

SALMON FRITTERS

 2   30 mins

Ingredients:

6 oz. salmon, canned
1 tbsp. flour
1 garlic clove, crushed
½ red onion, finely chopped
2 eggs
2 tsp. olive oil
Salt and pepper to taste
2 cups arugula

Directions:

Separate egg whites from yolks and beat them until very stiff. In a separate bowl, mix salmon, flour, salt, pepper, onion, garlic, and yolks.

Add egg whites and mix slowly. Heat a pan on medium-high. Add 1 tsp. oil and, when hot, form salmon fritters with a spoon.

Cook until brown (around 4 minutes per side) and serve with arugula salad seasoned with salt, pepper, and 1 tsp. olive oil.

NUTRITION FACTS: CALORIES 320KCAL FAT 7 G CARBOHYDRATE 18 G PROTEIN 27 G

SEARED TUNA IN SOY SAUCE AND BLACK PEPPER

 1   35 mins

Ingredients:

5 ounces tuna, 1-inch thick
1 red onion, chopped
2 tbsp. soy sauce
¼ tsp. ground black pepper
½ tbsp. grated ginger
1 tsp. sesame seeds
2 tsp. extra-virgin olive oil
2 cups baby spinach
1 tbsp. orange juice

Directions:

Marinate tuna with 1 tbsp. soy sauce, oil, and black pepper for 30 minutes. Place a skillet over high heat and, when very hot, add tuna and quickly cook 1 minute per side.

Cut the tuna into slices, dress them with 1 tbsp. soy sauce mixed with grated ginger. Add green onion and sesame seeds on top.

Serve with a baby spinach salad dressed with 1 tsp olive oil, salt, pepper, and orange juice.

NUTRITION FACTS: CALORIES 154KCAL FAT 4.1 G CARBOHYDRATE 3 G PROTEIN 15 G

SERRANO HAM & ARUGULA

 2   🕐 10 mins

Ingredients:
6 oz. Serrano ham
4 oz. arugula leaves
2 tbsp. olive oil
1 tbsp. orange juice

Directions:
Pour the oil and juice into a bowl and toss the arugula in the mixture. Place the arugula mixture on plates and top off with the ham.

NUTRITION FACTS: CALORIES 220KCAL FAT 7 G CARBOHYDRATE 7 G PROTEIN 33.5 G

SESAME TUNA WITH ARTICHOKE HEARTS

 2   🕐 35 mins

Ingredients:
8 oz. tuna steaks
2 tbsp. white sesame
2 tbsp. black sesame
1 tsp. sesame oil
2 artichokes
2 tsp. extra-virgin olive oil
½ lemon, juiced
1 garlic clove
1 handful parsley

Directions:
Discard the outer leaves, and then slice artichokes very fine. Heat a pan with olive oil, add garlic and cook for a couple of minutes, then remove the clove. Add artichokes, lemon, salt, and pepper. Cook 5-10 minutes until tender. Set aside.

Mix sesame seeds and press them on tuna until it is completely covered.

Heat a pan and add sesame oil. When the oil is very hot, cook tuna for 1-2 minutes per side.

Serve tuna alongside artichokes.

NUTRITION FACTS: CALORIES 353KCAL FAT 4.8 G CARBOHYDRATE 28.1 G PROTEIN 28.3 G

SESAME GLAZED CHICKEN WITH GINGER AND CHILI GREENS

⊖ 2   🕐 35 mins

Ingredients:

1 tbsp mirin

1 tbsp. miso paste

10 oz. chicken breast

1 oz. celery

2 oz. red onion

2 zucchini

1 Thai chili

2 garlic cloves

1 tsp. fresh ginger

1 cup spinach

2 tsp. sesame seeds

3 oz. buckwheat

1 tsp. ground turmeric

1 tsp. extra-virgin olive oil

1 tsp. tamari

Directions:

Heat the oven to 400 F. Line a roasting pan with parchment-paper Mix in the mirin and the miso. Cut the chicken lengthwise and marinate it with the miso mix for 15 minutes.

Place the chicken in the roasting pan, sprinkle it with the sesame seeds, and roast in the oven for 15-20 minutes until it has been beautifully caramelized.

Wash the buckwheat in a sieve, and then place it along with the turmeric in a saucepan of boiling water. Cook 25-30 minutes until done, and then drain. Chop celery, red onion, and zucchini into medium pieces. Chop the chili, garlic, and ginger very thinly, and set aside.

Heat the oil in a frying pan; add the celery, onion, zucchini, chili, garlic, and ginger. Fry over high heat for 1-2 minutes, then reduce to medium heat for 3-4 minutes until the vegetables are cooked through but are still crunchy.

If the vegetables begin to stick to the pan, you can add a cup of water. Add the tamari and spinach, and cook for 2 minutes. Serve with chicken and buckwheat.

NUTRITION FACTS: CALORIES 417KCAL FAT 6.5 G CARBOHYDRATE 34.8 G PROTEIN 32.1 G

SHREDDED CHICKEN BOWL

2   40 mins

Ingredients:
8 oz. chicken breast
1 tsp. onion powder
1 tsp. garlic powder
2 cups broth
2 cups baby spinach
½ lime
2 tsp. extra-virgin olive oil
2 ripe avocados
1 cup cherry tomatoes

Directions:
Put the chicken breasts in a saucepan with salt, pepper, onion, and garlic powder. Add the broth, bring to a boil, and cook 30-40 minutes with a lid until the meat starts to shred.

Remove the chicken from the broth, and shred it with a fork. Place the baby spinach as a base in a serving bowl.

Add the shredded chicken into the bowl, with sliced avocado and cherry tomatoes.

Prepare the dressing with lime, oil, salt, and pepper and drizzle it over the salad just before serving.

NUTRITION FACTS: CALORIES 420KCAL FAT 5.6 G CARBOHYDRATE 12.5 G PROTEIN 21.4 G

SHRIMP TOMATO STEW

1   40 mins

Ingredients:
8 oz. shrimps
1 tbsp. extra-virgin olive oil
2 leeks, finely chopped
1 carrot, finely chopped
1 celery stick, finely chopped
1 Garlic clove, finely chopped
1 Bird's eye chili, thinly sliced
2 tbsp. red wine
2 cups tomatoes
2 cups stock
1 tbsp. parsley, chopped

Directions:
Fry garlic, onion, celery, carrot, and chili in oil over low heat for 5 minutes. Add the leeks. Turn up the heat to medium, add the red wine, and let evaporate.

Add tomatoes and cook for 5 minutes, then add the stock and let simmer for 20 minutes.

Add shrimps and let cook for 4-5 minutes until they become opaque. Don't overcook it.

Serve warm.

NUTRITION FACTS: CALORIES 213KCAL FAT 13.1 G SUGAR 51.7 G PROTEIN 80.6 G

SIRTFOOD CAULIFLOWER COUSCOUS AND TURKEY STEAK

 2   🕐 35 mins

Ingredients:

5 ¼ oz. cauliflower, roughly chopped
1 garlic clove, finely chopped
1 ½ oz. red onion, finely chopped
1 Bird's Eye chili, finely chopped
1 tsp. fresh ginger, finely chopped
2 tbsp. extra-virgin olive oil
2 tsp. ground turmeric
1 oz. sun-dried tomatoes, finely chopped
⅜ oz. parsley
5 ¼ oz. turkey steaks
1 tsp. sage
½ lemon, juiced
1 tbsp. capers

Directions:

Put the cauliflower in the food processor and blend it in 1-2 pulses until it has a breadcrumb-like consistency.

In a skillet, fry garlic, chili, ginger, and red onion in 1 tsp. olive oil for 2 to 3 minutes.

Throw in the turmeric and cauliflower, then cook for another 1 to 2 minutes. Remove from heat and add tomatoes and parsley.

Marinate the turkey steak with sage, capers, lemon juice, and olive oil for 10 minutes.

In a skillet, over medium heat, fry the turkey steak, turning occasionally.

Serve with the couscous.

NUTRITION FACTS: CALORIES 462KCAL FAT 39.8 G CARBOHYDRATE 9.9 G PROTEIN 16.8 G

SMOKED SALMON OMELET

  1   🕐 25 mins

Ingredients:

2 eggs
4 oz. smoked salmon, chopped
1/2 tsp. capers
½ cup arugula, chopped
1 tsp. parsley, chopped
1 tsp. extra-virgin olive oil

Directions:

Crack the eggs into a bowl and whisk well. Add the salmon, capers, arugula, and parsley. Heat the olive oil in a skillet.

Add the egg mixture and, with a spatula, move the mix around the pan until it's even.

Reduce the heat and allow the omelet to cook. Twist the spatula around the edges to lift them, add salmon and arugula and fold the omelet in 2.

NUTRITION FACTS: CALORIES 303KCAL FAT 22 G CARBOHYDRATE 12 G PROTEIN 23 G

SLOPPY JOE SCRAMBLE STUFFED SPUDS

🍴 6   🕐 1h

Ingredients:

1 tbsp. vegetable oil
1 lb. extra-firm tofu, crumbled
¼ tsp fine sea salt
¼ tsp ground black pepper
¾ cup onion, finely chopped
¼ cup yellow bell pepper, finely chopped
3 cloves garlic, finely chopped
1 tbsp. ground cumin
2 tsp chili powder
1 can (15 oz.) tomato sauce
2 tbsp. ketchup
1 tbsp. tamari
1 tbsp. Worcestershire sauce
1 tbsp. yellow mustard
¾ cup water
3 baked potatoes, cooled
1 tbsp. extra-virgin olive oil

Directions:

Heat 1 tbsp. of vegetable oil in a skillet over medium-high heat. If the skillet is not well-seasoned, add the remaining tbsp. of oil.

Add the tofu, salt, and pepper. Cook for 8 to 10 minutes, occasionally stirring until the tofu is firm and golden. Stir in the onion, bell pepper, garlic, cumin, and chili powder.

Reduce the heat to medium and cook for 3 minutes, occasionally stirring, until fragrant.

Add the tomato sauce, ketchup, tamari, Worcestershire sauce, mustard, and dill pickle. Bring to a boil, and then reduce the heat to simmer. Swish the water in the tomato sauce can to clean the sides.

Simmer for 30 minutes, occasionally stirring, adding the tomato sauce's water can as needed for the desired consistency. Preheat the oven to broil. Cut the baked potatoes in half lengthwise.

Scoop the insides from the potatoes, leaving about 1 inch of the skin intact.

Brush both the inside and the outside of the potato skins with the olive oil and place them on a baking sheet.

Broil for 3 to 4 minutes until lightly browned. Remove from the oven and divide the filling evenly in the potatoes, using about ¼ cup in each.

NUTRITION FACTS: CALORIES 306KCAL FAT 21 G CARBOHYDRATE 6 G PROTEIN 23 G

SMOKY BEAN AND TEMPEH PATTIES

 4   50 mins

Ingredients:

1 cup cooked cannellini beans
8 oz. tempeh
¼ cup cooked bulgur
2 cloves garlic, pressed
¼ tsp. onion powder
1 tsp liquid smoke
1 tsp. smoked paprika
2 tbsp. organic ketchup
2 tbsp. agave syrup
2 tbsp. vegetable oil
3 tbsp. tamari.
¼ cup chickpea flour

Directions:

Mash the beans in a bowl: it's okay if a few small pieces of beans are left. Crumble the tempeh into small pieces on top. Add the bulgur and garlic.

In a bowl, whisk together the remaining ingredients, except the flour and cooking spray. Stir into the crumbled tempeh preparation. Add the flour and mix until well combined. Chill for 1 hour before shaping into patties.

Preheat the oven to 350°F. Line a baking tray with parchment paper. Scoop out 1/3 cup per patty, shaping into an approximately 3-inch circle and flattening slightly on the tray. You should get eight 3.5-inch patties in all. Lightly coat the top of the patties with cooking spray.

Bake for 15 minutes, carefully flip, lightly coat the top of the patties with cooking spray, and bake for another 15 minutes until lightly browned and firm.

Leftovers can be stored in an airtight container in the refrigerator for up to 4 days.

The patties can also be frozen, tightly wrapped in foil, for up to 3 months. If you don't eat all the patties at once, reheat the leftovers on low heat in a skillet lightly greased with olive oil or cooking spray for about 5 minutes on each side until heated through.

NUTRITION FACTS: CALORIES 200KCAL FAT 9 G CARBOHYDRATE 18 G PROTEIN 14 G

SPICY CHICKEN STEW

 2   🕐 40 mins

Ingredients:

2 red peppers, chopped
2 white onions, sliced
2 garlic cloves, minced
1 ½ cups vegetable broth
3 tsp. extra-virgin olive oil
½ tsp. ground nutmeg
1 tbsp. paprika
1 Bird's Eye chili, sliced
1 tomato, chopped
4 chicken thighs
4 oz. buckwheat
1 tbsp. parsley

Directions:

Boil the buckwheat for 25 minutes, then drain it and set it aside.

Put the oil in a pan and heat, add onion, garlic, chili and spices and cook for 5 minutes until soft. Add the chicken and let it turn golden brown on medium-high heat for 5 minutes.

Add the peppers and the tomato, salt, and pepper and cook another 3-5 minutes until they start softening. Add the stock, turn the heat down and let simmer for 25 minutes. Add the buckwheat and let it absorb all the spicy flavors for 2-3 minutes. Serve hot.

NUTRITION FACTS: CALORIES 305KCAL FAT 9.5 G CARBOHYDRATE 14.2 G PROTEIN 3.7 G

SPICY INDIAN LENTILS WITH BASMATI RICE

 1   🕐 35 mins

Ingredients:

1 tsp. of extra-virgin olive oil
2 oz. onion, nicely chopped
2 garlic cloves, nicely chopped
1 tsp. fresh ginger
1 Bird's Eye chili, nicely chopped
1 tsp. of mild curry powder
1 tsp. of ground turmeric
1 tsp. cinnamon stick
½ tsp. cardamom seeds
½ tsp. cumin seeds
1 cup red lentils
1 tomato, chopped
1 oz. basmati rice
1 tsp. extra-virgin olive oil

Directions:

Cook the lentils in boiling water for 20 to 25 minutes until almost done. In the meantime, cook the rice in a separate pot for 20 minutes and drain.

Put cinnamon, onion, garlic, ginger, and chili in a hot pan with olive oil. Cook until tender, for about 5 minutes, then discard the cinnamon stick. Drain the lentils and put them in the pan.

Add tomato, turmeric, curry, cardamom, and cumin and cook for a few minutes until all the flavors have mixed.

NUTRITION FACTS: CALORIES 272KCAL FAT 4.3 G CARBOHYDRATE 26.8 G PROTEIN 23.6 G

SPICY SALMON WITH TURMERIC AND LENTILS

 4 35 mins

Ingredients:

20 oz. salmon fillets
1 tsp. extra-virgin olive oil
1 tsp. turmeric
1/4 juice of a lemon
½ red onion, finely chopped
3 oz. lentils, canned
1 garlic clove, finely chopped
1 bird's eye chili, finely chopped
5 oz. celery cut into 2cm sticks
1 tsp. Mild curry powder
1 tomato, cut into 8 wedges
1 cup chicken or vegetable stock
1 tbsp. parsley, chopped

Directions:

Heat the oven to 400°F. Heat a frying pan over medium-low heat; add the olive oil, then onion, garlic, ginger, chili, and celery. Fry gently for 2–3 minutes or until softened, then add the curry powder and cook for another minute.

Add the tomatoes, then stock and lentils, and simmer gently for 10 minutes. You may want to increase or decrease the cooking time, depending on how crunchy you like your celery.

Meanwhile, mix the turmeric, oil, and lemon juice and rub over the salmon. Place on a baking tray and cook for 8–10 minutes. To finish, spread parsley on top of the celery and serve with the salmon.

NUTRITION FACTS: CALORIES 177KCAL CARBOHYDRATE 4 G PROTEIN 12 G

SPICY STEW WITH POTATOES AND SPINACH

 2 40 mins

Ingredients:

2 sweet potatoes
2 tsp. extra-virgin olive oil
1 red onion, finely chopped
½ Bird's Eye chili
2 tbsp. paprika
1 cup tomatoes, chopped
1 cup stock
1 cup spinach
8 oz. chicken breast

Directions:

Peel and cut sweet potatoes into 1-inch cubes and boil them for 12 minutes. Drain and set aside.

Heat a pan on medium-high heat, add onion and cook for 5 minutes.

Add chicken cubes and spices and let the meat color on all sides for 5 minutes.

Add tomatoes and stock and let cook 15 minutes on low heat.

Add sweet potatoes and spinach, let the flavors mix for 5 minutes, then turn the heat off.

Let rest 10 minutes, then serve.

NUTRITION FACTS: CALORIES 213KCAL FAT 13.1 G SUGAR 51.6 G PROTEIN 80.6 G

SPINACH QUICHE

 2   🕐 50 mins

Ingredients:

5 oz. all purposes flour
2 oz. buckwheat flour
3 oz. almond flour
½ cup water
2 tbsp. extra-virgin olive oil
1 small pinch of baking soda
3 cups spinach
3 eggs
1 cup ricotta cheese
1 tbsp. parmesan

Directions:

Mix the flours, salt, and baking soda. Add the water and mix until you get a dough. If needed, add some more water. Let the dough rest for 30 minutes.

Heat the oven to 350°F. Heat a pan with oil, put spinach and salt, and cook 5 minutes on low heat. Set aside.

When the dough is ready, roll the dough to 1/8 inch thickness and put it in a baking tin. Mix ricotta, eggs, salt, pepper, and spinach and put the filling in the tin.

Remove the excess dough with a knife. Bake 35 minutes. Let cool 10 minutes and serve.

The remaining dough can be stored in the fridge or freezer in an airtight container.

NUTRITION FACTS: CALORIES 353KCAL FAT 4.8 G CARBOHYDRATE 28.1 G PROTEIN 28.3 G

SWEET AND SOUR PAN WITH CASHEW NUTS

 4   30 mins

Ingredients:

2 tbsp. coconut oil
2 red onion
2 yellow bell pepper
12 oz. white cabbage
6 oz. bok choy
1 ½ oz. mung bean sprouts
4 pineapple slices
1 ½ oz. cashew nuts
¼ cup apple cider vinegar
4 tbsp. coconut sugar
1 1/2 tbsp. tomato paste
1 tsp. coconut-aminos
2 tsp. arrowroot powder
¼ cup water

Directions:

Roughly cut the vegetables. Mix the arrowroot with five tbsp. of cold water into a paste.

Then put all the other ingredients for the sauce in a saucepan and add the arrowroot paste for binding.

Melt the coconut oil in a pan and fry the onion. Add the bell pepper, cabbage, bok choy, and bean sprouts and stir-fry until the vegetables become a little softer.

Add the pineapple and cashew nuts and stir a few more times. Pour a little sauce over the wok dish and serve.

NUTRITION FACTS: CALORIES 573KCAL FAT 27.8 G CARBOHYDRATE 77.9 G PROTEIN 15.3 G

SWEET POTATO AND SALMON PATTIES

 2   40 mins

Ingredients:

3 tbsp. buckwheat flour
8 oz. wild salmon, cooked or tinned
8 oz. sweet potato cooked and mashed
1 tbsp. dill
1 head red endive
1 tbsp. extra-virgin olive oil
1 tbsp. balsamic vinegar

Directions:

Preheat the oven up to 325°F.

Mix the sweet potato, salmon, dill, salt, and pepper. Take a small handful of the mixture and shape it into a ball. Flatten into the shape of a burger, then dip into the flour on each side. Place it on a lined baking tray. Repeat until the blend is used up.

Bake only turning once for 20 minutes. Serve with a salad made with finely sliced red endive seasoned with a vinaigrette made with olive oil, salt, pepper, and vinegar.

NUTRITION FACTS: CALORIES 316KCAL FAT 6.3 G CARBOHYDRATE 18.3 G PROTEIN 19.2 G

TOFU SCRAMBLE WITH MUSHROOMS

2   25 mins

Ingredients:
3 tbsp. extra-virgin olive oil
½ yellow onion, diced
3 cloves garlic, finely chopped
1 tsp. soy sauce
12 oz. firm tofu, cubed
½ red bell pepper, diced
¾ cup mushrooms, cut
3 green onions, diced
2 tomatoes, cleaved
½ tsp. ground ginger
½ tsp. bean stew powder
¼ tsp. cayenne pepper

Directions:
Gently sauté onion and garlic in the olive oil for 3 to 5 minutes, until they are soft. Add the remaining ingredients, except salt and pepper.

Sautee for another 6 to 8 minutes, until veggies are done, and tofu absorbed the liquid. Add salt and pepper to taste.

NUTRITION FACTS: CALORIES 330KCAL FAT 9 G CARBOHYDRATE 36 G PROTEIN 18 G

TOMATO & GOAT'S CHEESE PIZZA

2   55 mins

Ingredients:
10 oz. buckwheat flour
2 tsp. dried yeast
Pinch of salt
5 fl. oz. water
1 tsp. extra-virgin olive oil
3 oz. feta cheese, crumbled
3 oz. tomato sauce
1 tomato, sliced
1 red onion, finely chopped
1 oz. arugula leaves, chopped

Directions:
In a bowl, combine all the ingredients for the pizza dough and allow it to stand for at least an hour until it has doubled in size.

Roll the dough out to a size to suit you. Spoon the passata onto the base and add the rest of the toppings. Bake in the oven at 400°F for 15 to 20 minutes or until browned at the edges and crispy and serve.

NUTRITION FACTS: CALORIES 387KCAL FAT 9.9 G CARBOHYDRATE 52 G PROTEIN 8.4 G

TOFU WITH CAULIFLOWER

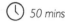 2   50 mins

Ingredients:

¼ cup red pepper, seeded
1 Thai chili, seeded
2 cloves of garlic
1 tsp. of olive oil
1 pinch of cumin
1 pinch of parsley
Juice of ½ lemon
8 oz. tofu
8 oz. cauliflower, chopped
1 ½ oz. red onions, finely chopped
1 tsp finely chopped ginger
2 teaspoons turmeric
1 oz. sun-dried tomatoes, chopped
1 oz. parsley, chopped

Directions:

Preheat oven to 400 °F. Slice the peppers and put them in an ovenproof dish with chili and garlic.

Pour some olive oil over it, add the dried herbs, and put in the oven until the peppers are soft, about 20 minutes).

Let it cool down, put the peppers together with the lemon juice in a blender, and work it into a soft mass.

Cut the tofu in half and divide the halves into triangles.

Place the tofu in a casserole dish, cover with the paprika mixture, and place in the oven for about 20 minutes.

Chop the cauliflower until the pieces are smaller than a grain of rice. Then, in a saucepan, heat the garlic, onions, chili, and ginger with olive oil until they become transparent. Add turmeric and cauliflower, mix well, and heat again.

Remove from heat and add parsley and tomatoes. Mix well. Serve with the tofu in the sauce.

NUTRITION FACTS: CALORIES 298KCAL FAT 5 G CARBOHYDRATE 55 G PROTEIN 27.5 G

TROUT WITH ROASTED VEGETABLES

 2   🕐 45 mins

Ingredients:

2 turnips, peeled and chopped
Extra-virgin olive oil
Dill
1 lemon, juiced
2 carrots cut into sticks
2 parsnips, peeled and cut into wedges
2 tbsp. tamari
2 trout fillets

Directions:

Put the sliced vegetables into a baking tray. Sprinkle with a dash of tamari and olive oil. Set on gas mark 7 in the oven. Take the vegetables out of the oven after 25 minutes, and stir well.

Place fish on vegetables. Sprinkle with the dill and lemon juice. Cover with foil, and go back to the oven.

Turn down the oven to 375°F and cook till the fish is cooked through for 20 minutes.

NUTRITION FACTS: CALORIES 154KCAL FAT 2.2 G CARBOHYDRATE 14.5 G PROTEIN 23.6 G

TUNA AND KALE

🍲 4   🕐 25 mins

Ingredients:

1 lb. tuna fillets, skinless and cubed
A pinch of salt and black pepper
2 tbsp. olive oil
1 cup kale
½ cup cherry tomatoes, cubed
1 redonion, chopped

Directions:

Steam kale for 6 minutes, drizzle 1tbsp. olive it and a pinch of salt, and mix well.

Heat a pan with the remaining oil over medium heat; add the onion and sauté for 5 minutes.

Add tuna and cherry tomatoes and cook for 5 minutes.

Serve the tuna with the kale on the side.

NUTRITION FACTS: CALORIES 251KCAL FAT 4 G CARBOHYDRATE 14 G PROTEIN 7 G

TUNA AND TOMATOES

 4   🕐 25 mins

Ingredients:

1 red onion, chopped
1 tbsp. olive oil
1 lb. tuna fillets, skinless and cubed
1 cup tomatoes, chopped
1 red pepper, chopped
1 tsp. sweet paprika
1 tbsp. parsley, chopped

Directions:

Heat a pan with the oil over medium heat, add the onions and the pepper and cook for 5 minutes. They have to be crispy and crunchy: don't overcook.

Add tuna, tomato, and paprika and cook 1 minute on high heat.

Add parsley and serve immediately.

NUTRITION FACTS: CALORIES 215KCAL FAT 4 G CARBOHYDRATE 14 G PROTEIN 7 G

TURKEY BACON FAJITAS

 2   🕐 25 mins

Ingredients:

3 eggs, lightly beaten
2 whole-grain tortillas
½ cup cherry tomatoes
1 red onion
2 turkey bacon slices
2 oz. cup shredded cheddar
1 tsp extra-virgin olive oil

Directions:

Sauté the onion with olive oil on medium heat for 5 minutes, add the eggs and stir continuously until they are done.

Add turkey bacon, finely sliced, and cheddar cheese on top so that it starts to melt.

Quick heat the tortillas on a pan (keep them soft), divide the egg mixture between them, and serve immediately.

NUTRITION FACTS: CALORIES 353KCAL FAT 4.8 G CARBOHYDRATE 28.1 G PROTEIN 28.3 G

TUNA, EGG & CAPER SALAD

 2   🕐 25 mins

Ingredients:

3½ oz. red endive
5 oz. tinned tuna, drained
3 ½ oz. cucumbers
1 oz. arugula
6 black olives, pitted
2 hard-boiled eggs, quartered
2 tomatoes, chopped
2 tbsp. fresh parsley, chopped
1 red onion, chopped
1 stalk of celery
1 tbsp. capers
2 tbsp. extra-virgin olive oil
1 tbsp. white vinegar
1 garlic clove, crushed

Directions:

Place the tuna, cucumber, olives, tomatoes, onion, endive, celery, and parsley, and arugula into a bowl.

Combine olive oil, vinegar, garlic, and a pinch of salt into a vinaigrette dressing.

Pour the vinaigrette on the salad, and toss. Serve on plates and scatter the eggs and capers on top.

NUTRITION FACTS: CALORIES 309KCAL FAT 12.2 G CARBOHYDRATE 25.7 G PROTEIN 26.7 G

TURKEY BREAST WITH PEPPERS

 2   ⏱ 30 mins

Ingredients:

4 oz. buckwheat
8 oz. turkey breast
1 tsp. ground turmeric
2 peppers, chopped
2 oz. red onion, sliced
1 oz. celery
1 tsp. chopped fresh ginger
1 lemon, juiced
2 tsp. extra-virgin olive oil
1 tomato
1 Bird's Eye chili, finely chopped
1 oz. parsley, finely chopped

Directions:

Boil the buckwheat for 25 minutes, then drain. Set aside. In the meantime, marinate the turkey breast with turmeric, 1 tsp oil, lemon juice, celery, and ginger.

Cook the marinated chicken in the oven for 10 to 12 minutes. Remove from the oven, cover with foil, and leave to rest for 5 minutes before serving.

Meanwhile, fry the red onions and the ginger in a 1 tsp oil until they become soft, then add peppers and fry on high heat for 6 minutes. They have to stay crunchy. Serve buckwheat alongside chicken and peppers.

NUTRITION FACTS: CALORIES 107KCAL FAT 2.9 G CARBOHYDRATE 20.6 G PROTEIN 2.1 G

VEGETARIAN CURRY

2   ⏱ 1h+ 15 mins

Ingredients:

4 carrots
2 sweet potatoes
1 red onion
3 cloves garlic
4 tbsp. curry powder
½ tsp. chili powder
1 pinch cinnamon
3 cups vegetable broth
1 can tomatoes
8 oz. sweet peas
2 tbsp. tapioca flour

Directions:

Roughly chop carrots, sweet potatoes, onions, potatoes, and garlic and put them all in a pot.

Mix tapioca flour with curry powder, cumin, chili powder, salt, and cinnamon and sprinkle this mixture on the vegetables.

Add tomato cubes. Pour the vegetable broth over it.

Close the pot with a lid, bring to a boil and let it simmer for 60 minutes on low heat. Stir in snap peas after 30 minutes. Cauliflower rice is an excellent addition to this dish.

NUTRITION FACTS: CALORIES 397KCAL FAT 6.1 G CARBOHYDRATE 81.6 G PROTEIN 9.4 G

TURMERIC BAKED SALMON

 I 45 mins

Ingredients:

6 oz. Salmon fillet, skinned
1 tsp. extra-virgin olive oil
1 tsp. Ground turmeric
¼ lemon, juiced
1 tsp. extra-virgin olive oil
1 oz. red onion, finely chopped
1 oz. tinned green peas
1 garlic clove, finely chopped
1-inch fresh ginger, finely chopped
1 Bird's Eye chili, thinly sliced
4 oz. celery cut into small cubes
1 tsp. mild curry powder
1 tomato, chopped
½ cup vegetable stock
1 tbsp. parsley, chopped

Directions:

Heat the oven to 400°F. Start cooking the sauce. Heat a skillet over moderate --low heat, then add the olive oil then the garlic, onion, ginger, chili, celery.

Stir lightly for 2 to 3 minutes until softened but not colored, then add the curry powder and cook for another minute.

Put in tomato, green peas, and stock and simmer for 10 to 15 minutes depending on how thick you enjoy your sauce.

Meanwhile, combine turmeric, oil, and lemon juice and rub the salmon.

Put on a baking tray and cook for 10 minutes in the oven. Serve the salmon with the celery sauce.

NUTRITION FACTS: CALORIES 360KCAL FAT 8 G CARBOHYDRATE 10 G PROTEIN 40 G

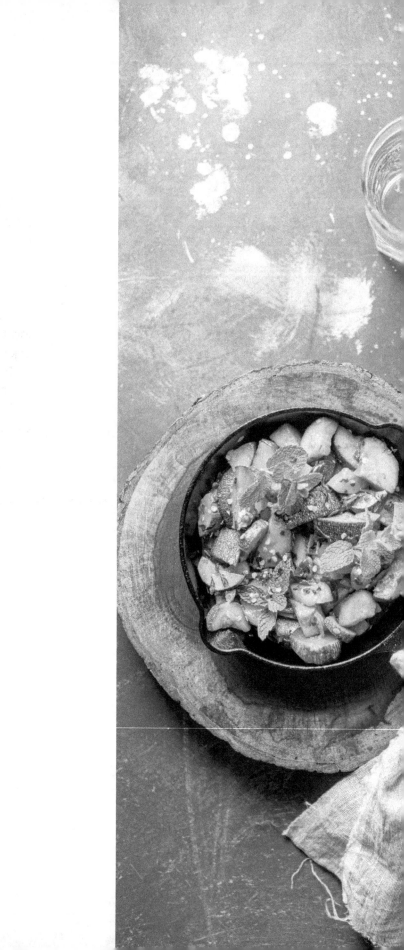

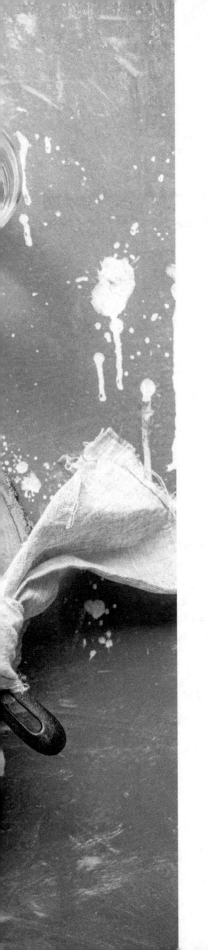

SIDE DISHES

APPLES AND CABBAGE MIX

🍳 4   🕐 10 mins

Ingredients:
2 cored and cubed green apples
2 tbsp. Balsamic vinegar
½ tsp. caraway seeds
2 tbsp. Olive oil
Black pepper
1 shredded red cabbage head

Directions:
In a bowl, combine the cabbage with the apples and the other ingredients, toss and serve.

NUTRITION FACTS: CALORIES 165KCAL FAT 7.4 G CARBOHYDRATE 26 G PROTEIN 2.6 G

ARUGULA WITH APPLES AND PINE NUTS

🍳 4   🕐 18 mins

Ingredients:
2 tbsp. extra-virgin olive oil
2 cloves garlic, slivered
2 tbsp. pine nuts
1 apple, peeled, cored, and chopped
10 oz. arugula
Salt and pepper to taste

Directions:
Heat the olive oil in a skillet or wok over low heat. Add the garlic, pine nuts, and apple.

Cook until the nuts and garlic are golden, and the apple is just starting to soften 3 to 5 minutes. Increase the heat to medium and add the arugula.

Stir and cook another 2 to 3 minutes. Season with salt and pepper to taste.

NUTRITION FACTS: CALORIES 121KCAL FAT 9 G CARBOHYDRATE 8 G PROTEIN 3 G

BAKED SWEET POTATO

 1   55 mins

Ingredients:
1 sweet potato
1 tsp. butter

Directions:
Heat the oven to 425°F.

Clean the potato very well under running water to get rid of the dirt.

Prick it several times and put it in the oven for 50 minutes. Always remember to test if it's done using a stick.

Cut the upper part and pour the butter over the sweet potato.

NUTRITION FACTS: CALORIES 353KCAL FAT 4.8 G CARBOHYDRATE 28.1 G PROTEIN 28.3 G

CARROT, TOMATO, AND ARUGULA QUINOA PILAF

 4   35 mins

Ingredients:
2 tsp. extra-virgin olive oil
½ red onion, chopped
1 cup quinoa, raw
2 cups vegetable or chicken broth
1 tsp. fresh lovage, chopped
1 carrot, chopped
1 tomato, chopped
1 cup arugula

Directions:
Heat the olive oil in a saucepan over medium heat and add the red onion. Cook and stir until translucent, about 5 minutes.

Lower the heat, stir in quinoa, and toast, continually stirring, for 2 minutes. Stir in the broth, black pepper, and thyme.

Raise the heat to high and bring to a boil. Cover, reduce heat to low and simmer for 5 minutes.

Stir in the carrots, cover, and simmer until all water is absorbed, about 10 more minutes.

Turn off the heat, add tomatoes, arugula and lovage and let sit for 5 minutes. Add salt and pepper to taste.

NUTRITION FACTS: CALORIES 165KCAL FAT 4 G CARBOHYDRATE 27 G PROTEIN 6 G

CHICKPEAS WITH CARAMELIZED ONION AND ENDIVE

 4 35 mins

Ingredients:

2 red endives
¼ cup extra-virgin olive oil
2 red onions, sliced thinly
2 tsp. sugar
¼ cup Medjool dates, chopped
Salt and pepper, to taste
2 cans of chickpeas

NUTRITION FACTS: CALORIES 288KCAL FAT 6 G
CARBOHYDRATE 52 G PROTEIN 10 G

Directions:

Prepare the endives discarding the outer leaves and the core. Wash them in a bowl of cold water, cut them into large pieces, and set aside.

Heat the oil over medium heat in a large skillet.

Add the onions and cook until translucent, about 5 minutes. Stir in the sugar, and continue cooking until the onions are golden brown, about 10 minutes.

Add the dates and the endive leaves.

Cook, occasionally stirring, until the leaves are tender, about 6 minutes. Season with salt and pepper to taste.

Stir in the chickpeas and let cook until the flavors have blended for about 5 minutes.

EASY CAJUN GRILLED VEGGIES

 4 40 mins

Ingredients:

¼ cup extra-virgin olive oil
1 tsp. Cajun seasoning
1/2 tsp. cayenne pepper
1 tbsp. Worcestershire sauce
2 zucchini cut into 1/2-inch slices
2 red onions, sliced into ½" wedges
2 yellow squash, cut into 1/2-inch slices

Directions:

In a bowl, mix olive oil, Cajun seasoning, cayenne pepper, and Worcestershire sauce. Place zucchinis, onions, yellow squash in a bowl and cover with the olive oil mixture. Salt to taste.

Cover the bowl and marinate vegetables in the refrigerator for at least 30 minutes.

Preheat an outdoor grill for high heat and lightly oil grate.

Place marinated vegetable pieces on skewers or directly on the grill. Cook 5 minutes until done.

NUTRITION FACTS: CALORIES 95KCAL FAT 7 G CARBOHYDRATE 8 G PROTEIN 2 G

JERUSALEM ARTICHOKE GRATIN

 3   35 mins

Ingredients:

1 lb. jerusalem artichoke
1 cup milk
3 tbsp. grated cheese
1 tbsp. crème Fraiche
1 tsp. butter
Curry, paprika powder, nutmeg, salt, pepper

Directions:

Wash and peel the Jerusalem artichokes and slice them into approx. ½ inch thick slices. Bring them to a boil with the milk in a saucepan. Then stir in the spices and crème Fraiche.

Grease a baking dish with butter and add the Jerusalem artichoke and milk mixture. Bake on the middle shelf in the oven for about half an hour at 325°F.

Sprinkle with grated cheese five minutes before the end of the baking time.

NUTRITION FACTS: CALORIES 133KCAL FAT 8.2 G CARBOHYDRATE 9.9 G PROTEIN 4.7 G FIBER 1.1

KALE GREEN BEAN CASSEROLE

 4   45 mins

Ingredients:

1 ½ cups milk
1 cup sour cream
1 cup mushrooms, chopped
2 cups green beans, chopped
2 cups kale, chopped
¼ cup capers, drained
¼ cup walnuts, crushed

Directions:

Preheat the oven to 375° F and lightly grease a casserole dish.

Whisk the milk and sour cream together in a bowl.

Add mushrooms, green beans, kale, and capers. Pour into the casserole dish and top with the crushed walnuts.

Bake uncovered in the preheated oven until bubbly and browned on top, about 40 minutes.

NUTRITION FACTS: CALORIES 130KCAL FAT 6 G CARBOHYDRATE 14 G PROTEIN 2 G

KALE SAUTÉ

 2   25 mins

Ingredients:

1 chopped red onion
3 tbsp. coconut aminos
2 tbsp. Olive oil
1 lb. kale
1 tbsp. chopped parsley
1 tbsp. lime juice
2 minced garlic cloves

Directions:

Heat a pan with the olive oil over medium heat; add the onion and the garlic and sauté for 5 minutes.

Add the kale and the other ingredients, toss, cook over medium heat for 10 minutes, divide between plates and serve.

NUTRITION FACTS: CALORIES 200KCAL FAT 7.1 G CARBOHYDRATE 6.4 G PROTEIN 6 G

KALE WALNUT BAKE

  4   40 mins

Ingredients:

1 red onion, finely chopped
¼ cup extra-virgin olive oil
2 cups kale
½ cup half-and-half cream
½ cup walnuts, coarsely chopped
1/3 cup breadcrumbs
½ tsp ground nutmeg
2 tbsp. extra-virgin olive oil

Directions:

Preheat oven to 350°F. In a skillet, sauté onion in olive oil until tender. In a bowl, combine cooked onion, kale, cream, walnuts, breadcrumbs, nutmeg, salt, and pepper to taste, mixing well.

Transfer to a greased 1-1/2-qt. baking dish. Combine topping ingredients and sprinkle over the kale mixture. Bake, uncovered, for 30 minutes or until lightly browned.

NUTRITION FACTS: CALORIES 555KCAL FAT 31 G CARBOHYDRATE 65 G PROTEIN 26 G

MINTY TOMATOES AND CORN

 2   10 mins

Ingredients:

2 cups corn

1 tbsp. rosemary vinegar

2 tbsp. mint, chopped

1 lb. sliced tomatoes

¼ tsp. black pepper

2 tbsp. olive oil

Directions:

In a salad bowl, combine the tomatoes with the corn and the other ingredients, toss and serve. Enjoy!

NUTRITION FACTS: CALORIES 230KCAL FAT 7.2 G CARBOHYDRATE 11.6 G PROTEIN 4 G

PESTO GREEN BEANS

2   20 mins

Ingredients:

2 tbsps. Extra-virgin olive oil

2 tsps. sweet paprika

Juice of 1 lemon

2 tbsp. basil pesto

1 lb. trimmed and halved green beans

¼ tsp. black pepper

1 sliced red onion

Directions:

Heat a pan with the oil over medium-high heat; add the onion, stir and sauté for 5 minutes.

Add the beans and the rest of the ingredients, toss, cook over medium heat for 10 minutes, divide between plates and serve.

NUTRITION FACTS: CALORIES 280KCAL FAT 10 G CARBOHYDRATE 13.9 G PROTEIN 4.7 G

PLANT-BASED STUFFED PEPPERS

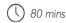 6   🕐 80 mins

Ingredients:

1 ½ cups brown rice, raw
6 green bell peppers
3 tbsp. soy sauce
3 tbsp. dry red wine
1 tsp. vegetarian Worcestershire sauce
1 ½ cups extra firm tofu
1/2 cup cranberries
¼ cup walnuts, chopped
½ cup parmesan, grated
2 cups tomato sauce
2 tbsp. brown sugar

Directions:

Preheat oven to 350°F. In a saucepan, bring 3 cups water to a boil. Stir in rice. Reduce heat, cover, and simmer for 40 minutes. Meanwhile, core and deseed green peppers, leaving bottoms intact.

Place peppers in a microwavable dish with about ½" of water in the bottom. Microwave on high for 6 minutes. In a saucepan, bring soy sauce, wine, and Worcestershire sauce to a simmer. Add tofu and simmer until the liquid is absorbed.

Combine rice, tofu, cranberries, nuts, cheese, salt, and pepper in a bowl and mix well. Pack rice firmly into peppers. Return peppers to the dish you first microwaved them in and bake for 25 to 30 minutes, or until lightly browned on top.

Meanwhile, in a saucepan over low heat, combine tomato sauce and brown sugar. Heat until hot.

Serve stuffed peppers with the tomato sauce spooned over each serving.

NUTRITION FACTS: CALORIES 250KCAL FAT 10 G CARBOHYDRATE 22 G PROTEIN 17 G

PURPLE POTATOES WITH ONIONS, MUSHROOMS, AND CAPERS

4   35 mins

Ingredients:

6 purple potatoes, scrubbed
3 tbsp. extra-virgin olive oil
1 red onion, chopped
8 oz. mushrooms, sliced
¼ tsp. chili pepper flakes
1 tbsp. capers, drained and chopped
1 tsp. fresh tarragon, chopped

Directions:

Cut each potato into wedges by quartering the potatoes, then cutting each quarter in half. Heat 1 tbsp. of olive oil over medium heat in a skillet and cook the onion and mushrooms until the mushrooms start to release their liquid, and the onion becomes translucent (about 5 minutes). Transfer the onion and mushrooms into a bowl and set aside.

Heat 2 more tbsp. olive oil over high heat in the same skillet and add the potato wedges into the hot oil. Sprinkle with salt and pepper, and allow to cook, occasionally stirring, until the wedges are browned on both sides, about 10 minutes.

Reduce heat to medium, sprinkle the potato wedges with red pepper flakes, and allow to cook until the potatoes are tender, about 10 more minutes. Stir in the onion and mushroom mixture, toss the vegetables together, and mix in the capers and fresh tarragon.

NUTRITION FACTS: CALORIES 215KCAL FAT 6 G CARBOHYDRATE 23 G PROTEIN 3 G

RICE WITH LEMON AND ARUGULA

 4   45 mins

Ingredients:

1 red onion, chopped
1 cup fresh mushrooms, sliced
2 cloves garlic, minced
1 tbsp. extra-virgin olive oil
3 cups long-grain rice, steamed
10 oz. fresh arugula
3 tbsp. lemon juice
¼ tsp. dill weed
Salt and pepper to taste
1/3 cup feta cheese, crumbled

Directions:

Preheat oven to 350°F. In a skillet, sauté the onion, mushrooms, and garlic in oil until tender. Stir in the rice, arugula, lemon juice, dill, and salt and pepper to taste.

Reserve 1 tbsp. cheese and stir the rest into skillet; mix well. Transfer to an 8-in. square baking dish coated with nonstick cooking spray. Sprinkle with reserved cheese. Cover and bake for 25 minutes.

Uncover and bake for an additional 5 to 10 minutes or until heated through, and cheese is melted.

NUTRITION FACTS: CALORIES 290KCAL FAT 6 G CARBOHYDRATE 55 G PROTEIN 13 G

ROASTED BEETS

 4   35 mins

Ingredients:

2 garlic cloves, minced
¼ tsp. black pepper
4 beets, peeled and sliced
¼ cup walnuts, chopped
2 tbsp. extra-virgin olive oil
¼ cup parsley, chopped

Directions:

In a baking dish, combine the beets with the oil and the other ingredients, toss to coat, put in the oven at 420°F, and bake for 30 minutes.

Divide between plates and serve.

NUTRITION FACTS: CALORIES 156KCAL FAT 11.8 G CARBOHYDRATE 11.5 G PROTEIN 3.8 G

ROASTED RED ENDIVE WITH CAPER BUTTER

🍴 4   🕐 35 mins

Ingredients:

2 red endives
2 tsp. extra-virgin olive oil
2 anchovy fillets, packed in oil
1 lemon, juiced
3 tbsp. capers, drained
5 tbsp. butter, cut into cubes
1 tbsp. fresh parsley, chopped
Salt and pepper as needed

Directions:

Preheat the oven to 425°F. Toss endives with olive oil, salt, and pepper, and spread out onto a baking sheet cut side down.

Bake for about 20 to 25 minutes or until caramelized.

While they're roasting, add the anchovies to a pan over medium heat and use a fork to mash them until broken up.

Add lemon juice and mix well, then add capers.

Lower the heat and slowly stir in the butter and parsley. Drizzle butter over roasted endives, season as necessary, and garnish with more fresh parsley.

NUTRITION FACTS: CALORIES 109KCAL FAT 8.6 G CARBOHYDRATE 4.9 G PROTEIN G FIBER 4G

ROSEMARY ENDIVES

🍴 2   🕐 30 mins

Ingredients:

2 tbsp. extra-virgin olive oil
1 tsp. rosemary
2 halved endives
¼ tsp. black pepper
½ tsp. turmeric powder

Directions:

In a baking pan, combine the endives with the oil and the other ingredients, toss gently, introduce in the oven and bake at 400°F for 20 minutes. Divide between plates and serve.

NUTRITION FACTS: CALORIES 66KCAL FAT 7.1 G CARBOHYDRATE 1.2 G PROTEIN 0.3 G

SAGE CARROTS

 4   🕐 35 mins

Ingredients:
2 tsp. sweet paprika
1 tbsp. sage, chopped
2 tbsps. Extra-virgin olive oil
1 lb. carrots, chopped
¼ tsp. black pepper
1 red onion, chopped

Directions:
In a baking pan, combine the carrots with the oil and the other ingredients, toss and bake at 380°F for 30 minutes. Divide between plates and serve.

NUTRITION FACTS: CALORIES 200KCAL FAT 8.7 G CARBOHYDRATE 7.9 G PROTEIN 4 G

SCALLOPS WITH ALMONDS AND MUSHROOMS

 4   🕐 15 mins

Ingredients:
1-lb. scallops
2 tbsp. olive oil
4 scallions, chopped
½ cup mushrooms, sliced
2 tbsp. almonds, chopped
1 cup coconut cream

Directions:
Heat a pan with the oil over medium heat; add the scallions and the mushrooms and sauté for 2 minutes.

Add the scallops, cook over medium heat for 8 minutes more, divide into bowls, and serve.

NUTRITION FACTS: CALORIES 322KCAL FAT 23.7 G CARBOHYDRATE 8.1 G PROTEIN 21.6 G

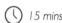

THYME MUSHROOMS

🍳 4   🕐 40 mins

Ingredients:

1 tbsp. thyme, chopped
2 tbsp. extra-virgin olive oil
2 tbsp. parsley, chopped
4 garlic cloves, minced
2 lbs. halved white mushrooms

Directions:

In a baking pan, combine the mushrooms with the garlic and the other ingredients, toss, put in the oven and cook at 400°F for 30 minutes.

Divide between plates and serve.

NUTRITION FACTS: CALORIES 251KCAL   FAT 9.3 G   CARBOHYDRATE 13.2 G   PROTEIN 6 G

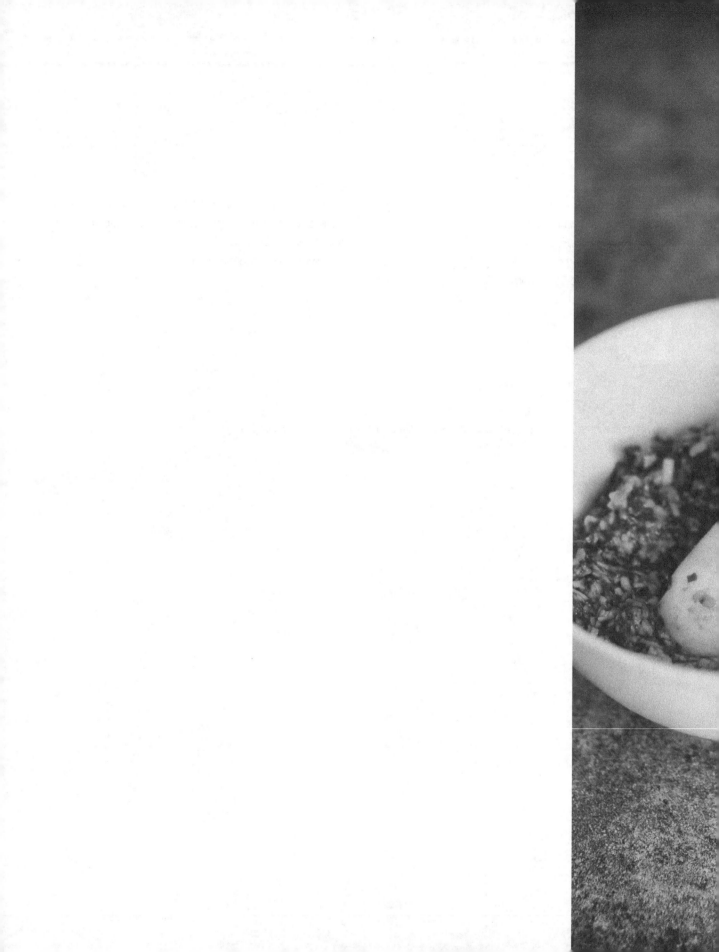

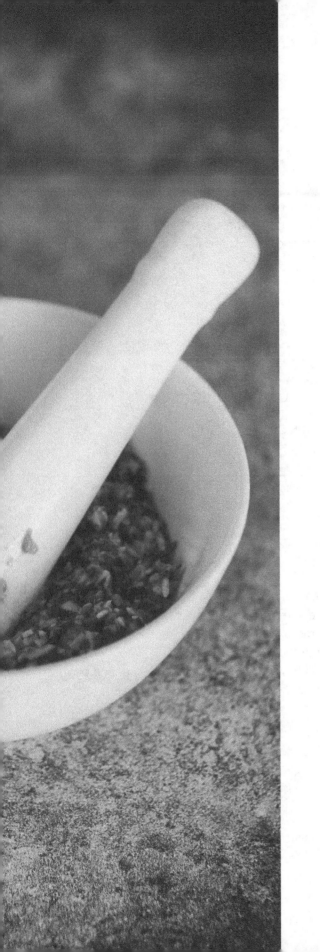

SAUCES AND DRESSINGS

AVOCADO CAESAR DRESSING

 4   ⏱ 10 mins

Ingredients:
1/3 cup avocado, mashed
2 cloves garlic, minced
1 tbsp. olive oil
2 anchovy fillets
3 tbsp. lemon juice
¼ cup parmesan cheese, shredded
2 tbsp. almond milk, unsweetened
2 teaspoons Worcestershire sauce
½ tsp. mustard
2 tbsp. water
¾ tsp. sea salt
¼ tsp. ground pepper

Directions:
Add all ingredients into a high-powered blender or food processor and blend until smooth.

Taste and add additional salt and pepper if needed.

NUTRITION FACTS: CALORIES 58KCAL FAT 5 G CARBOHYDRATE 2 G PROTEIN 2 G

GUACAMOLE

 4   ⏱ 15 mins

Ingredients:
2 ripe avocados
1 garlic clove
3 tbsp. olive oil
½ white onion
1 tomato, diced
5 1/3 tbsp. fresh parsley
½ lime, the juice

Directions:
Peel the avocados and mash with a fork. Grate or chop the onion finely and add to the mash. Squeeze the lime and add the juice.

Add tomato, olive oil, and finely chopped parsley. Season with salt and pepper and mix well.

Let the sauce sit in the refrigerator for at least 10 minutes for the flavors to develop.

NUTRITION FACTS: CALORIES 244KCAL FAT 25 G CARBOHYDRATE 5 G PROTEIN 3 G

ITALIAN VEGGIE SALSA

 4   🕐 20 mins

Ingredients:

2 red bell peppers, chopped
3 zucchini, sliced
½ cup garlic, minced
2 tbsp. olive oil
A pinch of black pepper
1 tsp. Italian seasoning

Directions:

Heat a pan with the oil over medium-high heat, add bell peppers and zucchini, toss and cook for 5 minutes.

Add garlic, black pepper, and Italian seasoning, toss, cook for 5 minutes more.

Blitz in a food processor until entirely smooth.

NUTRITION FACTS: CALORIES 132KCAL FAT 3 G CARBOHYDRATE 7 G PROTEIN 4 G

MUNG SPROUTS SALSA

🥣 2   🕐 10 mins

Ingredients:

1 red onion, chopped
2 cups mung beans, sprouted
A pinch of red chili powder
1 green chili pepper, chopped
1 tomato, chopped
1 tsp. chaat masala
1 tsp. lemon juice
1 tbsp. parsley, chopped

Directions:

In a salad bowl, mix onion with mung sprouts, chili pepper, tomato, chili powder, chaat masala, lemon juice, parsley, and pepper, toss well, divide into small cups and serve.

NUTRITION FACTS: CALORIES 100KCAL FAT 2 G CARBOHYDRATE 3 G PROTEIN 6 G

SALSA VERDE

 4   🕐 10 mins

Ingredients:

½ cup fresh parsley, finely chopped
3 tbsp. fresh basil, finely chopped
2 cloves garlic, crushed
¾ cup olive oil
2 tbsp. capers
½ lemon, the juice
½ tsp. ground black pepper
1 tsp. sea salt

Directions:

Add all of the ingredients to a deep bowl and mix with an immersion blender until the sauce has the desired consistency.

Store the sauce in the refrigerator for up to 4-5 days or in the freezer.

NUTRITION FACTS: CALORIES 323KCAL FAT 37 G CARBOHYDRATE 2 G PROTEIN 1 G

TZATZIKI

🍴 6   🕐 30 mins

Ingredients:

½ cucumber
1 cup Greek yogurt
1 tbsp. olive oil
2 cloves garlic
1 tbsp. fresh mint, finely chopped
Pinch of ground black pepper
1 tsp salt

Directions:

Rinse the cucumber, grate without peeling it. The green skin adds color and texture to the sauce.

Put the grated cucumber in a strainer and sprinkle salt on top. Mix well and let the liquid drain for 5 to 10 minutes. Wrap cucumber in a tea towel and squeeze out excess liquid.

Crush garlic and place it in a bowl. Add cucumber, oil, and fresh mint.

Stir in the yogurt and add black pepper and salt to taste. Let the sauce sit in the refrigerator for at least 10 minutes for the flavors to develop.

NUTRITION FACTS: CALORIES 81KCAL FAT 7 G CARBOHYDRATE 3 G PROTEIN 1 G

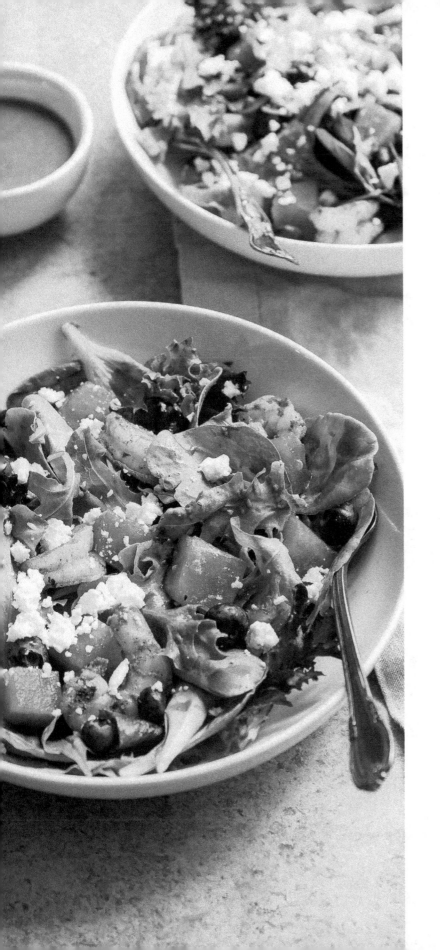

SALADS

ARUGULA SALAD WITH TURKEY
AND ITALIAN DRESSING

 2   20 mins

Ingredients:

8 oz. turkey breast
1 cup arugula
1 cup lettuce
2 tsp. Dijon mustard
1 tbsp. cumin
1/2 cup celery, finely diced
2 tsp. oregano
1/4 cup scallions, sliced
2 tsp. extra-virgin olive oil

Directions:

Grill the turkey and shred it. Set aside.

Mix lettuce and arugula on a plate. Evenly distribute shredded turkey, celery, and scallions.

In a bowl, mix all dressing ingredients: mustard, oil, lemon juice, oregano, salt, and pepper and pour it over the salad just before serving.

NUTRITION FACTS: CALORIES 165KCAL FAT 2.9 G CARBOHYDRATE 13.6 G PROTEIN 26.1 G

ARUGULA WITH FRUITS AND NUTS

 1   15 mins

Ingredients:

½ cup arugula
½ peach
½ red onion
¼ cup blueberries
5 walnuts, chopped
1 tbsp. extra-virgin olive oil
2 tbsp. red wine vinegar
1 spring of fresh basil

Directions:

Halve the peach and remove the seed. Heat a grill pan and grill it briefly on both sides. Cut the red onion into thin half-rings. Roughly chop the pecans.

Heat a pan and roast the pecans in it until they are fragrant.

Place the arugula on a plate and spread peaches, red onions, blueberries, and roasted pecans over it.

Put all the ingredients for the dressing in a food processor and mix to an even dressing. Drizzle the dressing over the salad.

NUTRITION FACTS: CALORIES 160KCAL FAT 7 G CARBOHYDRATE 25 G PROTEIN 3 G

BROCCOLI SALAD

  1   🕐 25 mins

Ingredients:
1 head of broccoli
1/2 red onion
2 carrots, grated
¼ cup red grapes
2 1/2 tbsp. Coconut yogurt
1 tbsp. Water
1 tsp. mustard
1 pinch salt

Directions:
Cut the broccoli into florets and cook for 8 minutes. Cut the red onion into thin half-rings. Halve the grapes. Mix coconut yogurt, water, and mustard with a pinch of salt to make the dressing.

Drain the broccoli and rinse with ice-cold water to stop the cooking process.

Mix the broccoli with the carrot, onion, and red grapes in a bowl. Serve the dressing separately on the side.

NUTRITION FACTS: CALORIES 230KCAL FAT 18 G CARBOHYDRATE 35 G PROTEIN 10 G

BRUNOISE SALAD

  1   🕐 10 mins

Ingredients:
1 tomato
1 zucchini
½ red bell pepper
½ yellow bell pepper
½ red onion
3 springs fresh parsley
½ lemon
2 tbsp. olive oil

Directions:
Finely dice tomatoes, zucchini, peppers, and red onions to get a brunoise. Mix all the cubes in a bowl. Chop parsley and mix in the salad. Squeeze the lemon over the salad and add the olive oil. Season with salt and pepper.

NUTRITION FACTS: CALORIES 30KCAL FAT 4 G CARBOHYDRATE 3 G

BRUSSELS SPROUTS AND RICOTTA SALAD

 2   15 mins

Ingredients:

1 ½ cups Brussels sprouts, thinly sliced
1 green apple cut "à la julienne."
½ red onion
8 walnuts, chopped
1 tsp. extra-virgin olive oil
1 tbsp. lemon juice
1 tbsp. orange juice
4 oz. ricotta cheese

Directions:

Put the red onion in a cup and cover it with boiling water. Let it rest 10 minutes, then drain and pat with kitchen paper. Slice Brussels sprouts as thin as you can, cut the apple à la julienne (sticks).

Mix Brussels sprouts, onion, and apple and season them with oil, salt, pepper, lemon juice, and orange juice and spread it on a serving plate.

Spread small spoonfuls of ricotta cheese over Brussels sprouts mixture and top with chopped walnuts.

NUTRITION FACTS: CALORIES 353KCAL FAT 4.8 G CARBOHYDRATE 28.1 G PROTEIN 28.3 G

CELERY AND RAISINS SNACK SALAD

 4   10 mins

Ingredients:

½ cup raisins
4 cups celery, sliced
¼ cup parsley, chopped
½ cup walnuts, chopped
Juice of ½ lemon
2 tbsp. olive oil
Salt and black pepper to taste

Directions:

In a salad bowl, mix celery with raisins, walnuts, parsley, lemon juice, oil, and black pepper, toss, divide into small cups and serve as a snack.

NUTRITION FACTS: CALORIES 120KCAL FAT 1 G CARBOHYDRATE 6 G PROTEIN 5 G

CORONATION CHICKEN SALAD

  15 mins

Ingredients:
3 oz. natural yogurt
Juice of 1/4 of a lemon
1 tsp. parsley, chopped
1 tsp. ground turmeric
½ tsp. mild curry powder
4 oz. cooked chicken breast
6 walnut halves, finely chopped
2 Medjool dates, thinly sliced
1/2 red onion, diced
1 bird's eye chili
2 oz. arugula

Directions:
Cut the chicken breast into bite-sized pieces

On a serving plate, use the arugula as a base, then sprinkle the chicken, walnuts, dates, onion.

Mix yogurt, lemon juice, spices, and parsley in a small bowl and drizzle it over the salad.

NUTRITION FACTS: CALORIES 364KCAL FAT 12 G CARBOHYDRATE 45 G PROTEIN 15 G

DIJON CELERY SALAD

 4 10 mins

Ingredients:
½ cup lemon juice
1/3 cup Dijon mustard
2/3 cup olive oil
Black pepper to taste
2 apples, cored, peeled, and cubed
1 bunch celery roughly chopped
¾ cup walnuts, chopped

Directions:
In a salad bowl, mix celery and its leaves with apple pieces and walnuts.

Add black pepper, lemon juice, mustard, and olive oil, whisk well, add to your salad, toss, divide into small cups and serve.

NUTRITION FACTS: CALORIES 125KCAL FAT 2 G CARBOHYDRATE 7 G PROTEIN 7 G

FRESH ENDIVE SALAD

 1 10 mins

Ingredients:
½ red endive
1 orange
1 tomato
½ cucumber
½ red onion

Directions:
Cut off the hard stem of the endive and remove the leaves. Peel the orange and cut the pulp into wedges.

Cut the tomatoes and cucumbers into small pieces. Cut the red onion into thin half-rings.

Place the endive boats on a plate; spread the orange wedges, tomato, cucumber, and red onion over the boats. Drizzle some olive oil and fresh lemon juice and serve.

NUTRITION FACTS: CALORIES 112KCAL FAT 11 G CARBOHYDRATE 2 G

FRESH SALAD WITH ORANGE DRESSING

 2  10 mins

Ingredients:
½ cup lettuce
1 yellow bell pepper
1 red pepper
4 oz. carrot, grated
10 almonds
4 tbsp. extra-virgin olive oil
½ cup orange juice
1 tbsp. apple cider vinegar

Directions:
Clean the peppers and cut them into long thin strips. Tear off the lettuce leaves and cut them into smaller pieces.

Mix the salad with the peppers and the carrots in a bowl. Roughly chop the almonds and sprinkle over the salad.

Mix all the ingredients for the dressing in a bowl. Pour over the salad just before serving.

NUTRITION FACTS: CALORIES 150KCAL FAT 10 G CARBOHYDRATE 11 G PROTEIN 2 G

GREEK SALAD SKEWERS

 2   10 mins

Ingredients:
8 big black olives
8 cherry tomatoes
1 yellow pepper, cut into 8 squares
½ red onion, split into 8 wedges
1 cucumber, cut into 8 pieces
4 oz. feta, cut into 8 cubes
1 tbsp. extra-virgin olive oil
Juice of 1/2 lemon
1 tsp. balsamic vinegar
1/2 tsp. garlic, crushed

Directions:
Put the salad ingredients on the skewers following this order: cherry tomato, yellow pepper, red onion, cucumber, feta, black olive.

Repeat for each skewer and put on a serving plate.

As a dressing, put in a bowl: olive oil, a pinch of salt and pepper, lemon juice, balsamic vinegar, and crushed garlic. Whisk well and drizzle on the skewers.

NUTRITION FACTS: CALORIES 236KCAL FAT 21 G CARBOHYDRATE 14 G PROTEIN 7 G

HAWAII SALAD

 1   15 mins

Ingredients:
1 cup arugula
1 / 2 pieces red onion
1-piece winter carrot
1 cup pineapple
3 oz. ham, diced
1 pinch salt
1 pinch black pepper

Directions:
Cut the red onion into thin half-rings. Remove the peel and hardcore from the pineapple and cut the pulp into thin pieces. Clean the carrot and use a spiralizer to make strings.

Mix arugula and carrot in a bowl. Spread this over a plate. Spread red onion, pineapple, and diced ham over the arugula.

Drizzle the olive oil and balsamic vinegar on the salad to your taste.

Season with salt and pepper.

NUTRITION FACTS: CALORIES 200KCAL FAT 6 G CARBOHYDRATE 28 G PROTEIN 8 G

LEMON GINGER SHRIMP SALAD

 2   ⏱ 20 mins

Ingredients:

1 cup endive leaves
½ cup arugula
½ cup baby spinach
2 tsp. of extra-virgin olive oil
6 walnuts, chopped
1 avocado, sliced
Juice of ½ lemon
8 oz. shrimp
1 pinch chili

Directions:

Mix endive, baby spinach, and arugula and put them on a plate.

Heat a skillet on medium-high, add 1 tbsp. oil and cook shrimp with garlic, chili, salt, and pepper until they are no longer transparent (5 minutes).

Blend avocado with oil, lemon juice with a pinch of salt and pepper and distribute the dressing on top. Chop the walnuts, put them on the plate as the last ingredient, and serve.

NUTRITION FACTS: CALORIES 353KCAL FAT 4.8 G CARBOHYDRATE 28.1 G PROTEIN 28.3 G

MOROCCAN LEEKS SNACK SALAD

 4   ⏱ 10 mins

Ingredients:

1 bunch radishes, sliced
3 cups leeks, chopped
1 ½ cups olives, pitted and sliced
A pinch of turmeric powder
1 cup parsley, chopped
2 tbsp. extra-virgin olive oil

Directions:

In a bowl, mix radishes with leeks, olives, and parsley. Add black pepper, oil, and turmeric, toss to coat, and serve.

NUTRITION FACTS: CALORIES 135KCAL FAT 1 G CARBOHYDRATE 18 G PROTEIN 9 G

MUNG BEANS SNACK SALAD

 6   🕐 10 mins

Ingredients:

2 cups tomatoes, chopped
2 cups cucumber, chopped
2 cups mung beans, sprouted
2 cups clover sprouts
1 tbsp. cumin, ground
1 cup dill, chopped
4 tbsp. lemon juice
1 avocado, pitted and roughly chopped
1 cucumber, roughly chopped

Directions:

In a salad bowl, mix tomatoes with 2 cups cucumber, greens, clover, and mung sprouts.

In your blender, mix cumin with dill, lemon juice, 1 cup of cucumber, and avocado, blend well, add this to your salad, toss well and serve.

NUTRITION FACTS: CALORIES 120KCAL FAT 3 G CARBOHYDRATE 10 G PROTEIN 6 G

RAINBOW SALAD

 1   🕐 10 mins

Ingredients:

1 cup lettuce
½ pieces avocado
1 egg
¼ green pepper
¼ red bell pepper
2 tomatoes
½ red onion
½ carrot, grated
2 tbsp. olive oil
1 tbsp. red wine vinegar

Directions:

Boil the egg until done (6 minutes for soft boiled, 8 minutes for hard-boiled). Cool it under running water, peel it and cut into slices.

Remove the seeds from the peppers and cut them into thin strips. Cut the tomatoes into small cubes. Cut the red onion into thin half-rings.

Cut the avocado into thin slices.

Place the salad on a plate and distribute all the vegetables in colorful rows.

Drizzle the vegetables with olive oil and red wine vinegar. Season with salt and pepper.

NUTRITION FACTS: CALORIES 40KCAL FAT 1 G CARBOHYDRATE 5 G PROTEIN 2 G

ROASTED BUTTERNUT AND CHICKPEAS SALAD

 4   🕐 50 mins

Ingredients:

1 cup chickpeas, drained
2 cups kale
2 tsp. oil
½ lemon, juiced
2 cloves of garlic
1 lb. butternut squash
1 green apple
½ tsp. honey

Directions:

Heat the oven to 400°F.

Cut the squash into medium cubes, put them in a baking tray, add drained chickpeas, garlic, 1 tbsp. oil, salt, and pepper and mix. Cook for 25 minutes.

Mix the kale with the dressing: salt, pepper, lemon, olive oil, and honey so that while the squash is cooking, it becomes softer and more pleasant to eat.

When squash and chickpeas are done, put them aside 10 minutes, and in the meantime, chop the apple and mix it with kale.

Add squash and chickpeas on top and serve warm.

NUTRITION FACTS: CALORIES 353KCAL FAT 4.8 G CARBOHYDRATE 28.1 G PROTEIN 28.3 G

SALAD WITH BACON, CRANBERRIES, AND APPLE

 2   🕐 50 mins

Ingredients:

½ cup arugula
4 slices bacon
½ apple
2 tbsp. cranberries
½ red onion
½ red bell pepper
10 Walnuts
1 tsp. mustard yellow
1 tsp. honey
3 tbsp. extra-virgin olive oil

NUTRITION FACTS: CALORIES 70KCAL FAT 3 G
CARBOHYDRATE 6 G PROTEIN 7 G

Directions:

Heat a pan over medium heat and fry the bacon until crispy. Place the bacon on a piece of kitchen towel so that the excess fat is absorbed. Cut half the red onion into thin rings. Cut the bell pepper into small cubes. Cut the apple into four pieces and remove the core. Then cut into thin wedges. Drizzle some lemon juice on the apple wedges so that they do not change color.

Roughly chop walnuts. Mix the ingredients for the dressing in a bowl. Season with salt and pepper. Spread the lettuce on a plate and season with red pepper, red onions, apple wedges, and walnuts.

Sprinkle bacon and cranberries over the salad. Drizzle the dressing over the salad and serve.

SESAME CHICKEN SALAD

 2 *12 mins*

Ingredients:

1 tbsp. sesame seeds
1 cucumber, chopped
4 oz. baby spinach
2 oz. bok choi, really finely chopped
1/2 red onion, very finely chopped
6 oz. cooked chicken, shredded
1 tbsp. extra-virgin olive oil
1 tsp. sesame oil
Juice of 1 lime
1 tsp. clear honey
2 tsp. soy sauce

Directions:

Toast the sesame seeds in a dry skillet for two minutes until lightly browned and aromatic. Transfer to a plate to cool. In a bowl, mix the olive oil, sesame oil, lime juice, honey, and soy sauce to create the dressing.

Put the cucumber, peeled, halved lengthways, deseeded using a teaspoon, and chopped in a bowl. Add spinach, bok choi, red onion, and mix. Pour on the dressing and mix.

Divide the salad between 2 plates and top with the shredded chicken. Add the sesame seeds just before serving.

NUTRITION FACTS: CALORIES 391KCAL FAT 15 G CARBOHYDRATE 20 G PROTEIN 39 G

SIRT FRUIT SALAD

 1 *10 mins*

Ingredients:

½ cup matcha green tea
1 tsp. honey
1 orange, halved
1 apple, cored and roughly chopped
10 red seedless grapes
10 blueberries

Directions:

Stir the honey into half a cup of green tea and let it chill.

When chilled, add the juice of half an orange.

Slice the other half and put in a bowl with the chopped apple, blueberries, and grapes.

Cover with tea and let rest in the fridge for 30 minutes before serving.

NUTRITION FACTS: CALORIES 110KCAL FAT 0 G CARBOHYDRATE 17 G PROTEIN 2 G

SIRT SALMON SALAD

 2   15 mins

Ingredients:
1 Medjool date, thinly chopped
1 cup endive leaves
½ cup arugula
1 tsp. of extra-virgin olive oil
1 tbsp. parsley, chopped
3 oz. celery, sliced
6 walnuts, chopped
1 tbsp. capers
2 oz. red onion-sliced
½ avocado, sliced
Juice of ¼ lemon
6 oz. smoked salmon

Directions:
Mix endive and arugula and put them on a plate. Evenly distribute on top finely sliced onion, avocado, walnuts, capers, celery, and parsley.

Mix oil, lemon juice with a pinch of salt and pepper and distribute the dressing on top.

NUTRITION FACTS: CALORIES 353KCAL FAT 4.8 G CARBOHYDRATE 28.1 G PROTEIN 28.3 G

SPINACH SALAD WITH ASPARAGUS AND SALMON

  2   25 mins

Ingredients:
2 cups spinach
2 eggs
4 oz. smoked salmon
1 cup asparagus tips
4 oz. cherry tomatoes
Lemon cut in ½ pieces
1 tsp olive oil

Directions:
Boil the eggs until they are done (6 minutes for soft boiled, 8 minutes for hard-boiled). Heat a pan with a little oil and fry the asparagus tips. Halve cherry tomatoes.

Place the spinach on a plate and spread the asparagus tips, cherry tomatoes, and smoked salmon on top.

Peel and halve the eggs. Add them to the salad. Squeeze the lemon and drizzle some olive oil over it.

Season the salad with a little salt and pepper.

NUTRITION FACTS: CALORIES 552KCAL FAT 40 G CARBOHYDRATE 6 G PROTEIN 39 G

SPROUTS AND APPLES SNACK SALAD

 4   🕐 10 mins

Ingredients:
1 lb. Brussels sprouts, shredded
1 cup walnuts, chopped
1 apple, cored and cubed
1 red onion, chopped
3 tbsp. red vinegar
1 tbsp. mustard
½ cup olive oil
1 garlic clove, crushed
Black pepper to the taste

Directions:
In a salad bowl, mix sprouts with apple, onion, and walnuts.

In another bowl, mix vinegar with mustard, oil, garlic, and pepper, whisk well, add this to your salad, toss well and serve as a snack.

NUTRITION FACTS: CALORIES 120KCAL FAT 2 G CARBOHYDRATE 8 G PROTEIN 6 G

STEAK SALAD

 4   1h + 10 mins

Ingredients:
2 4 oz. beefsteak
2 cloves garlic
1 red onion
2 eggs
1 cup cherry tomatoes
2 tbsp. extra-virgin olive oil
1 ripe avocado
½ cucumber
1 tbsp. red wine vinegar

Directions:
Place the steaks in a tray. Pour the olive oil over the steaks and crush the garlic over. Turn the steaks a few times so that they are covered with oil and garlic. Cover the meat and let it marinate for at least 1 hour. Boil eggs until done, rinse, and let cool.

Heat a grill pan and fry the steaks. When done, let them rest 5 minutes wrapped in aluminum foil. Spread the lettuce on the plates. Cut the steaks into slices and place them in the middle of the salad.

Cut the eggs into wedges, the cucumber into half-moons, the red onion into thin half-rings, the cherry tomatoes into halves, and the avocado into slices.

Spread this on the steaks. Drizzle the olive oil and red wine vinegar and season with a little salt and pepper.

NUTRITION FACTS: CALORIES 513KCAL FAT 15 G
CARBOHYDRATE 1 G PROTEIN 47 G

TOMATO AND AVOCADO SALAD

 1 10 mins

Ingredients:

1 tomato
4 oz. cherry tomatoes
½ red onion
1 ripe avocado
1 tsp. fresh oregano
1 tbsp. extra-virgin olive oil
1 tsp. red wine vinegar
1 pinch Celtic sea salt

Directions:

Cut the tomato into thick slices. Cut half of the cherry tomatoes into slices and the remaining in half. Cut the red onion into super-thin half rings. (if you have it, use a mandolin for this)

Cut the avocado into 6 parts. Spread the tomatoes on a plate, place the avocado on top.

Sprinkle red onion and oregano and drizzle olive oil, vinegar, and a pinch of salt on the salad.

NUTRITION FACTS: CALORIES 165KCAL FAT 14 G CARBOHYDRATE 7 G PROTEIN 5 G

TUNA SALAD AND RED ENDIVE

 2 20 mins

Ingredients:

2 pieces red endive
5 oz. tuna
1 orange
1 tbsp. fresh parsley, finely chopped
5 pieces radish
1 tsp Olive oil

Directions:

Drain the tuna. Cut the orange into wedges and then into small pieces.

Cut radishes into small pieces too.

Mix all the ingredients (except the red endive) in a bowl. Season with salt and pepper

Spread the tuna mix on the red endive leaves and serve.

NUTRITION FACTS: CALORIES 93KCAL FAT 6 G CARBOHYDRATE 2 G PROTEIN 9 G

ZUCCHINI SALAD WITH LEMON CHICKEN

 1   1h + 15 mins

Ingredients:

2 zucchini, sliced
4 oz. cherry tomatoes
5 oz. chicken breast
1 lemon
2 tbsp. olive oil
1 tbsp. rosemary
1 clove of garlic, crushed

Use a meat mallet or a heavy pan to make the chicken fillets as thin as possible. Put the fillets in a bowl. Squeeze the lemon over the chicken and add the olive oil, salt, pepper, rosemary, and garlic.

Cover and let marinate for at least 1 hour. Heat a pan over medium-high heat and fry the chicken until cooked through and browned.

Quarter the tomatoes and slice the zucchini, and put everything on a serving plate. Slice the chicken fillets diagonally and place them on the salad.

Drizzle the salad with a little olive oil and season with salt and pepper.

Directions:

NUTRITION FACTS: CALORIES 268KCAL   FAT 8 G   CARBOHYDRATE 4 G   PROTEIN 0 G

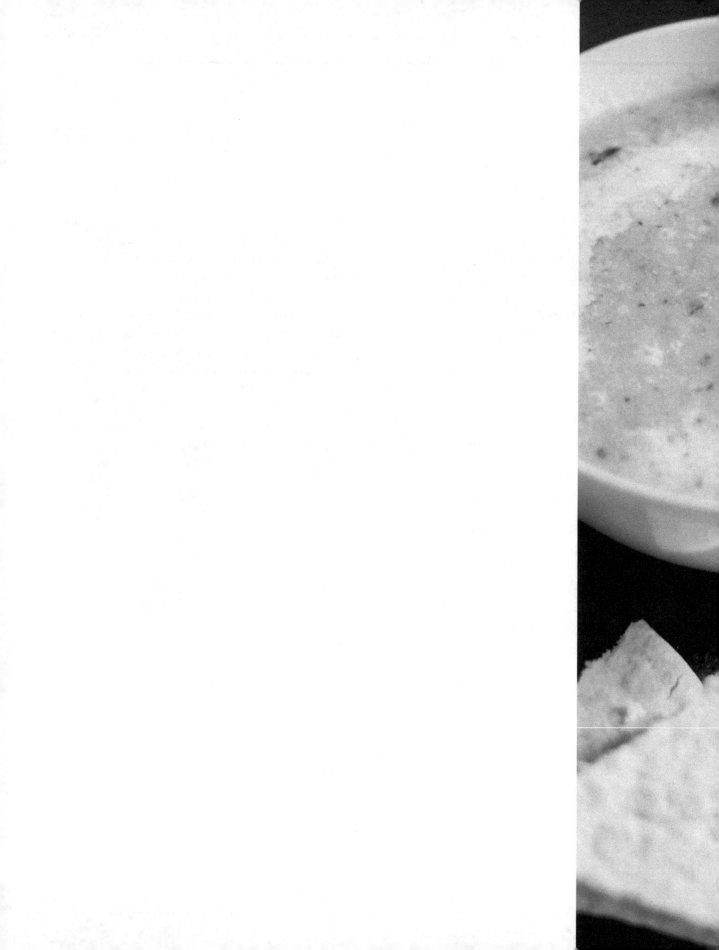

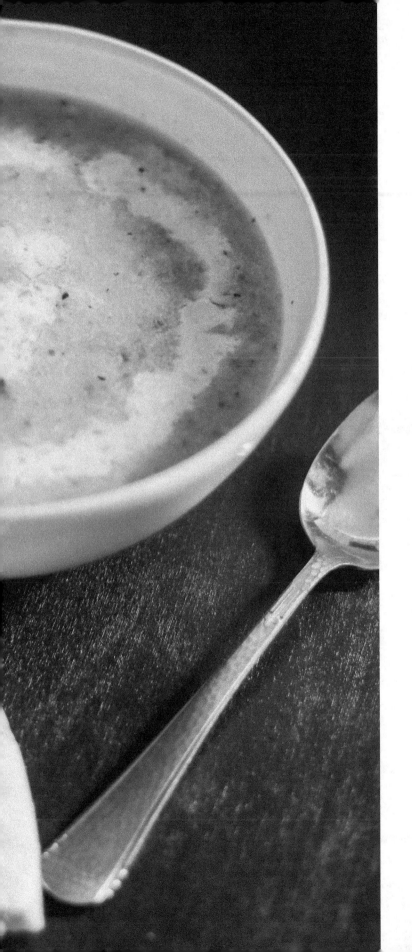

SOUPS

CAULIFLOWER AND WALNUT SOUP

 4   20 mins

Ingredients:

1 lb. cauliflower, chopped
8 walnut halves, chopped
1 red onion, chopped
2 cups vegetable stock
3½ fl. oz. double heavy cream
½ tsp. turmeric
1 tbsp. olive oil

Directions:

Heat the oil in a saucepan, add the cauliflower and red onion and cook for 4 minutes, stirring continuously. Pour in the stock, bring to a boil and cook for 15 minutes. Stir in double heavy cream and turmeric.

Using a food processor, blitz the soup until smooth and creamy.

Serve in bowls and top off with a sprinkling of chopped walnuts.

NUTRITION FACTS: CALORIES 240KCAL FAT 5 G CARBOHYDRATE 2 G PROTEIN 3 G

CELERY AND BLUE CHEESE SOUP

 3   30 mins

Ingredients:

4 oz. blue cheese
1 oz. butter
1 head of celery
1 red onion, chopped
1½ pints chicken stock
5 fl. oz. single cream

Directions:

Heat the butter in a saucepan, add the onion and celery and cook until the vegetables have softened.

Pour in the stock, bring to a boil, then reduce the heat and simmer for 15 minutes.

Pour in the cream and stir in the cheese until it has melted.

Serve and eat straight away.

NUTRITION FACTS: CALORIES 340KCAL FAT 16 G CARBOHYDRATE 41 G PROTEIN 31 G

CHICKEN, KALE, AND LENTIL SOUP

 3   30 mins

Ingredients:

5 cups vegetable stock
1 chicken breast, cooked and shredded
1 red onion
2 cups of kale, finely chopped
1 cup of spinach, chopped
1 cup of lentils
1 celery stick, chopped
1 carrot, chopped
1 Bird's Eye chili pepper
A dash of salt
1 tsp. of extra-virgin olive oil

Directions:

Boil the lentils according to the package but taking them out just a few minutes before they would be done. Set aside.

Add all the vegetables to a pot, sauté in a bit of the oil on medium heat. Stir until the vegetables are softer but not cooked through.

Add the chicken and the lentils you had set aside, and cook for 3 to 5 minutes more.

Add a dash of the salt. Add the stock, turn down to low, and simmer for 20 minutes. Remove from heat. Serve when cooled.

NUTRITION FACTS: CALORIES 199KCAL FAT 5 G CARBOHYDRATE 20 G PROTEIN 18 G

CREAM OF BROCCOLI & KALE SOUP

 4   40 mins

Ingredients:

9 oz. broccoli
9 oz. kale
1 potato, peeled and chopped
1 red onion, chopped
1-pint vegetable stock
½ pint milk
1 tbsp. olive oil

Directions:

Heat the olive oil in a saucepan, add the onion and cook for 5 minutes. Add in the potato, kale, and broccoli and cook for 5 minutes.

Pour in stock and milk and simmer for 20 minutes.

Using a food processor, blitz the soup until smooth and creamy. Season with salt and pepper. Serve immediately.

NUTRITION FACTS: CALORIES 207KCAL FAT 12 G CARBOHYDRATE 17 G PROTEIN 9 G

CREAMY BROCCOLI AND POTATO SOUP

 4   🕐 35 mins

Ingredients:

3 cups broccoli, chopped
2 potatoes, peeled and chopped
1 red onion, chopped
3 garlic cloves, minced
1 cup cashews
3 cups vegetable broth
3 tsp. extra-virgin olive oil
½ tsp. ground nutmeg

NUTRITION FACTS: CALORIES 305KCAL FAT 9.5 G
 CARBOHYDRATE 14.2 G PROTEIN 3.7 G

Directions:

Soak cashews in a bowl with boiling water and let rest for at least 4 hours.

Drain them and blend them with 1 cup of vegetable broth until smooth. Set aside. This will make the soup super creamy.

Gently heat olive oil in a saucepan over medium-high heat. Cook onion and garlic for 3-4 minutes until tender. Add in broccoli, potato, nutmeg, and water.

Cover and bring to boil, then reduce heat and simmer for 20 minutes, stirring from time to time. Remove from heat and stir in cashew mixture.

Blend until smooth, return to pan and cook until heated through.

CREAMY MUSHROOM SOUP WITH CHICKEN

🍲 2   🕐 50 mins

Ingredients:

2 cups vegetable stock
8 oz. mixed mushrooms, sliced
1 red onion, finely diced
1 carrot, finely diced
1 stick celery, finely diced
4 oz. chicken breast, cubed
1 tbsp. extra-virgin olive oil
3 sage leaves

Directions:

Put 1 tbsp. oil in a skillet and cook chicken until lightly brown. Set aside.

Put the mushrooms in a hot pan with 1 tbsp. oil, celery, carrot, onion, and sage. Cook for 3 to 5 minutes.

Add the stock and let it simmer for another 5 minutes. Then using a hand blender, blend the soup until smooth.

Add the chicken and cook for another 8 to 10 minutes until creamy.

NUTRITION FACTS: CALORIES 302KCAL FAT 3.5 G CARBOHYDRATE 16.3 G PROTEIN 15 G

FRENCH ONION SOUP

 4   30 mins

Ingredients:

2 lbs. red onions, thinly sliced
2 oz. cheddar cheese, grated
½ oz. butter
2 tsp. flour
2 slices whole-wheat bread
1 ½ pints beef stock
1 tbsp. olive oil

Directions:

Heat the butter and oil in a pan.

Add the onions and gently cook on low heat for 25 minutes, stirring occasionally. Add in the flour and mix well. Pour in the stock and keep stirring. Bring to the boil, reduce the heat and simmer for 30 minutes.

Cut the slices of bread into triangles, sprinkle with cheese and place them under a hot grill until the cheese has melted. Serve the soup into bowls and add two triangles of cheesy toast on top and enjoy.

NUTRITION FACTS: CALORIES 210KCAL   FAT 10 G   CARBOHYDRATE 18 G   PROTEIN 13 G

KALE AND SHIITAKE SOUP

4   45 mins

Ingredients:

1 cup kale
3 garlic cloves, minced
2 cups red onions, chopped
3 tbsp. extra-virgin olive oil
4 cups vegetable broth
2 lbs. dry shiitake mushrooms

Directions:

Put oil, garlic, onion, and kale in pan on medium heat, let them soften a few minutes.

Add mushrooms and sauté for 2 minutes.

Add stock, bring to a boil and let simmer for 30 minutes.

Serve immediately.

NUTRITION FACTS: CALORIES 124KCAL   FAT 2 G   CARBOHYDRATE 17 G   PROTEIN 9 G

KALE, APPLE AND FENNEL SOUP

 4   🕐 25 mins

Ingredients:
1 lb. kale, chopped
7 oz. fennel, chopped
2 apples, chopped
2 tbsp. fresh parsley, chopped
1 tbsp. olive oil

Directions:
Heat the oil in a saucepan, add the kale and fennel and cook for 5 minutes until the fennel has softened. Stir in the apples and parsley. Cover with hot water, bring it to a boil, and simmer for 10 minutes.

Blitz in a food processor until the soup is smooth. Season with salt and pepper.

NUTRITION FACTS: CALORIES 165KCAL FAT 9 G CARBOHYDRATE 21 G PROTEIN 3 G

LENTIL SOUP

  4   🕐 30 mins

Ingredients:
6 oz. red lentils
1 red onion, chopped
1 clove of garlic, chopped
2 sticks of celery, chopped
2 carrots, chopped
½ Bird's Eye chili
1 tsp. ground cumin
1 tsp. ground turmeric
2 pints vegetable stock
2 tbsp. extra-virgin olive oil

Directions:
Heat the oil in a saucepan and add the onion and cook for 5 minutes. Add in the carrots, lentils, celery, chili, cumin, turmeric, and garlic and cook for 5 minutes.

Pour in the stock, bring it to the boil, reduce the heat and simmer for 45 minutes.

Blitz in a food processor until the soup is smooth Season with salt and pepper and serve.

NUTRITION FACTS: CALORIES 196KCAL FAT 4 G CARBOHYDRATE 3 G PROTEIN 3.4 G

SPICY SQUASH SOUP.

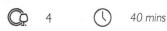 4   40 mins

Ingredients:

5 oz. kale
1 butternut squash, chopped
1 red onion, chopped
3 chilies, chopped
3 cloves of garlic
2 tsp. turmeric
1 tsp. ground ginger
2 cups vegetable stock
2 tbsp. olive oil

Directions:

Heat the olive oil in a saucepan, add the chopped butternut squash and onion and cook for 6 minutes until softened.

Stir in the kale, garlic, chili, turmeric, ginger, and cook for 2 minutes, stirring constantly.

Pour in the vegetable stock, bring it to the boil and cook for 20 minutes. Using a food processor, blitz the soup until smooth. Serve immediately.

NUTRITION FACTS: CALORIES 298KCAL FAT 9 G CARBOHYDRATE 24 G PROTEIN 5 G

TOFU AND SHITAKE MUSHROOM SOUP

  4   35 mins

Ingredients:

½ oz. dried wakame seaweed
4 cups vegetable stock
8 oz. shiitake mushrooms, sliced
2 oz. miso paste
16 oz. firm tofu, diced
2 green onion, trimmed and diagonally chopped
1 Bird's Eye chili, finely chopped

Directions:

Soak the wakame in lukewarm water for 10 to 15 minutes before draining.

In a saucepan, add the vegetable stock and bring to a boil. Toss in the mushrooms and simmer for 2to 3 minutes.

Mix the miso paste with 3-4 tbsp. of vegetable stock from the saucepan, until the miso is entirely dissolved.

Pour the miso-stock back into the pan and add the tofu, wakame, green onions, and chili, then serve immediately.

NUTRITION FACTS: CALORIES 203KCAL FAT 5 G CARBOHYDRATE 32 G PROTEIN 8 G

SPICY ASIAN NOODLE SOUP

 2 30 mins

Ingredients:

1 package buckwheat noodles
1 red onion
2 stalks of celery, chopped
1 chunk of ginger, diced
1 clove of garlic, minced
1 cup of arugula
¼ cup basil leaves, chopped
¼ cup of walnuts
1 tsp. of sesame seeds
2 tbsp. blackcurrants
½ Bird's Eye chili pepper
5 cups of vegetable stock
Juice of ½ lime
1 tsp. extra-virgin olive oil
1 tbsp. of soy sauce

Directions:

Cook the noodles as instructed and set aside. In a pan, sauté all of the vegetables, ginger, garlic, chili, and nuts for about 10 minutes on very low heat.

Add the stock, and simmer for another 5 minutes.

Cut the noodles so that they are a size small enough to eat in a soup comfortably. Add these to the soup, toss in the sesame seeds, lime juice and remove from heat. Serve warm.

NUTRITION FACTS: CALORIES 220KCAL FAT 3 G CARBOHYDRATE 23 G PROTEIN 25 G

TOMATO SOUP WITH MEATBALLS

2   45 mins

Ingredients:
8 oz. lean mince
1 egg
1 tbsp. parmesan
1 tbsp. breadcrumbs
2 tsp. of extra-virgin olive oil
1 red onion finely chopped
1 yellow pepper, chopped
1 red pepper, chopped
3 ripe tomatoes, chopped
2 cups stock
1 clove of garlic, crushed
1 Bird's Eye chili, finely sliced
4 oz. buckwheat

Directions:
Put mince, egg, breadcrumbs, parmesan, salt, and pepper in a bowl and mix well, then create small meatballs.

Heat a pan, add oil and gently sauté onion and garlic until transparent.

Add the meatballs and cook another 5 minutes.

Add peppers and chili, let flavors mix, add the tomatoes, add the broth, and let it simmer for 20-25 minutes.

While the soup cooks, boil buckwheat for 25 minutes, drain it, and add it to the soup right before serving it.

NUTRITION FACTS: CALORIES 348KCAL FAT 7.6 G CARBOHYDRATE 28.4 G PROTEIN 23.2 G

TURMERIC ZUCCHINI SOUP

 2   ⏱ 20 mins

Ingredients:

1 tbsp. extra-virgin olive oil
1 red onion, diced
1 tbsp. mild curry powder
3 cloves garlic, diced
3 zucchini, cubed
1 tbsp. fresh parsley
¼ tsp. white pepper
2 tsp. turmeric powder
2 tbsp. lime juice
1 tsp. fish sauce
1 cup coconut milk
1 cup vegetable stock

Directions:

Place a saucepan over medium heat with olive oil. Once hot, add the onion and sauté for 5 minutes, occasionally stirring, until golden and soft.

Add the garlic, zucchini, and salt. Stir to mix with the onion.

Add pepper, curry powder, and turmeric and stir for some seconds to release the aromas. Now add the fish sauce, coconut milk, and vegetable stock and stir again.

Allow to boil, then reduce the heat to low. Cover with a lid and simmer for 10 minutes.

Add the lime juice and stir through. Garnish with a few fresh parsley leaves.

NUTRITION FACTS: CALORIES 141KCAL FAT 11 G CARBOHYDRATE 7 G PROTEIN 4 G

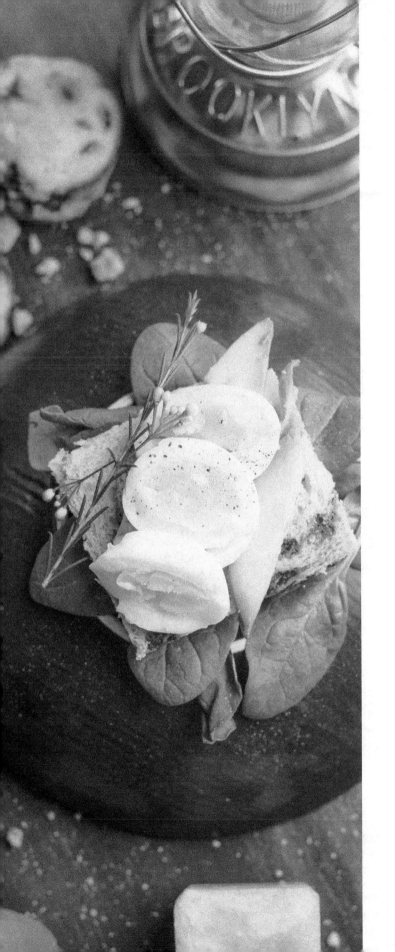

SNACKS

BLACK BEAN SALSA

 6  10 mins

Ingredients:

1 tbsp. coconut aminos
½ tsp. cumin, ground
1 cup canned black beans, drained
1 cup salsa
6 cups romaine lettuce leaves, torn
½ cup avocado pitted and cubed

Directions:

In a bowl, combine the beans with the aminos, cumin, salsa, lettuce, and avocado, toss, divide into bowls, and serve as a snack.

NUTRITION FACTS: CALORIES 181KCAL FAT 4 G CARBOHYDRATE 14 G PROTEIN 7 G

CHICKPEA FRITTERS

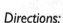 4 35 mins

Ingredients:

1 can chickpeas, drained
2 chicken breasts, cooked and shredded
2 egg whites
½ cup parsley, chopped
1 tsp. ginger
2 tbsp. coconut oil, for frying

Directions:

Blend the chickpeas in a food processor, combine them with the chicken, egg whites, parsley, and ginger into a smooth batter.

Heat the oil in a frying pan over medium heat. Using a spoon, scoop the batter into fritters.

Cook each one for 2-3 minutes each side or until golden and cooked through.

NUTRITION FACTS: CALORIES 207KCAL FAT 3.1 G CARBOHYDRATE 35.6 G PROTEIN 10.3 G

CACAO-COATED ALMONDS

🔥 10   🕐 25 mins

Ingredients:

¼ cup cocoa nibs
¼ cup light brown sugar
1 tsp. instant espresso powder
Pinch of salt
2 tsp. cornstarch
2 tsp. warm water
1 tbsp. pure agave syrup
1 tsp. pure vanilla extract, unsweetened
2 cups roasted whole almonds

Directions:

Preheat the oven to 325°F. Line a baking tray with parchment paper.

Place the cocoa nibs, sugar, espresso powder, and salt in a coffee grinder. Grind to turn into a fine powder.

In a bowl, whisk the cornstarch with the warm water until thoroughly combined. Stir the agave syrup and vanilla into the mixture. Add the almonds on top and fold until thoroughly coated.

Add the ground cacao mixture and combine until the almonds are thoroughly coated.

Place the almonds evenly on the baking tray. Toast for 10 minutes. Remove from the oven and stir gently. Toast for another 5 minutes or until the coating looks mostly dry. Be careful not to burn them. Let cool on the sheet. The coating will further harden once cooled. Store in an airtight container in the refrigerator for up to 2 weeks.

NUTRITION FACTS: CALORIES 132KCAL FAT 1 G CARBOHYDRATE 6 G PROTEIN 5 G

CHOC CHIP GRANOLA

  45 mins

Ingredients:

8 oz. jumbo oats
2 oz. pecans
3 tbsp. olive oil
1 oz. butter
1 tbsp. brown sugar
2 tbsp. rice malt syrup
2 oz. 70% chocolate chips

Directions:

Preheat the oven to 325°F. Line a baking tray with parchment paper.

Mix the oats and pecans in a bowl. In a skillet, gently warm the olive oil, butter, brown sugar, and rice malt butter till the butter has melted and the sugar and butter have simmered. Pour the syrup over the mix and stir thoroughly until the oats are fully covered.

Put the mix in a baking tray and bake it in the oven for about 30 minutes until golden brown at the edges. Remove from the oven and leave to cool entirely.

Once cool, gently divide lumps with your hands and mix in the chocolate chips. Put the granola in an airtight jar or tub. It will last around two weeks.

NUTRITION FACTS: CALORIES 220KCAL   FAT 8 G   CARBOHYDRATE 35 G   PROTEIN 6 G

CINNAMON APPLE CHIPS

 4   2h + 10 mins

Ingredients:
Cooking spray
2 teaspoons cinnamon powder
2 apples, cored and thinly sliced

Directions:
Arrange apple slices on a lined baking sheet, spray them with cooking oil, sprinkle cinnamon, introduce in the oven, and bake at 250°F for 2 hours. Divide into bowls and serve as a snack.

NUTRITION FACTS: CALORIES 80KCAL FAT 0.5 G CARBOHYDRATE 7 G PROTEIN 4 G

CINNAMON-SCENTED QUINOA

4   20 mins

Ingredients:
Chopped walnuts
1 ½ cup water
Agave syrup
2 cinnamon sticks
1 cup quinoa

Directions:
Add the quinoa to a bowl and wash it until the water is clear. Use a fine-mesh sieve to drain it.

Prepare your pressure cooker with a trivet and steaming basket. Place the quinoa and the cinnamon sticks in the basket and pour the water.

Close and lock the lid. Cook at high pressure for 6 minutes. When the cooking time is up, release the pressure using the quick-release method.

Fluff the quinoa with a fork and remove the cinnamon sticks. Divide the cooked quinoa among serving bowls and top with agave syrup and chopped walnuts.

NUTRITION FACTS: CALORIES 30KCAL FAT 0.4 G CARBOHYDRATE 4.5 G PROTEIN 1 G

COCOA BARS

🍽 12   🕐 10 mins + 12h

Ingredients:

1 cup dark chocolate chips
2 cups rolled oats
1 cup low-fat peanut butter
½ cup chia seeds
½ cup raisins
¼ cup of coconut sugar
½ cup of coconut milk

Directions:

Put 1 cup oats in the blender, pulse, and transfer to a bow.

Add the rest of the oats, cocoa chips, chia seeds, raisins, sugar, and milk, stir well, spread into a square pan, press well, keep in the refrigerator for 12 hours, slice into 12 bars, and serve.

Bars can also be put in the freezer.

NUTRITION FACTS: CALORIES 198KCAL FAT 5 G CARBOHYDRATE 10 G PROTEIN 89 G

CRUNCHY AND CHEWY GRANOLA

🍽 20   🕐 65 mins

Ingredients:

1 tbsp. flax seeds
¼ tsp. salt
½tsp. cinnamon
½ cup honey
2 tbsp. brown-sugar
¾ cup rolled oats
½ cup almonds, slivered
½ cup golden raisins
½ cup cranberries

Directions:

Pre-heat oven to 300°F. Line baking tray with parchment paper.

Mix flax seeds, cinnamon, honey, sugar oats, and almonds. Insert 1 cup hot water, then mix with hands. Spread into a thin layer over the baking tray.

Bake for 50 to 60 minutes until golden brown. Remove from the oven and let cool.

Stir in dried raisins and cranberries Put the granola in an airtight container. It will last around two weeks.

NUTRITION FACTS: CALORIES 233KCAL FAT 13 G CARBOHYDRATE 31 G PROTEIN 5 G

BELL PEPPER SNACK BOWLS

4   10 mins

Ingredients:

2 tbsp. dill, chopped
1 red onion, chopped
1 lb. bell peppers, cut into thin strips
3 tbsp. extra-virgin olive oil
2 ½ tbsp. red wine vinegar

Directions:

In a salad bowl, mix bell peppers with onion, dill, pepper, oil, and vinegar; toss to coat, divide into small bowls and serve as a snack.

NUTRITION FACTS: CALORIES 120KCAL FAT 3 G CARBOHYDRATE 2 G PROTEIN 3 G

HONEY CHILI NUTS

20   35 mins

Ingredients:

5 oz. walnuts
5 oz pecan nuts
2 oz. butter, softened
1 tbsp. honey
½ Bird's Eye chili, very finely chopped

Directions:

Preheat the oven to 360°F. Combine butter, honey, and chili in a bowl, then add the nuts and stir them well.

Spread the nuts onto a lined baking sheet and roast them in the oven for 10 minutes, stirring once halfway through. Remove from the oven and allow them to cool before eating.

NUTRITION FACTS: CALORIES 260KCAL FAT 15 G CARBOHYDRATE 20 G PROTEIN 6 G

NO-BAKE CHOCO CASHEW CHEESECAKE

 8   12h + 25 mins

Ingredients:

2 cups cashews
¼ cup coconut cream
¼ cup cocoa powder
¼ cup agave syrup
1 tsp. vanilla extract
1 ¼ cups walnuts
¼ cup chopped dates
¼ tsp. ground cinnamon
¼ cup almond meal

NUTRITION FACTS: CALORIES 168KCAL FAT 11 G
CARBOHYDRATE 11 G PROTEIN 7 G

Directions:

Line the bottom of four 4-inch springform pans with a parchment paper circle.

Place cashews, coconut cream, cocoa powder, agave syrup, and vanilla in a high-speed food processor. Repeat the process until it is entirely smooth, occasionally scraping the pieces with a rubber spatula. Transfer the mixture to a medium bowl and set aside. Clean the food processor or blender with a paper towel. This is the cream.

Place walnuts, dates, and cinnamon in the same food processor and blend quickly. This is the base.

Put the base mix in a baking tin. Create an even layer by pressing well. Pour in the cream and put it in the refrigerator for 12 hours before enjoying it.

POTATO BITES

 2   30 mins

Ingredients:

1 potato, sliced
2 bacon slices, cooked and crumbled
1 avocado, pitted and cubed
Cooking spray

Directions:

Spread potato slices on a lined baking sheet, spray with cooking oil, introduce in the oven at 350°F, bake for 20 minutes, arrange on a platter, top each slice with avocado and crumbled bacon, and serve as a snack.

NUTRITION FACTS: CALORIES 180KCAL FAT 4 G CARBOHYDRATE 8 G PROTEIN 6 G

PEAR, CRANBERRY, AND CHOCOLATE CRISP

 8   55 mins

Ingredients:

½ cup flour
½ cup brown sugar
1 tsp. cinnamon
⅛ tsp. salt
¾ cup yogurt
¼ cup apples
⅓ cup butter, melted
1 tsp. vanilla
1 tbsp. brown sugar
¼ cup cranberries
1 tsp. lemon juice
1 pear, diced
2 handfuls of dark chocolate chips

Directions:

Pre-heat oven to 375°F. Spray a casserole dish with a cooking spray. Put flour, sugar, cinnamon, salt, apple, yogurt, and butter into a bowl and mix. Pour it on a baking tray lined with parchment paper.

In a bowl, combine sugar, lemon juice, vanilla, pear, and cranberries. Pour this fruit mix along with chocolate chips over the baking tray. Bake for 45 minutes until golden. Cool before serving.

NUTRITION FACTS: CALORIES 239KCAL FAT 5 G CARBOHYDRATE 46 G PROTEIN 3 G

POWER BALLS

🍽 20   🕐 2h + 25 mins

Ingredients:
1 cup oats
¼ cup quinoa cooked using 3/4 cup orange juice
¼ cup shredded coconut
⅓ cup cranberry/raisin blend
⅓ cup dark chocolate chips
¼ cup slivered almonds
1 tbsp. peanut butter

Directions:
Cook quinoa in orange juice. Bring to boil and simmer for approximately 15 minutes. Let cool. Combine quinoa and the remaining ingredients in a bowl.

Wet hands and combine ingredients and roll into ball sized chunks. Put in a container and let cool in the fridge for at least 2 hours before eating them.

NUTRITION FACTS: CALORIES 189KCAL FAT 11 G CARBOHYDRATE 22 G PROTEIN 5 G

ROSEMARY & GARLIC KALE CHIPS

🍽 6   🕐 25 mins

Ingredients:
9 oz. kale chips, chopped
2 sprigs of rosemary
2 cloves of garlic
2 tbsp. olive oil

Directions:
Gently warm the olive oil, rosemary, and garlic over low heat for 10 minutes. Remove it from the heat and set aside to cool.

Take the rosemary and garlic out of the oil and discard them.

Toss the kale leaves in the oil, making sure they are well coated. Season with salt and pepper. Spread the kale leaves onto 2 baking sheets and bake them in the oven at 325°F for 10 minutes, until crispy.

NUTRITION FACTS: CALORIES 187KCAL FAT 13 G CARBOHYDRATE 14 G PROTEIN 6 G

SEED CRACKERS

🍽 20　　🕐 38 mins

Ingredients:

3 tbsp. white chia seeds
1/3 cup water
1/3 cup amaranth, cooked
1/3 cup whole-wheat flour,
3 tbsp. shelled hemp seeds
3 tbsp. golden roasted flaxseeds
2 tbsp. almond flour
1 1/2 tsp. nutritional yeast
1/3 tsp. fine sea salt
2 tbsp. olive oil

Directions:

Combine the chia seeds with the water in a bowl. Let stand 2 minutes to thicken.

Add flour, amaranth, hemp seeds, flaxseed, almond flour, yeast, and salt. Add the thick mixture of chia and oil on top. Use a blender to mix and form a very sticky dough.

Wrap it tightly in a plastic wrap and refrigerate for 2 hours or (better) overnight.

Heat the oven to 400°F. Line two baking trays with parchment paper. Divide the dough into 4 parts. Roll out one part, super-thin (0.5 inches), directly onto the baking tray. Use a cutter to cut the dough in rectangles.

Put the tray in the oven and bake for 8 minutes. Repeat until you cooked all the dough. Allow cooling on a rack before stacking in an airtight container at room temperature. They will last for 5 days.

NUTRITION FACTS: CALORIES 150KCAL FAT 8 G CARBOHYDRATE 15 G PROTEIN 4 G

SIRT MUESLI

 1   15 mins

Ingredients:
½ oz. buckwheat flakes
½ oz. buckwheat puffs
½ oz. shredded coconut
2 Medjool dates, pitted and chopped
4 walnuts, chopped
1 tbsp. cocoa nibs
4 oz. strawberries, hulled and chopped
4 oz. plain Greek yogurt

Directions:
Simply mix the dry ingredients and place them in an airtight container so that they are ready to eat. If you want, you can make it in bulk by multiplying the quantities.

To enjoy the sirt muesli, put the yogurt in a bowl, put strawberries on top, and then add the muesli.

NUTRITION FACTS: CALORIES 368KCAL FAT 16 G CARBOHYDRATE 54 G PROTEIN 26 G

SIRTFOOD BITES

 2   35 mins

Ingredients:
4 oz. walnuts
1 oz. 85% dark chocolate
8 oz. Medjool dates, pitted
1 tbsp. cocoa powder
1 tbsp. ground turmeric
1 tbsp. extra-virgin olive oil
1 tsp. vanilla extract, unsweetened
2 tbsp. water

Directions:
Put the walnuts and chocolate in a food processor and process until you have an even mixture.

Add all the remaining ingredients except water and combine until the mixture forms a disc.

Depending on the mixture's consistency, you may or may not have to add the water; you don't want it to be too sticky.

Shape the mixture into bite-sized balls using wet hands and roll them in cocoa powder.

Refrigerate for at least 1 hour in an airtight container before eating them.

They last up to 1 week in the refrigerator.

NUTRITION FACTS: CALORIES 127KCAL FAT 6 G CARBOHYDRATE 14 G PROTEIN 4 G

SIRTFOOD GRANOLA

  | ⏱ 55 mins

Ingredients:

7 oz. oats
9 oz. buckwheat flakes
3 ½ oz. walnuts, chopped
3 ½ oz. almonds, chopped
3 ½ oz. dried strawberries
1 ½ tsp. ground ginger
1 ½ tsp. ground cinnamon
4 fl. oz. extra-virgin olive oil
2 tbsp. honey (optional)

Directions:

Preheat oven to 300°F. Line a tray with parchment paper. Stir together walnuts, almonds, buckwheat flakes, and oats with ginger and cinnamon. In a pan, warm olive oil and honey, heating until the honey has dissolved.

Pour the honey-oil over the other ingredients, stirring to ensuring an even coating. Distribute the granola evenly over the lined baking tray and roast for 50 minutes, or until golden.

Remove from the oven and leave to cool. Once cooled, add the berries and store them in an airtight container. Eat dry or with milk and yogurt. It stays fresh for up to 1 week.

NUTRITION FACTS: CALORIES 178KCAL FAT 10.9 G CARBOHYDRATE 22 G PROTEIN 6.7 G

WALNUT ENERGY BAR

⊘ 4   ⏱ 35 mins

Ingredients:

4 oz. rolled oats
1 oz. shredded coconut
8 walnuts, chopped
½ cup almond milk, unsweetened
3 tbsp. agave syrup
1 pinch salt
½ tsp vanilla extract
1 tbsp. peanut butter

Directions:

Mix all the ingredients, put them on a baking tin lined with parchment paper, and cook 20-25 minutes at 325°F until golden and crisp.

NUTRITION FACTS: CALORIES 192KCAL FAT 4.3 G CARBOHYDRATE 32.8 G PROTEIN 6.6 G

SPELT AND SEED ROLLS

 9 3h +30 mins

Ingredients:

1 cup almond milk, unsweetened,
2 tsp apple cider vinegar
⅓ cup water, lukewarm
2 tbsp. neutral-flavored oil
2 tbsp. agave syrup
⅓ cup whole spelt flour
¼ cup oat flour or finely ground oats
¼ cup vital wheat gluten
3 tbsp. shelled hemp seeds
3 tbsp. sunflower seeds
2 tbsp. golden roasted flaxseeds
2 tbsp. chia seeds
1 tbsp. poppy seeds
1 tsp. fine sea salt
2 tsp. instant yeast

Directions:

Combine milk and vinegar in a measuring cup. Allow 5 minutes to curdle. Filter curd, add water, oil, and agave, and set aside. In a bowl, place flour, wheat gluten, seeds, salt, and yeast.

Mix them and then pour the wet mixture made with curd over the top.

Knead the dough with a stand mixer for 10 minutes until it becomes soft and not too dry or too sticky. If necessary, gently add 1 tbsp. of water until you get the desired result.

Cover and let it rest for 2 hours until doubled.

Divide the dough into 9 parts, give them the form of a roll, and put them on a tray to rest for 25 minutes.

While the rolls rise, heat the oven to 400°F. When hot, cook the rolls for 20 to 22 minutes.

Let cool on a rack.

NUTRITION FACTS: CALORIES 140KCAL FAT 6 G CARBOHYDRATE 14 G PROTEIN 10 G

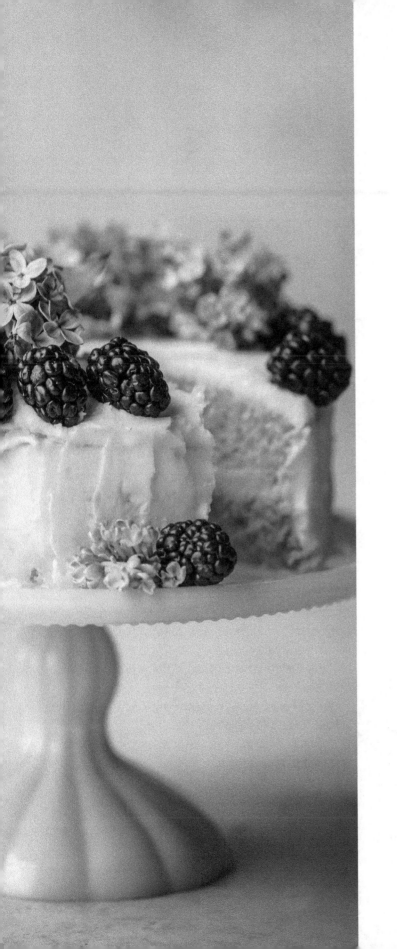

DESSERTS

BANANA AND BLUEBERRY MUFFINS

 12   50 mins

Ingredients:

4 ripe bananas, mashed
¾ cup of sugar
1 egg, lightly beaten
½ cup of peanut butter,
2 cups of blueberries
1 tsp. baking powder
1 tsp. baking soda
½ tsp. salt
1 cup of coconut, shredded
½ cup of flour
½ cup applesauce
Dab of cinnamon

Directions:

Add mashed banana to a mixing bowl. Insert sugar and egg and mix well. Add peanut butter and blueberries.

Add the dry ingredients into the wet mix and mix lightly.

Set into 12 greased muffin cups and bake for 20 to 25min at 350°F.

NUTRITION FACTS: CALORIES 250KCAL FAT 9 G CARBOHYDRATE 39 G PROTEIN 4 G

BANANA PECAN MUFFINS

8   45 mins

Ingredients:

3 tbsp. butter softened
4 ripe bananas
1 tbsp. honey
⅛ cup orange juice, unsweetened
1 tsp. cinnamon
2 cups flour
1 tbsp. instant yeast
2 pecans, sliced
1 tbsp. vanilla
2 eggs

Directions:

Preheat the oven to 350°F. Lightly oil sides and bottom of a muffin tin and dust with flour. Tap to remove any excess flour.

Peel the bananas and mash them in a bowl. Add flour and mix.

Add orange juice, butter, eggs, vanilla, yeast, and cinnamon and stir to combine.

Roughly chop the pecans onto a chopping board, add to the mix.

Fill each muffin tin 3/4 full and bake in the oven for approximately 40 minutes, or until golden.

NUTRITION FACTS: CALORIES 233KCAL FAT 9 G CARBOHYDRATE 31 G PROTEIN 7 G

BOUNTY BARS

 4   🕐 45 mins

Ingredients:

2 cups desiccated coconut
3 coconut oil - melted
1 cup of coconut cream - full fat
4 tsp. of honey
1 tsp. ground vanilla bean

Coating

Pinch of sea salt
½ cup cacao powder
2 tsp. honey
1/3 cup of coconut oil (melted)

Directions:

Mix coconut oil, coconut cream, and honey, vanilla, and salt. Pour over desiccated coconut and mix well.

Mold coconut mixture into balls and freeze. Or pour the whole mixture into a tray, freeze, and cut into small bars when frozen.

Prepare the coating by mixing salt, cocoa powder, honey, and coconut oil. Dip frozen coconut balls/bars into the chocolate coating, put on a tray, and freeze again.

NUTRITION FACTS: CALORIES 120KCAL FAT 4.3 G CARBOHYDRATE 16.7 G PROTEIN 1 G

CHOCOLATE BALLS

 6   🕐 15 mins

Ingredients:

2 oz. peanut butter (or almond butter)
1 oz. cocoa powder
1 oz. desiccated (shredded) coconut
1 tbsp. honey
1 tbsp. cocoa powder for coating

Directions:

Place the ingredients into a bowl and mix. Using a tsp, scoop out a little of the mixture and shape it into a ball.

Roll the ball in a bit of cocoa powder and set aside. Repeat for the remaining mixture.

It can be eaten straight away or stored in the refrigerator.

NUTRITION FACTS: CALORIES 240KCAL FAT 15 G CARBOHYDRATE 21 G PROTEIN 4 G

CHOCOLATE BROWNIES

 14   45 mins

Ingredients:

7 oz. dark chocolate (min 85% cocoa)
7oz. Medjool dates, pitted
3½ oz. walnuts, chopped
3 eggs
1 fl. oz. melted coconut oil
2 tsp. vanilla essence
½ tsp. baking soda

Directions:

Place the dates, chocolate, eggs, coconut oil, baking soda, and vanilla essence into a food processor and mix until smooth.

Stir the walnuts into the mixture. Pour the mixture into a lined baking tray and bake at 350°F for 25 to 30 minutes.

Allow it to cool. Cut into pieces and serve.

NUTRITION FACTS: CALORIES 188KCAL FAT 12 G CARBOHYDRATE 19 G PROTEIN 3 G

CHOCOLATE CASHEW TRUFFLES

 4   15 mins

Ingredients:

1 cup ground cashews
1 tsp. of ground vanilla bean
½ cup of coconut oil
¼ cup honey
2 tsp. flax meal
2 hemp hearts
2 tsp. cacao powder

Directions:

Mix all ingredients and make truffles by rolling small amounts of mixture into balls. Sprinkle coconut flakes on top.

NUTRITION FACTS: CALORIES 187KCAL FAT 16.5 G CARBOHYDRATE 6 G PROTEIN 2.3 G

CHOCOLATE CREAM

 4   5 mins

Ingredients:
1 avocado
2 tsp. coconut oil
2 tsp. honey
2 tsp. cacao powder
1 tsp. ground vanilla bean
Pinch of salt
¼ cup almond milk
¼ cup goji berries

Directions:
Blend all the ingredients in the food processor until smooth and thick.

Distribute in four cups, decorate with goji berries, and put the refrigerator overnight.

NUTRITION FACTS: CALORIES 200KCAL FAT 4.3 G CARBOHYDRATE 25.2 G PROTEIN 12.8 G

CHOCOLATE FONDUE

4   10 mins

Ingredients:
4 oz. dark chocolate
11 oz strawberries
7 oz. cherries
2 apples, peeled, cored, and sliced
3½ fl. oz. double cream

Directions:
Place the chocolate and cream into a saucepan and warm it until smooth and creamy. Serve in the fondue pot or transfer it to a serving bowl. Scatter the fruit on a serving plate, ready to be dipped into the chocolate..

NUTRITION FACTS: CALORIES 350KCAL FAT 10 G CARBOHYDRATE 23 G PROTEIN 2 G

CHOCOLATE CUPCAKES WITH MATCHA ICING

 12   35 mins

Ingredients:

5 oz. self-rising flour
5 oz. caster sugar
2 oz. 60g cocoa
½ tsp salt
½ tsp. espresso coffee
½ cup milk
½ tsp. vanilla extract, unsweetened
¼ cup vegetable oil
1 egg
⅜ cup boiling water

For the icing:

2 oz. butter at room temperature
2 oz. icing sugar
1 tbsp. matcha green tea powder
½ tsp. vanilla bean paste
2 tbsp. soft cream cheese

Directions:

Preheat the oven to 350°F. Line a cupcake tin with silicone or paper muffin cups. Put the flour, cocoa, sugar, salt, and espresso powder in a big bowl and mix.

Add the vanilla, vanilla extract, vegetable oil, and egg into the dry ingredients beat with an electric mixer until well blended. Add the boiling water gradually until thoroughly blended.

Keep mixing to add air bubbles to the batter. The batter will create more liquid than a standard cake mixture.

Spoon the batter evenly in the cupcake tin. Remember that each place must not be fuller than 3/4. Bake in the oven for about 15 to 18 minutes until the mix bounces back when exploited.

Remove from the oven and let it cool completely before icing.

To make the icing, cream the butter and icing sugar together until smooth and soft. Add matcha powder vanilla and stir. Ice the cupcakes.

NUTRITION FACTS: CALORIES 220KCAL FAT 8 G CARBOHYDRATE 33 G PROTEIN 4 G

CHOCOLATE HAZELNUTS TRUFFLES

🍽 12   🕐 15 mins

Ingredients:
1 cup ground almonds
1 tsp. ground vanilla bean
½ cup of coconut oil
½ cup mashed pitted dates
12 hazelnuts
2 tsp. cacao powder

Directions:
Mix all ingredients and make truffles with one hazelnut in the middle.

NUTRITION FACTS: CALORIES 70KCAL FAT 2.8 G CARBOHYDRATE 16.9 G PROTEIN 2.2 G

CHOCOLATE PIE

🍽 4   🕐 40 mins

Ingredients:
2 cups flour
1 cup dates, soaked and drained
1 cup dried apricots, chopped
1½ tsp. ground vanilla bean
2 eggs
1 banana, mashed
5 tsp. cocoa powder
3 tsp. honey
1 ripe avocado, mashed
2 tbsp. organic coconut oil
½ cup almond milk

Directions:
In a bowl, add flour, apricots, and dates finely chopped and mix. Add the banana and the eggs lightly beaten and mix.

Add vanilla, cocoa, honey, avocado, and coconut oil and mix.

Add almond milk bit by bit. You may need less than ½ cup to get the right "cake consistency."

Put in a greased baking tin and cook for 30 to 35 minutes at 350°F. Always check the cake and allow a few more minutes if it's not done.

Allow cooling before serving.

NUTRITION FACTS: CALORIES 380KCAL FAT 18.4 G CARBOHYDRATE 50.2 G PROTEIN 7.2 G

CHOCOLATE PUDDING WITH FRUIT

 2   2h + 5 mins

Ingredients:
1 avocado
2 tsp. honey
2 tbsp. coconut oil
3 tsp. cacao powder
1 tsp. ground vanilla bean
Pinch of sea salt
¼ cup of coconut milk

Fruits:
1 chopped banana
1 cup pitted cherries
1 tbsp. coconut flakes

Directions:
Blend all chocolate cream ingredients and divide them into two cups.

Put fruit chunks on top and sprinkle shredded coconut on top.

Place in the refrigerator at least 2 hours before serving.

NUTRITION FACTS: CALORIES 106KCAL FAT 5 G CARBOHYDRATE 20.4 G PROTEIN 14 G

CHOCOLATE WALNUT TRUFFLES

 4   15 mins

Ingredients:
1 cup ground walnuts
1 tsp. cinnamon
½ cup of coconut oil
¼ cup honey
2 tsp. chia seeds
2 tsp. cacao powder

Directions:
Mix all ingredients and make truffles. Coat with cinnamon, coconut flakes, or chopped almonds.

NUTRITION FACTS: CALORIES 120KCAL FAT 4.4 G CARBOHYDRATE 10.2 G PROTEIN 5.2 G

CRÈME BRÛLÉE

 4   13 mins

Ingredients:

14 oz. strawberries
11 oz. plain low-fat yogurt
4 oz. Greek yogurt
3½ oz. brown sugar
1 tsp. vanilla extract

Directions:

Divide the strawberries between 4 ramekin dishes.

In a bowl, combine the plain yogurt with the vanilla extract. Spoon the mixture onto the strawberries.

Scoop the Greek yogurt on top. Sprinkle the sugar over each dish, completely covering the top.

Place the dishes under a hot grill (broiler) for around 3 minutes or until the sugar has caramelized.

NUTRITION FACTS: CALORIES 311KCAL FAT 25 G CARBOHYDRATE 16 G PROTEIN 5 G

DARK CHOCOLATE MOUSSE

 4   2h + 5 mins

Ingredients:

1 (16 oz.) package silken tofu, drained
½ cup pure agave syrup
1 tsp. pure vanilla extract
¼ cup of soy milk
½ cup unsweetened cocoa powder
Mint leaves

Directions:

Place the tofu, agave syrup, and vanilla in a food processor or blender. Process until well blended.

Add remaining ingredients and process until the mixture is thoroughly blended.

Pour into small dessert cups or espresso cups. Chill for at least 2 hours. Garnish with fresh mint leaves just before serving.

NUTRITION FACTS: CALORIES 175KCAL FAT 24 G CARBOHYDRATE 18 G PROTEIN 5 G

DOUBLE ALMOND RAW CHOCOLATE TART

Co 4   45 mins

Ingredients:
1 ½ cups of almonds
¼ cup of coconut oil, melted
1 tbsp. honey
8 oz. dark chocolate, chopped
1 cup of coconut milk
½ cup unsweetened shredded coconut

Directions:
Crust:
Ground almonds and add melted coconut oil, honey, and combine. Using a spatula, spread this mixture into a pie pan.

Filling:
Put the chopped chocolate in a bowl, heat coconut milk and pour over chocolate and whisk together. Pour filling into tart shell. Refrigerate. Toast almond slivers chips and sprinkle over tart.

NUTRITION FACTS: CALORIES 291KCAL FAT 9.4 G CARBOHYDRATE 23.4 G PROTEIN 12.4 G

FROZEN BLACKBERRY CAKE

Co 4   55 mins

Ingredients:
¾ cup shredded coconut
15 dates
⅓ cup pumpkin seeds
¼ cup of coconut oil
Coconut whipped cream
1 lb. of frozen blackberries
¾ cup agave syrup
¼ cup of coconut cream
2 egg whites

Directions:
Grease the cake tin with coconut oil and mix all base ingredients in the blender until you get a sticky ball. Press the base mixture in a cake tin. Freeze. Make coconut whipped cream. Freeze.

Blitz berries and then add honey, coconut cream, and egg whites.

Pour middle filling - Coconut whipped cream in and spread evenly. Freeze. Pour top filling berries mixture-in the tin, spread, decorate with blueberries and almonds and return to freezer.

NUTRITION FACTS: CALORIES 472KCAL FAT 18 G CARBOHYDRATE 15.8 G PROTEIN 33.3 G

FRUIT SKEWERS & STRAWBERRY DIP

 6 　　 15 mins

Ingredients:
5 oz. red grapes
2 lb. pineapple, peeled and diced
14 oz. strawberries

Directions:
Place 3½ oz. of the strawberries into a food processor and blend until smooth. Pour the dip into a serving bowl. Skewer the grapes, pineapple chunks, and remaining strawberries onto skewers. Serve alongside the strawberry dip.

NUTRITION FACTS: CALORIES 131KCAL FAT 1 G CARBOHYDRATE 30 G PROTEIN 2 G

MANGO MOUSSE WITH CHOCOLATE CHIPS

 1 　　 5 mins

Ingredients:
1 cup mango
½ cup Greek yogurt
¼ tsp. vanilla extract
2 squares dark chocolate, chopped

Directions:
Blend mango, yogurt, and vanilla together. Add chocolate chips, and serve immediately.

NUTRITION FACTS: CALORIES 87KCAL FAT 1.1 G CARBOHYDRATE 11.8 G PROTEIN 1.6 G

MATCHA AND CHOCOLATE DIPPED STRAWBERRIES

 5   🕐 50 mins

Ingredients:

4 tbsp. cocoa butter
4 squares of dark chocolate,
¼ cup of coconut oil
1 tsp. matcha green tea powder
20 – 25 strawberries, stems on

Directions:

Melt cocoa butter, dark chocolate, coconut oil, and matcha until smooth. Remove from heat and continue stirring until chocolate is completely melted.

Pour into a glass bowl and continuously stir until the chocolate thickens and starts to lose its sheen, about 2 to 5 minutes.

One at a time, hold the strawberries by stems and dip into chocolate matcha mixture to coat. Let excess drip back into the bowl.

Place on a parchment-lined baking sheet and chill dipped berries in the fridge until the shell is set, 20 to 25 minutes.

NUTRITION FACTS: CALORIES 188KCAL FAT 5.3 G CARBOHYDRATE 10.9 G PROTEIN 0.2 G

MATCHA GREEN TEA MOCHI

 12 pieces   🕐 30 mins

Ingredients:

2 tbsp. matcha powder
1 cup superfine white rice flour
1 tsp. baking powder
1 cup coconut milk
½ cup sugar
2 tbsp. butter melted

Directions:

Heat your oven to 325 ° F. Grease your baking tin with a non-stick spray. Mix all the dry ingredients plus the sugar.

Whisk to blend, then add the coconut milk and melted butter. Stir well.

Place the mixture into a muffin baking tin and place in the oven to bake for approximately 20 minutes.

NUTRITION FACTS: CALORIES 100KCAL FAT 8 G CARBOHYDRATE 13 G PROTEIN 2 G

WALNUT CUPCAKES WITH MATCHA GREEN TEA ICING

🍽 24   🕐 45 mins

Ingredients:

For the Cupcakes:
2 cups of all-purpose flour
½ cup buckwheat flour
2 ½ tsp. baking powder
½ tsp. salt
1 cup of cocoa butter
1 cup white sugar
1 tbsp. pure agave syrup
3 eggs
2/3 cup milk
¼ cup walnuts, chopped

For the Icing:
3 tbsp. coconut oil, thick at room temperature
3 tbsp. icing sugar
1 tbsp. matcha green tea powder
½ tsp. vanilla bean paste
3 tbsp. cream cheese, softened

Directions:

Preheat oven to 350°F. Place paper baking cups into muffin tins for 24 regular-sized muffins. In a medium bowl, mix flours, baking powder, and salt.

In a separate bowl, mix sugar, butter, syrup, and eggs with a mixer. Add to the dry ingredients, mix, and add milk. Pour batter into muffin cup until 2/3 full.

Bake for 20 to 25 minutes or until an inserted toothpick comes out clean. Cool completely before icing. To Make the Icing: Add the coconut oil and icing sugar to a bowl and use a hand-mixer to cream until it's pale and smooth.

Fold in the matcha powder and vanilla. Finally, add the cream cheese and beat until smooth. Pipe or spread over the cupcakes once they are cold.

NUTRITION FACTS: CALORIES 164KCAL FAT 6 G CARBOHYDRATE 21 G PROTEIN 2 G

PEANUT BUTTER TRUFFLES

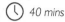 4   40 mins

Ingredients:
5 tbsp. peanut butter
1 tbsp. coconut oil
1 tbsp. honey
1 tsp. ground vanilla bean
¾ cup almond flour

<u>Coating</u>
Pinch of salt
1 tsp. cocoa butter
½ cup 70% chocolate

Directions:

Mix all ingredients into a dough.

Roll the dough into 1-inch balls, place them on parchment paper and refrigerate for half an hour (yield about 12 truffles).

Melted chocolate and cocoa butter, add a pinch of salt. Dip each truffle in the melted chocolate, one at the time. Place them back on the pan with parchment paper and place in the refrigerator.

NUTRITION FACTS: CALORIES 194KCAL FAT 8 G CARBOHYDRATE 13.1 G PROTEIN 4 G

SPICED POACHED APPLES

 4   20 mins

Ingredients:
4 apples
2 tbsp. honey
4-star anise
2 cinnamon sticks
1 cup green tea
¼ cup Greek yogurt

Directions:

Place the honey and green tea into a saucepan and bring to a boil. Add apples, star anise, and cinnamon. Reduce the heat and simmer gently for 15 minutes. Serve the apples with a dollop of Greek yogurt.

NUTRITION FACTS: CALORIES 180KCAL FAT 0.5 G CARBOHYDRATE 25 G PROTEIN 5 G

STRAWBERRY FROZEN YOGURT

🍳 4   🕐 3h + 5 mins

Ingredients:
1 lb. plain yogurt
6 oz. strawberries
Juice of 1 orange
1 tbsp. honey (optional)

Directions:
Place strawberries and orange juice in a food processor and blitz until smooth.

Filter the mixture through a sieve into a bowl to remove seeds. Stir in the honey and yogurt.

Transfer the mixture to an ice-cream maker and follow the manufacturer's instructions. Alternatively, pour the mixture into a container and place in the freezer for 1 hour.

Use a fork to whisk it and break up ice crystals and freeze for another 2 hours.

NUTRITION FACTS: CALORIES 100KCAL FAT 0.6 G CARBOHYDRATE 21 G PROTEIN 4 G

STRAWBERRY RHUBARB CRISP

🍳 8   🕐 55 mins

Ingredients:
1 cup white sugar
½ cup buckwheat flour + 3 tbsp.
3 cups strawberries, sliced
3 cups rhubarb, diced
½ lemon, juiced
1 cup packed brown sugar
1 cup coconut oil, melted
¾ cup rolled oats
¼ cup buckwheat groats
¼ cup walnuts, chopped

Directions:
Preheat oven to 375°F. In a bowl, mix white sugar, 3 tbsp. flour, strawberries, rhubarb, and lemon juice. Place the mixture in a 9x13 inch baking tray.

In a separate bowl, mix ½ cup flour, brown sugar, coconut oil, oats, buckwheat groats, and walnuts until crumbly.

Crumble on top of the rhubarb and strawberry mixture. Bake 45 minutes in the preheated oven, or until crisp and lightly browned.

NUTRITION FACTS: CALORIES 167KCAL FAT 3.1 G CARBOHYDRATE 58.3 G PROTEIN 3.5 G

WALNUT & DATE LOAF

 12   55 mins

Ingredients:
9 oz self-rising flour
4 oz. Medjool dates, chopped
2 oz. walnuts, chopped
8 fl. oz. milk
3 eggs
1 banana, mashed
1 tsp. baking soda

Directions:
Sift baking soda and flour into a bowl. Add in banana, eggs, milk, and dates and mix well. T ransfer the mixture to a lined loaf tin and smooth it out. Scatter the walnuts on top. Bake the loaf in the oven at 360°F for 45 minutes.

Transfer to a wire rack to cool before serving.

NUTRITION FACTS: CALORIES 186KCAL FAT 5 G CARBOHYDRATE 33 G PROTEIN 2 G

WARM BERRIES & CREAM

 4   15 mins

Ingredients:
9 oz. blueberries
9 oz. strawberries
3½ oz. redcurrants
3½ oz. blackberries
4 tbsp. whipped cream
1 tbsp. honey
Zest and juice of 1 orange

Directions:
Place all of the berries into a pan along with the honey and orange juice.

Gently heat the berries for around 5 minutes until warmed through.

Serve the berries into bowls and add a dollop of whipped cream on top.

NUTRITION FACTS: CALORIES 217KCAL FAT 2 G CARBOHYDRATE 30 G PROTEIN 2 G

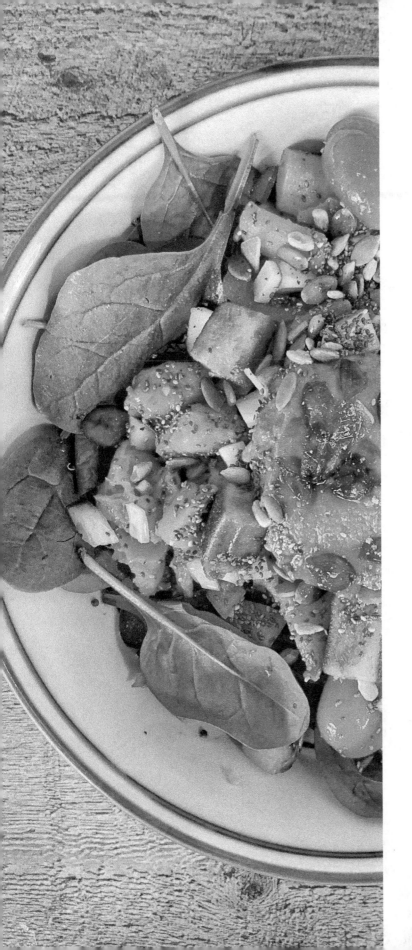

PLANT-BASED RECIPES

SMOOTHIES

APPLE AND AVOCADO SMOOTHIE

 2   5 mins

Ingredients:
1 apple, cored
½ avocado
2 cups baby spinach
8 oz. water
1 date

Directions:
Add all ingrediets to a high-power blender and pulse until smooth.

Pour the smoothie into two glasses and serve immediately.

It can be stored in the refrigerator in an airtight container for up to 3 days.

NUTRITION FACTS: CALORIES 108KCAL FAT 0.8 G CARBOHYDRATE 18.5 G PROTEIN 1.6 G

APPLE AND BERRIES SMOOTHIE

🥤 2   🕐 5 mins

Ingredients:

1 cup mixed berries (like raspberries, strawberries, and blueberries)
1 apple
2 cups greens
1 cup water
1 date

Directions:

Add all ingredients to a high-power blender and pulse until smooth.

Pour the smoothie into two glasses and serve immediately.

It can be stored in the refrigerator in an airtight container for up to 3 days.

NUTRITION FACTS: CALORIES 118KCAL FAT 0.8 G CARBOHYDRATE 19 G PROTEIN 3 G

APPLE AND BANANA SMOOTHIE

🥤 2   🕐 5 mins

Ingredients:

½ apple, cored
½ banana, peeled
1 and ½ cups baby spinach
1 tsp. ground cinnamon
1 date
8 oz. unsweetened almond milk

Directions:

Add all ingredients to a high-power blender and pulse until smooth.

Pour the smoothie into two glasses and serve immediately.

It can be stored in the refrigerator in an airtight container for up to 3 days.

NUTRITION FACTS: CALORIES 120KCAL FAT 0.6 G CARBOHYDRATE 19 G PROTEIN 2 G

APPLE JUICE MIX SMOOTHIE

🥤 2   🕐 5 mins

Ingredients:
1 ½ cups apple juice
2 cups kale
1 apple, peeled
½ avocado

Directions:
Add all ingredients to a high-power blender and pulse until smooth.

Pour the smoothie into two glasses and serve immediately.

It can be stored in the refrigerator in an airtight container for up to 3 days.

NUTRITION FACTS: CALORIES 106KCAL FAT 0.8 G CARBOHYDRATE 17 G PROTEIN 3 G

BANANA BERRY KALE SMOOTHIE

🥤 2   🕐 5 mins

Ingredients:
1 banana
1 cup strawberries
1 cup kale
1 cup ice

Directions:
Add all ingredients to a high-power blender and pulse until smooth.

Pour the smoothie into two glasses and serve immediately.

It can be stored in the refrigerator in an airtight container for up to 3 days.

NUTRITION FACTS: CALORIES 98KCAL FAT 0.5 G CARBOHYDRATE 15 G PROTEIN 2 G

BANANA-BERRY OATS SMOOTHIE

 2   5 mins

Ingredients:
½ banana, peeled
¼ cup rolled oats
½ cup raspberries
1 ½ cups kale
8 oz. unsweetened almond milk

Directions:
Add all ingredients to a high-power blender and pulse until smooth.

Pour the smoothie into two glasses and serve immediately.

It can be stored in the refrigerator in an airtight container for up to 3 days.

NUTRITION FACTS: CALORIES 139KCAL FAT 2 G CARBOHYDRATE 19 G PROTEIN 4 G

BANANA FLAX SMOOTHIE

 2   5 mins

Ingredients:
2 cups kale
½ cup blueberries
1 frozen banana
1 tbsp. flax seeds
1 cup water

Directions:
Add all ingredients to a high-power blender and pulse until smooth.

Pour the smoothie into two glasses and serve immediately.

It can be stored in the refrigerator in an airtight container for up to 3 days.

NUTRITION FACTS: CALORIES 138KCAL FAT 4 G CARBOHYDRATE 18 G PROTEIN 4 G

FRESH GREENS SMOOTHIE

🍽 2   🕐 5 mins

Ingredients:
1 handful of greens, including kale
½ lime, peeled
1-inch ginger, fresh
½ cucumber, peeled
1 cup coconut water
1 date

Directions:
Add all ingredients to a high-power blender and pulse until smooth.

Pour the smoothie into two glasses and serve immediately.

It can be stored in the refrigerator in an airtight container for up to 3 days.

NUTRITION FACTS: CALORIES 105KCAL FAT 0.8 G CARBOHYDRATE 14 G PROTEIN 2 G

KALE BERRY DELIGHT SMOOTHIE

🍽 2   🕐 5 mins

Ingredients:
1 cup blueberries
1 apple
2 cups kale
1 cup strawberries
1 cup coconut milk

Directions:
Add all ingredients to a high-power blender and pulse until smooth.

Pour the smoothie into two glasses and serve immediately.

It can be stored in the refrigerator in an airtight container for up to 3 days.

NUTRITION FACTS: CALORIES 109KCAL FAT 0.9 G CARBOHYDRATE 17 G PROTEIN 2 G

LOW-CARB CHOCOLATE SMOOTHIE

🍹 2   🕐 5 mins

Ingredients:
1 banana, peeled
¼ avocado
1 tbsp. cacao powder
2 cups baby spinach
1 date
8 oz. almond milk, unsweetened

Directions:
Add all ingredients to a high-power blender and pulse until smooth.

Pour the smoothie into two glasses and serve immediately.

It can be stored in the refrigerator in an airtight container for up to 3 days.

NUTRITION FACTS: CALORIES 124KCAL FAT 1 G CARBOHYDRATE 20 G PROTEIN 3 G

MANGO BANANA SMOOTHIE

🍹 2   🕐 5 mins

Ingredients:
1 mango
½ banana
2 cups greens, including kale
1 cup water

Directions:
Add all ingredients to a high-power blender and pulse until smooth.

Pour the smoothie into two glasses and serve immediately.

It can be stored in the refrigerator in an airtight container for up to 3 days.

NUTRITION FACTS: CALORIES 126KCAL FAT 1 G CARBOHYDRATE 23 G PROTEIN 1 G

PEANUT BUTTER CUP SMOOTHIE

 2   5 mins

Ingredients:

1 pear, cored
1 tbsp. all-natural peanut butter
½ tbsp. cacao powder
2 cups baby spinach
8 oz. almond milk, unsweetened

Directions:

Add all ingredients to a high-power blender and pulse until smooth.

Pour the smoothie into two glasses and serve immediately.

It can be stored in the refrigerator in an airtight container for up to 3 days.

NUTRITION FACTS: CALORIES 202KCAL FAT 4 G CARBOHYDRATE 21 G PROTEIN 9 G

RASPBERRY GREENS SMOOTHIE

 2   5 mins

Ingredients:

1 handful leafy greens
1 cup raspberries , frozen
2 tbsp. lime juice
1 cup coconut milk

Directions:

Add all ingredients to a high-power blender and pulse until smooth.

Pour the smoothie into two glasses and serve immediately.

It can be stored in the refrigerator in an airtight container for up to 3 days.

NUTRITION FACTS: CALORIES 110KCAL FAT 0.7 G CARBOHYDRATE 16 G PROTEIN 1 G

SUMMERTIME REFRESH SMOOTHIE

🍶 2   🕐 5 mins

Ingredients:
1 peach, pitted
1 cup strawberries
1 ½ cups kale
8 oz. almond milk, unsweetened

Directions:
Add all ingredients to a high-power blender and pulse until smooth.

Pour the smoothie into two glasses and serve immediately.

It can be stored in the refrigerator in an airtight container for up to 3 days.

NUTRITION FACTS: CALORIES 124KCAL FAT 0.7 G CARBOHYDRATE 21 G PROTEIN 1 G

STRAWBERRY-FIG SMOOTHIE

🍶 2   🕐 5 mins

Ingredients:
½ banana, peeled
2 fresh figs
4 strawberries
2 cups baby spinach
8 oz. almond milk, unsweetened

Directions:
Add all ingredients to a high-power blender and pulse until smooth.

Pour the smoothie into two glasses and serve immediately.

It can be stored in the refrigerator in an airtight container for up to 3 days.

NUTRITION FACTS: CALORIES 136KCAL FAT 0.5 G CARBOHYDRATE 23 G PROTEIN 2 G

MAIN DISHES

ASPARAGUS SEITAN WITH BLACK BEAN SAUCE 5 *35 mins*

Ingredients:

½ cup veggie broth
1 tbsp. soy sauce
1 tbsp. cornstarch
2 cups seitan, sliced
2 tsp. red wine
1 tsp. water
1 tsp. cornstarch
1 tsp. soy sauce
1 tbsp. extra-virgin oil
2 cloves garlic, diced or crushed
2 tsp. black beans, mashed
1 lb. asparagus, into 1-inch pieces

Directions:

Add the cooking sauce in a bowl and set aside

Stir the seitan slices with the sherry, 1 tsp. water, 1 tsp. cornstarch and 1 tsp. soy sauce in a bowl.

Heat a skillet over high heat with oil. When hot, add the garlic and black beans, mash, and sauté for 1 minute. Add the seitan and cook for another 4 minutes until golden on all sides.

Add the asparagus and the onion to the pan and stir-fry for 2 minutes. Add 2 tbsps. water, cover, and cook for another 2 minutes.

Add back the seitan stir-fry and cook until the juices of the veggies have thickened thanks to cornstarch.

Serve hot.

NUTRITION FACTS: CALORIES 340KCAL FAT 5 G CARBOHYDRATE 20 G PROTEIN 18 G

BAKED CABBAGE WITH BUCKWHEAT AND WALNUTS

🍲 4   🕐 32 mins

Ingredients:

1 lb. white or green cabbage, finely chopped
1 onion, finely chopped
2 cups buckwheat, cooked
1 cup vegetable stock
1 cup boiling water
2 oz. walnuts
2 tbsp. extra-virgin olive oil
2 oz. raisins

Directions:

Cook the finely chopped onion in some olive oil until it is transparent. Add the cabbage, then add the stock season with salt and pepper to taste.

Simmer for 20 minutes on low heat until the cabbage is still crunchy.

Move the cabbage to an ovenproof dish. While the cabbage is cooking, boil buckwheat in salted water, drain, and stir in the walnuts and raisins.

Spread the buckwheat over the cabbage, and cook for 20 minutes in the oven at 350°F.

NUTRITION FACTS: CALORIES 199KCAL FAT 5 G CARBOHYDRATE 20 G PROTEIN 18 G

BROUSSARD BLACK-EYED PEAS

🍲 4   🕐 25 mins

Ingredients:

1 red onion, diced
1 bell pepper, diced
2 stalks celery, diced
1 tbsp. extra-virgin olive oil
2 cups black-eyed peas, cooked
1/3 cup green onions, diced
1/3 cup fresh parsley, chopped
3/4 tsp. salt
1/4 tsp. cayenne
8 cups water

Directions:

Sauté the celery, onion, and bell peppers in a pot with the oil. Add the water, black-eyed peas, green onions, salt, pepper, and cayenne, bring to a boil, and lower the heat to a simmer.

Cook for about 45 minutes until the liquid becomes creamy. Serve hot.

NUTRITION FACTS: CALORIES 199KCAL FAT 5 G CARBOHYDRATE 20 G PROTEIN 18 G

BEEFLESS STEW

 4　　　🕐 55mins

Ingredients:

1 cup dry soy "beef" protein chunks
1 tsp. lemon juice
1 red onion, chopped
1 garlic clove, diced
1 tbsp. extra-virgin olive oil
4 cups water
14 oz. tomatoes
1 tsp. vegan Worcestershire sauce
1 bay leaf
10 oz. peas
6 carrots, chopped
1 stalk celery
3 potatoes, chopped into bite-sized pieces
2 tbsp. cornstarch

Directions:

Put the textured vegetable protein chunks in boiling water and lemon juice. Set aside for 15 minutes. Heat a pan with the oil and sautè the onion and garlic. Add the soy chunks and cook for another 5 minutes.

Add 4 cups of water, tomatoes, Worcestershire sauce, bay leaf, salt, pepper, and simmer for 5 minutes. Add the peas, potatoes, and carrots, and cook 30 minutes.

Thicken with the cornstarch dissolved in a few drops of water.

NUTRITION FACTS: CALORIES 199KCAL FAT 5 G CARBOHYDRATE 20 G PROTEIN 18 G

CABBAGE ROLLS

🍽 4   🕐 1h + 15 mins

Ingredients:

½ red onion, diced
2 tbsp. extra-virgin olive oil
6 tomatoes, diced
2 tsp. paprika
¼ tsp. cayenne
½ tsp. turmeric
1 head cabbage, shredded
2 tbsp. extra-virgin olive oil
3 green onions, diced
2 cloves garlic, diced
1 cup tofu, crumbled
2 tomatoes, diced
4 cups rice, cooked
⅓ cup fresh parsley, chopped
2 tsp. salt
2 tsp. paprika
¼ tsp. cayenne

NUTRITION FACTS: CALORIES 350KCAL FAT 7 G CARBOHYDRATE 20 G PROTEIN 22 G

Directions:

Sautè tomatoes with onions, add 1 cup boiling water, and let simmer for 30 minutes.

Remove the cabbage's core and steam the whole head in a pot with the core side down for 20 minutes. Let cool.

Heat a skillet with oil, and when hot, sauté the onion for 5 minutes. Add the salt, paprika, cayenne, green onions, garlic, tofu, water, and simmer for 15 minutes on low heat. Add the rice and stir well.

Preheat the oven to 350°F.

Carefully separate cabbage leaves, pain attention to keep them whole. Put some of the rice stir-fry on each leaf but leave enough room to fold the sides inward create a roll.

Place the cabbage rolls onto a baking tray and cover with the tomato sauce.

Bake for 30 minutes.

CAJUN TOFU

 4   🕐 35 mins

Ingredients:

2 stalks celery, thinly chopped
1 red onion, thinly chopped
2 bell peppers, thinly chopped
2 lbs. firm tofu, diced
2 tomatoes, diced
3 tsp. paprika
3/4 tsp. thyme
¼ tsp. cayenne
½ cup parsley, chopped
3 tbsp. extra-virgin olive oil
⅓ cup water

Directions:

Sauté the onion, bell pepper, and celery in a saucepan with oil for 5 minutes. Add the tofu and sauté until it begins to brown on all sides.

Add tomatoes, paprika, thyme, cayenne, and water and simmer on low heat for 25 minutes. Top with parsley.

It can be served over rice or as a side dish.

NUTRITION FACTS: CALORIES 199KCAL FAT 5 G CARBOHYDRATE 20 G PROTEIN 18 G

CHICKPEA PITA POCKETS

 4   🕐 15 mins

Ingredients:

1 16 oz. can chickpeas, cooked
⅓ cup celery, chopped
1 tbsp. red onion, chopped
2 tbsp. pickle relish
2 tbsp. vegan mayonnaise
1 tsp. mustard
Dash of garlic powder
4 whole-wheat pitas
4 leaves lettuce
1 tomato, sliced
1 carrot, grated

Directions:

Mash the chickpeas with a potato masher or quickly blend them in a blender without making them too smooth.

Add the mash to a bowl and add celery, onion, relish, mayonnaise, mustard, and garlic powder. Stir well, then season with salt and pepper to taste.

Cut the pitas in half and fill them with 1/4 of the chickpea spread, top with lettuce, tomato, and carrot and serve immediately.

NUTRITION FACTS: CALORIES 199KCAL FAT 5 G CARBOHYDRATE 20 G PROTEIN 18 G

CARIBBEAN YELLOW AND GREEN SPLIT PEA BUCKWHEAT

 4   40 mins

Ingredients:

3 cups buckwheat
4 oz. yellow split peas
4 oz. green split peas
½ a red pepper, diced
½ a green pepper, diced
3 cardamom pods
2 garlic cloves, chopped
1 pinch of saffron
1 vegetable stock cube
1 ½ pints vegetable stock
1 red onion, chopped
1 handful parsley, chopped
2 tbsp. extra-virgin olive oil

Directions:

Heat a saucepan with oil and sauté the onion and garlic for 3 minutes. Add the split peas, buckwheat, peppers, and continue to sauté for a few minutes more.

Pour in the stock and add the cardamom pods, a saffron pinch for color, salt, and pepper to taste. Cook on medium for 35 minutes, then remove the cardamom and mix the rice with a fork to make the rice light and fluffy.

A nice idea for serving is using bowls filled with rice to turn onto plates or serving dish. Trim with parsley leaves.

Serve hot.

NUTRITION FACTS: CALORIES 199KCAL FAT 5 G CARBOHYDRATE 20 G PROTEIN 18 G

COLORFUL QUINOA SALAD

 4   🕐 25 mins

Ingredients:

1 cup dried red quinoa
2 cups of water
2 scallions, chopped
2 carrots, grated
1 stalk celery
1 beet, grated
1/3 cup fresh parsley, chopped
1/3 cup cranberries
1/3 cup walnuts, chopped
2 tbsp. olive oil
1 tsp. toasted sesame oil
2 tsp. lemon juice

Directions:

Cook the quinoa in salted water (1 cup quinoa and 2 cups of water) for about 25 minutes until the water is absorbed. Make it fluffy by mixing it gently with a fork.

Add scallions, carrots, beet, parsley, cranberries, and walnuts, tossing to mix.

In a separate bowl, prepare the dressing. Whisk the olive oil, sesame oil, lemon juice, and salt and pepper to taste. Pour over quinoa and toss to distribute it evenly.

Serve immediately, or refrigerate for a couple of hours.

NUTRITION FACTS: CALORIES 230KCAL FAT 3 G CARBOHYDRATE 24 G PROTEIN 13 G

CREOLE TOFU

 6   🕐 25 mins

Ingredients:

2 lbs. tofu, chopped 1/4 inch thick
2 tbsp. extra-virgin olive oil
1 red onion diced
3 cloves garlic, crushed
1 bell pepper diced
2 stalks celery, diced
1/4 tsp. cayenne
1/4 tbsp. chili powder
1/4 cup garlic powder
2 bay leaves
6 tomatoes, diced
1/2 lemon, thinly chopped
1/4 cup parsley, chopped

Directions:

Heat a saucepan with 1 tbsp. oil and sauté the tofu until golden. Set aside. Add garlic, onion, celery, bell pepper, cayenne, chili, garlic powder in the remaining oil and sauté for 5 minutes. Add the tomatoes with a splash of water and cook for 15 minutes. Add the tofu, lemon, parsley, heat through.

Very good when served over hot rice or steamed buckwheat.

NUTRITION FACTS: CALORIES 199KCAL FAT 5 G CARBOHYDRATE 20 G PROTEIN 18 G

CRISPY TOFU CUBES

 4   🕐 35 mins

Ingredients:
1 lb. firm tofu
2 tbsp. nutritional yeast
2 tbsp. flour
1 tbsp. garlic powder
1 tsp. pepper
2 tbsp. extra-virgin olive oil

Directions:
Cut the tofu into 1/4-inch cubes. Do not pat dry. Put the flour in a bowl, add the nutritional yeast, garlic, pepper, mix with a fork, add the tofu, and coat it well on all sides.

Heat the oil in a saucepan. Cook the tofu over medium heat, turning it after 2-3 minutes until crispy.

NUTRITION FACTS: CALORIES 192KCAL FAT 5 G CARBOHYDRATE 20 G PROTEIN 18 G

DELICIOUS JAMAICA

 4   35 mins

Ingredients:
1 lb. yams
2 medium carrots
1 stick celery, diced
1 red onion, chopped
1 tbsp. sweet pepper, seeded and chopped
1 tsp. hot pepper, seeded and chopped
1 sprig fresh thyme
6 pimento grains
2 cloves garlic, crushed and chopped
3 tomatoes, chopped
1 cup coconut milk peel,

Directions:
Preheat the oven to 350°F. Cut the yams and carrots. Boil the yams until firm and tender. Stir together the onion, celery, salt, sweet pepper, hot pepper, thyme, and garlic

Grease a casserole and place in it alternating layers of yams, carrots, tomatoes, and seasoning stir

Cover the casserole with coconut milk and bake until done (about 25 minutes).

NUTRITION FACTS: CALORIES 316KCAL FAT 5.2 G CARBOHYDRATE 13.1 G PROTEIN 7 G

EGGPLANT, TOMATO, AND ONION GRATIN

 6 35 mins

Ingredients:

3 red onions, chopped
3 cloves garlic, crushed
3 tbsp. extra-virgin olive oil
3 sprigs thyme
3 eggplants, sliced
3 ripe tomatoes, sliced

NUTRITION FACTS: CALORIES 316KCAL FAT 5.2 G
CARBOHYDRATE 13.1 G PROTEIN 7 G

Directions:

Fry onion and garlic in 1 tbsp. oil over medium heat for about 5 minutes until soft, then add thyme, salt, and pepper to taste.

Preheat oven to 400°F. Use 1 tbsp. oil to grease a gratin dish and spread the onions on it.

Alternate tomato and eggplant slices, overlapping them by 2/3, and season with salt and pepper.

Drizzle the remaining 1 tbsp. olive oil on top, and cook, covered with tin foil, until the eggplant is soft enough to be cut with a fork, about 30 minutes.

Uncover and cook for another 15 minutes or more until the liquid is absorbed. The time depends on the vegetables and on the juices they release.

FAVA BEANS AND TOMATOES

 4 75 mins

Ingredients:

4 tbsp. extra-virgin olive oil
2 onions, finely chopped
2 cloves garlic, crushed
2 cups fava beans, shelled
2 tbsps. parsley, chopped
2 cups tomatoes, diced
¼ tsp. chili flakes
½ tsp. cumin

Directions:

Stir fry onions and garlic in a saucepan with oil until they begin to brown, about 5 minutes. Add the fava beans and parsley and cook 5 more minutes.

Add tomatoes, chili, cumin, and enough water to cover beans and bring to a boil. Turn heat to low and simmer for about an hour until fava beans are tender.

Serve hot or cold.

NUTRITION FACTS: CALORIES 189KCAL FAT 5 G CARBOHYDRATE 18 G PROTEIN 14 G

FAVA BEAN RAGOUT WITH POTATO GNOCCHI

 6   55 mins

Ingredients:

2,2 lbs. Desiree potatoes
4 oz. plain flour
1 tsp. turmeric
3 lbs. fava beans, shelled
1 garlic clove, crushed
1 sprig of rosemary
2 tbsp. extra-virgin olive oil
½ lemon

Directions:

Cook the potatoes, whole, for 25 minutes or until tender (it depends on the size of the potatoes, so be sure to prick them to check them before draining them).

Drain the potatoes, then mash them in a big bowl. Let cool for 5 minutes, then add the flour and season. Work the mixture into a dough, divide it into 6 parts and roll them into sausages. Let sit for 5 minutes, then cut into 1-inch pieces.

Put the fava beans in a saucepan, add half the oil, rosemary, salt, pepper, and enough water to cover them.

Bring to a simmer, and cook for 10 minutes until the beans are tender. Crush them with a fork or blend quickly to leave some chunks.

Cook the gnocchi in salted boiling water until they rise to the surface. When this happens, remove them immediately from the water and set them aside until all of them have cooked.

Stir the gnocchi with the beans and finish with a squeeze of lemon juice and another grind or two of the pepper.

NUTRITION FACTS: CALORIES 387KCAL FAT 5 G CARBOHYDRATE 28 G PROTEIN 15 G

FRIED RICE WITH HOT LEEK SAUCE

 4   55 mins

Ingredients:

1 tbsp. cornstarch
2 tsp. extra-virgin olive oil
1 leek diced
1-inch ginger, peeled and diced
1 Bird's Eye chili, chopped
3 tbsp. garlic, chopped
¼ cup teriyaki sauce
2 tbsp. extra-virgin olive oil
6 scallions, diced
16 oz. firm tofu, cubed
½ cup cashews
½ cup walnuts
2 carrots, shredded
2 celery stalks, thinly chopped
1 cup mushrooms, chopped
15 oz. baby corn
2 broccoli, cut into florets
3 cups rice, cooked

Directions:

Heat oil in a saucepan over medium heat. Add the leek, ginger, and chili and sauté for 5 to 7 minutes, or until the leek is golden brown. Add the teriyaki sauce and cornstarch dissolved in a little water and cook for 2 to 3 minutes until the sauce thickens. Set aside.

Heat 2 tbsp. oil in another pan. Add the ginger, scallions, and garlic and sauté for 3 minutes. Add the tofu and cook for 8 to 10 minutes, until brown on all sides.

Add the cashews, walnuts, celery, mushrooms, broccoli, baby corn, and carrots and sauté for 10 minutes over high heat. Add teriyaki sauce and cooked rice. Stir well and sauté for 7 to 10 minutes or until the veggies are cooked and crispy.

Serve fried rice with the sauce on the side.

NUTRITION FACTS: CALORIES 402KCAL FAT 6 G CARBOHYDRATE 30 G PROTEIN 17 G

GRILLED ASPARAGUS WITH TAPENADE TOAST

 4   🕐 45 mins

Ingredients:

1 scallion
2 blood oranges
1 ½ tsp. balsamic vinegar
½ tsp. red wine vinegar
4 tsp. extra-virgin olive oil
1 ½ lbs. asparagus (25 –30 spears)
4 slices bread
2 cups black olives,
1 garlic clove

NUTRITION FACTS: CALORIES 199KCAL FAT 5 G
CARBOHYDRATE 20 G PROTEIN 18 G

Directions:

Blend olives, garlic, olive oil together to prepare the tapenade.

Peel and cut the scallion fine and macerate for 30 minutes in the juice of ½ orange and the balsamic and red wine vinegar. Add the olive oil with salt and pepper to taste and whisk to make a vinaigrette.

Grate the zest of 1 orange and add it to the vinaigrette.

Peel the oranges and slice them. Cut the bottom ends of the asparagus spears, brush them with olive oil and grill them for 5 minutes, until evenly brown.

Toast bread, cut it diagonally, and put the tapenade on top. Arrange asparagus on a platter with the orange cuts on top and the tapenade toasts on the side.

Drizzle vinaigrette over and serve.

HOT GARBANZO BEANS WITH SUN-DRIED TOMATOES

 2   🕐 37 mins

Ingredients:

2 tbsp. olive oil
4 sun-dried tomatoes, thinly chopped
2 garlic cloves, thinly chopped
½ red onion, thinly chopped
1 tsp. chili flakes
16 oz. garbanzo beans, cooked

Directions:

Sautè the onion, garlic, chili flakes, and sun-dried tomatoes in a hot pan with oil.

Add the garbanzo beans and cook for 5 minutes. Add 1 cup and simmer for 10 minutes, until the liquid is almost gone.

Add salt and black pepper to taste and serve immediately.

NUTRITION FACTS: CALORIES 268KCAL FAT 5 G CARBOHYDRATE 29 G PROTEIN 12 G

HOT CURRY

 6   50 mins

Ingredients:

19 oz. chickpeas, cooked
10 oz. frozen spinach
1 Bird's Eye chili, diced
2 garlic cloves, diced
3 white onions, diced
2 carrots, chopped
1 yellow bell pepper, chopped
½ cup almonds
½ cup golden raisins
2 tsp. ground cumin
1 tsp. ground parsley
1 tsp. turmeric
1 tbsp. paprika
3 tbsp. extra-virgin olive oil
¼ tsp. ground ginger
1 cup water
1 cup coconut milk
3 cups buckwheat

Directions:

Boil buckwheat in salted water for 35 minutes, then drain and set aside.

In a saucepan, allow the spinach to thaw on medium heat for 10 minutes. Set aside. In the same pan, add the oil, and when hot, add chili, garlic, and onions and sauté for 3 minutes. Add the carrots and sauté for 5 minutes.

Add the golden raisins, almonds, and garbanzo beans and stir well. Sauté for 1 minute. Add the turmeric, cumin, ginger, and paprika and. sauté for 1 minute. Add the spinach and cook for 5 minutes. Add coconut milk and the bell pepper, reduce heat to low, and simmer for 15 minutes.

Serve hot with buckwheat.

NUTRITION FACTS: CALORIES 199KCAL   FAT 5 G   CARBOHYDRATE 20 G   PROTEIN 18 G

GREEK-STYLE MACARONI CASSEROLE

 8   🕐 1h

Ingredients:

1 lb. seitan
16 oz. buckwheat macaroni
3 tbsp. olive oil
1 ½ tsp. soy sauce
1 cup buckwheat breadcrumbs
1 ½ tbsp. arrowroot
1 ½ cups water
1 ½ cups plain soymilk
1 tbsp. tahini
2 tbsp. capers
2 tbsp. black olives, pitted and chopped

Directions:

Pulse the seitan in a blender to crumble it.
Preheat oven to 400°F.

Cook the pasta al dente in salted boiling water for 8 minutes, then drain it and put it in a bowl.

Heat a skillet with oil, then add the seitan and fry it for 3 to 4 minutes, then add the soy sauce. Add the seitan to the pasta bowl, mix well, and set aside.

Dissolve the arrowroot in a few spoons of water. In a saucepan, heat the soymilk, 1/2 cup water, tahini, olives, capers, salt, and pepper to taste.

Add the arrowroot dissolved in a few spoons of water and cook 2 to 3 minutes until the sauce thickens.

Grease a baking dish with 1 tsp. oil and assemble the casserole by creating 2 layers.

First, spread half the pasta-seitan mix on the dish. Then pour half the sauce on top. Cover with the pasta and spread the remaining sauce. Spread breadcrumbs on top.

Bake for 35 to 40 minutes until the crust is brown and crispy. Serve hot.

NUTRITION FACTS: CALORIES 199KCAL FAT 5 G CARBOHYDRATE 20 G PROTEIN 18 G

INDIAN PLANT-BASED MEATBALLS

 2   35 mins

Ingredients:

1 cup cauliflower
1 cup brown rice
¼ cup breadcrumbs
2 tbsp. chickpea flour
½ tsp. turmeric
1 tsp. smoked paprika
1 tsp. of extra-virgin olive oil
1 cloves garlic crushed
1 cup tomato sauce
Broth (if needed)
1 tbsp. extra-virgin olive oil
1 ½ tbsp. garam masala
1 tsp ginger
1 tbsp. parsley, chopped
1 red onion-diced
6 oz. full-fat coconut milk

Directions:

Whisk chickpea flour with 4 tbsp. water and let sit 5 minutes. Steam cauliflower for 5 minutes, then blend it with rice. Use pulse to get a result similar to mince. Add chickpea batter, breadcrumbs, 1 garlic clove, salt, pepper, turmeric, paprika, and finely chopped parsley.

Mix well until you can form meatballs. Note: if it's too dry, add 1 tbsp. egg white and mix. If it's too runny, add 1 tbsp. breadcrumbs and mix. Spray a pan with cooking spray, heat it, and gently cook the meatballs for 5 minutes until golden. Be careful when you turn them so that they don't break. Put them aside

In a different pan, put oil, onion, ginger, garlic, salt, and pepper and cook on low heat until the onion is done. Add tomato sauce and coconut milk and let it simmer around 15 minutes until thickened. Put the meatballs in the sauce and cook another 5 minutes before serving.

NUTRITION FACTS: CALORIES 412KCAL FAT 7.8 G CARBOHYDRATE 39.1 G PROTEIN 18.3 G

LAFAYETTE LIMA BEANS

 4   95 mins

Ingredients:

1 red onion diced
2 tbsp. extra-virgin olive oil
8 cups water
2 cups dry lima beans, soaked overnight
1 bell pepper diced
4 cloves garlic, diced
¼ tsp. cayenne

Directions:

Sauté the onion for 10 minutes on low heat in a pan with oil. Add bell pepper, garlic, cayenne, beans, and water. Bring to a boil and cook for 75 minutes on low heat. Season with salt and pepper and cook for another 15 minutes.

Serve with cornbread.

NUTRITION FACTS: CALORIES 298KCAL FAT 5 G CARBOHYDRATE 31 G PROTEIN 12 G

LENTILS AND CHICKPEAS STEW

6   50 mins

Ingredients:

4 tbsp. extra-virgin olive oil
2 red onions, chopped
4 cloves garlic, finely chopped
1/2 cup parsley, finely chopped
1 cup lentils, soaked overnight
3 cups chickpeas, cooked
4 tomatoes, chopped
1 tsp. cumin
1/2 tsp. thyme
1/8 tsp. cayenne
3 cups water
1/4 cup green olives, chopped
2 tbsp. lemon juice

Directions:

Heat oil in a saucepan and sauté onion, garlic for 6 minutes. Add lentils, chickpeas, tomatoes, cumin, thyme, cayenne, and water. Bring to a boil and simmer for 35 minutes.

Add olives, lemon juice, and parsley, stir and serve.

NUTRITION FACTS: CALORIES 199KCAL FAT 5 G CARBOHYDRATE 20 G PROTEIN 18 G

LOUISIANA-STYLE VEGGIE SAUSAGES

 4    75 mins

Ingredients:

3 cups chickpeas, soaked overnight
2 cups flour
2 garlic cloves, crushed
1 cup rolled oats
1 cup nutritional yeast flakes
¾ cups extra-virgin olive oil
1 cup soymilk
½ tsp. salt
2 tsp. garlic powder
2 tsp. oregano
1 tsp. fennel seeds
¼ cup soy sauce

Directions:

Drain the chickpeas, wash them in running water, and then grind them in a food processor until very fine.

In a bowl, mix flour, rolled oats, nutritional yeast, salt, garlic powder, oregano, fennel seed. In a separate bowl, mix soy milk, soy sauce, and chickpeas. Mix and add to the flour. Stir well to create a dough.

Cut 4 pieces of aluminum foil 14 x 12 inches. Divide the mixture into 4 parts, and roll it up in a sausage shape. Close the foil packages by rolling the ends. Steam for 55 minutes and let cool before opening.

It can be served like this, with some arugula salad as a side, or they can be chopped and sautéed in 1 tsp oil until brown.

NUTRITION FACTS: CALORIES 368KCAL FAT 5 G CARBOHYDRATE 29 G PROTEIN 15 G

MOROCCAN CHICKPEAS

🍲 4   🕐 45 mins

Ingredients:

2 cups chickpeas, soaked overnight
1 carrot, chopped
1 red onion, chopped
1 celery stalk, chopped
1 handful parsley, chopped
2-inches ginger, peeled
1 cinnamon stick
1 pinch saffron
1 tsp. turmeric
½ tsp. cayenne
2 ripe tomatoes

Directions:

Wash the chickpeas and put them in a pot with 6 cups of fresh water. Add the carrot and the onion. Bring to a boil and simmer for 65 minutes.

Add the parsley stems, ginger, turmeric, cayenne, tomatoes, saffron, and cook for 30 minutes. Add salt and pepper to taste, and cook for another 20 minutes. Blend ½ cup of chickpeas until smooth and add them back in the pot to thicken the sauce.

Discard the cinnamon, ginger, and parsley stems.

Trim with chopped parsley leaves and serve.

NUTRITION FACTS: CALORIES 316KCAL FAT 5.2 G CARBOHYDRATE 13.1 G PROTEIN 7 G

MUSHROOM AND POTATO PIE

🍲 6   🕐 60 mins

Ingredients:

2 lbs. potatoes
2 cups soy milk
4 celery sticks, grated
1 red onion, chopped
1 lb. mushrooms, chopped
3 tbsp. extra-virgin olive oil
2 garlic cloves, crushed
1 ½ tbsp. arrowroot
1 handful parsley, chopped
1 tsp. thyme

Directions:

Wash the potatoes to remove any dirt. Cook them in boiling water for 25 to 30 minutes until tender (always check with a stick before draining).

Remove the skin and mash the potatoes. Add 1 tbsp. olive oil, ¼ cup soy milk, salt and pepper, and stir well to make it fluffy.

Sautè onion, garlic, mushrooms, and celery in a saucepan with oil over medium heat for 5 minutes.

Dissolve the arrowroot in a little soymilk, add to the mushrooms, then add the remaining milk and mix well. Add the parsley, thyme, and season with salt and pepper to taste. Simmer gently for 5 minutes.

Move the stir into an ovenproof dish creating two layers. Mushrooms spread on the bottom and mashed potato on top.

Cook at 375°F for about 15 minutes and broil the last 5 minutes to make the top golden and crispy.

NUTRITION FACTS: CALORIES 397KCAL FAT 6 G
CARBOHYDRATE 33 G PROTEIN 7 G

MUSHROOM AND TOMATO RISOTTO

Ingredients:

1 red onion, chopped
4 tsp. extra-virgin olive oil
4 cups mushrooms, chopped
2½ cups long-grain brown rice
7 cups boiling broth
2 cloves garlic, crushed
1 lb. tomatoes, peeled and chopped
1 tsp. thyme
1 tsp. oregano

Directions:

Warm a saucepan with 2 tsp. oil and sautè half the onion for 5 minutes. Add the rice and toast it for 2 to 3 minutes on high heat. Add the mushrooms, and cook for 5 minutes.

Add half boiling broth and simmer for around 50 minutes (time will depend on the variety of the brown rice). Keep adding 1 ladle of broth when the previous one has been absorbed. In this way, the rice will not overcook and will not be runny.

In another pan, sauté the remaining onion and garlic. Add the tomatoes, season with salt and pepper to taste, and simmer on low heat for at least 25 minutes, until the sauce thickens.

Add thyme and oregano right before removing the sauce from the heat, then add it to the rice.

Mix well and allow the flavors to combine for a few minutes, then serve.

NUTRITION FACTS: CALORIES 304KCAL FAT 5 G CARBOHYDRATE 30 G PROTEIN 14 G

NOODLES WITH WALNUT SAUCE

 4   🕐 25 mins

Ingredients:

½ lb. buckwheat spaghetti
½ cup walnuts
4 tbsp. soy sauce
2 tbsp. rice vinegar
1 tsp. chili powder
1 pinch cayenne
1-inch ginger, grated

Directions:

Bring a pot of salted water to a boil and cook the spaghetti al dente (around 8 minutes).

Put the walnuts in a blender with 1/2 cup lukewarm water and blend until smooth. Add the soy sauce, ginger, rice vinegar, chili powder, and cayenne pepper and mix again.

When the spaghetti is done, drain and place them in a bowl. Add the walnut sauce and toss well until the spaghetti is coated with the sauce.

Divide among four plates, sprinkle raisins over each one, and serve.

NUTRITION FACTS: CALORIES 316KCAL FAT 5.2 G CARBOHYDRATE 13.1 G PROTEIN 7 G

QUINOA SALAD

🍽 4   🕐 30 mins

Ingredients:

1 cup quinoa
¼ cup parsley, chopped
2 stems green onions, finely chopped
2 sprigs fresh basil, chopped
1 tomato, diced
½ red pepper, finely diced
¼ cup corn
2 tbsp. extra-virgin olive oil
⅛ cup red wine vinegar
1 pinch cumin

Directions:

Rinse quinoa in cold water thoroughly. Boil quinoa in 2 cups salted water for 25 minutes. Set aside.

Try not to over stir the quinoa as it makes it mushy. Add the cut vegetables.

Stir the remaining ingredients together and toss everything lightly.

NUTRITION FACTS: CALORIES 199KCAL FAT 5 G CARBOHYDRATE 20 G PROTEIN 18 G

ORANGE SESAME TOFU

 4   55mins

Ingredients:

28 oz. extra-firm tofu, cubed
¼ cup orange juice
2 tbsp. soy sauce
1 tsp. sesame oil
1 tbsp. rice vinegar
½ tbsp. cornstarch
3 cups brown rice
½ tbsp. salt
2 tbsp. scallions
1 tbsp. toasted sesame seeds

Directions:

Preheat oven to 200°F.

Put the tofu on a plate fixed with a few layers of paper towels; spread with extra paper towels and a subsequent plate. Put a plate on top. Let stand 30 minutes.

Put the tofu in a single layer in a pan, and cook at 375°F until firm and crisp, around 15 minutes, turning tofu blocks over part of the way through cooking

In the meantime, whisk together squeezed orange, soy sauce, nectar, sesame oil, rice vinegar, and cornstarch in a little pan over high, heat to the point of boiling, whisking continually, until sauce thickens, 2 to 3 minutes. Remove from heat; cover and set aside.

Get ready rice as indicated by package instructions. Mix in salt.

Toss tofu with soy sauce blend. Divide rice among 4 dishes; top with tofu. Sprinkle with scallions and sesame seeds.

NUTRITION FACTS: CALORIES 445KCAL FAT 20 G CARBOHYDRATE 46 G PROTEIN 23 G

SCALLOPED EGGPLANT

🍲 4   🕐 40 mins

Ingredients:

1 eggplant, diced
2 cups mushrooms, thinly chopped
1 red onion, thinly chopped
1 bell pepper, thinly chopped
3 tbsp. olive oil
½ cup soymilk
2 cups buckwheat breadcrumbs
½ tsp. paprika
1 tsp. turmeric
¼ tsp. cayenne

Directions:

Preheat oven to 350°F. In a skillet, sauté the eggplant, mushrooms, onion, and bell pepper in the oil until the eggplant becomes golden, about 10 minutes

Mix the milk, paprika, turmeric, cayenne, salt, and pepper with breadcrumbs. Put the veggie mix on a tray, cover with the breadcrumb mixture and bake for 25 minutes.

NUTRITION FACTS: CALORIES 360KCAL FAT 9 G CARBOHYDRATE 26 G PROTEIN 4 G

STIR-FRIED TOFU AND VEGETABLES IN GINGER SAUCE

🍲 4   🕐 55 mins

Ingredients:

¾ cup soy sauce
¾ cup lemon juice
1-2 tsp. ginger, grated
1 lb. extra firm tofu
2 tbsp. olive oil
1 cup broccoli florets
1 cup cauliflower florets
3 carrots, chopped
1 red onion, chopped
1 green pepper, chopped
1 cup snow peas
1 cup mushrooms, chopped
2 green onions, chopped
2 cups cooked rice

Directions:

Whisk the lemon juice, soy sauce, and ginger and add the marinade to the tofu.

Let marinate for 45 minutes. Drain the tofu saving the marinade. Heat the oil in a pan, and add the cauliflower, broccoli, carrots, onion, green pepper, and tofu.

Stir frequently, cooking evenly. Add the snow peas, mushrooms, and green onions.

Continue to stir frequently until the vegetables are cooked but still crunchy.

Serve over rice, topped with the marinade.

NUTRITION FACTS: CALORIES 358KCAL FAT 7 G CARBOHYDRATE 20 G PROTEIN 28 G

SMOKY TOFU STIR FRY

 4   28 mins

Ingredients:

3.75 oz. buckwheat noodles
2 broccoli, chopped
2 green onions
2 tbsp. extra-virgin olive oil
2 chilies
6 garlic cloves, chopped
1-inch ginger, peeled and diced
4 carrots peeled and chopped
3 celery stalks, chopped
1 lb. extra-firm tofu, cubed
1 zucchini, chopped
1 cup snow peas, trimmed
15 oz. baby corn
1 red bell pepper, chopped
1 dash liquid smoke

Directions:

Bring a pot of water to a boil. Add the bean threads, stir, remove from heat, and set aside to soak; they should be ready when the stir-fry is done.

Cut the white and light green sections of the green onions into 3/4-inch-thick cuts. Thinly cut the green sections.

Heat several tbsps. of oil in a skillet.

Put the chilies, garlic, and ginger into a wok. Stir-fry for 1 minute. Add the carrots and cook for 3 minutes. Add the celery and green onions and stir-fry for 2 minutes.

Place the tofu in a hot saucepan with oil and liquid smoke and cook until it begins to brown, 6 to 8 minutes.

Add the zucchini, snow peas, baby corn, and bell pepper to the sauté pan or wok. Stir in the broccoli, then stir-fry until the florets start to turn green, about 2 minutes.

Boil noodles for 5 minutes in salted water. Drain, mix with the stir fry, and serve immediately.

NUTRITION FACTS: CALORIES 472KCAL FAT 8 G CARBOHYDRATE 30 G PROTEIN 26 G

SPICY STUFFED TOMATOES

 4 45 mins

Ingredients:

8 Roma tomatoes
2 tbsp. extra-virgin olive oil
¾ cup red onion, finely sliced
1 tbsp. ginger, diced
1 Bird's Eye chili, chopped
¼ tsp. turmeric
2 tsp. chickpea flour
1 handful parsley
1 tbsp. finely chopped parsley

Directions:

Remove the stem end from 8 of the tomatoes.

Carefully hollow each tomato by removing the pulp and seeds; discard the seeds but save the pulp.

Cut enough of the remaining 2 tomatoes, discard the seeds, to make ¼ cup (60ml) together with the reserved pulp. Set aside.

Heat oil in a skillet over medium-low heat. When hot, add the red onion and fry it until it is richly browned, 8 to 10 minutes, stirring constantly.

Add ginger, green chili, and turmeric and stir a few times.

Stir in the chickpea flour. Lower the heat. Add the tomato pulp, salt, and parsley. Cook until the pulp becomes a sauce, about 12 minutes. Let cool for a few minutes.

Fill the tomatoes with the mixture and place them upright in a baking pan. If they don't stand, place a crumpled piece of aluminum foil on the baking pan's bottom and make small hollows in the foil to support the tomatoes upright.

Cook the tomatoes in the oven at 400°F until they are tender but retain their color and shape, about 10 to 14 minutes.

Serve immediately.

NUTRITION FACTS: CALORIES 316KCAL FAT 5.2 G CARBOHYDRATE 13.1 G PROTEIN 7 G

TOFU PATTIES WITH MUSHROOMS AND PEAS

 4   55 mins

Ingredients:

1 cup snow peas
1 cup mushrooms, chopped
8 green onions, chopped
1 ½-inch ginger
8 oz. chestnuts, chopped
2 tbsp. extra-virgin olive oil
2 cups fresh bean sprouts
1 ¾ lbs. tofu, mashed
2 tsp. baking powder
1 cup flour
3 tbsp. nutritional yeast
2 tbsp. soy sauce

Directions:

Heat a skillet with oil and sauté the onions, mushrooms, snow peas, and chestnuts for 5 to 6 minutes. Add the bean sprouts, mix, and set aside.

Remove from heat and set aside.

Preheat the oven to 325°F.

Blend the tofu and the soy sauce until smooth and creamy. Add flour, nutritional yeast, and baking powder and mix. Add onion, mushrooms, snow peas, and chestnuts.

On lined baking tray, form 6 1/2-inch-thick patties.

Bake for 30 minutes, flip over and bake for 15 more minutes.

NUTRITION FACTS: CALORIES 199KCAL FAT 5 G CARBOHYDRATE 20 G PROTEIN 18 G

ZUCCHINI BOATS

 5   50 mins

Ingredients:

3 zucchini
1 red onion, chopped
1 tbsp. olive oil
½ lb. tofu, crumbled
3 tbsp. nutritional yeast flakes
1 garlic clove, crushed
½ tsp. oregano
16 oz. tomato sauce

Directions:

Cut the zucchini lengthwise and scoop the pulp out. Heat a pan with oil, sauté the onion for 5 minutes, add the tofu, zucchini pulp, garlic salt, and oregano and cook for 10 more minutes. Let cool for 5 minutes, then add nutritional yeast.

Pour the tomato sauce into a 9x11-inch pan, place the zucchini 'boats' in the sauce and fill the boats with the tofu mixture.

Cook for 30 minutes at 400°F, then broil for 5 minutes until the top becomes golden brown.

NUTRITION FACTS: CALORIES 340KCAL FAT 7 G CARBOHYDRATE 20 G PROTEIN 18 G

VEGAN LASAGNA

🍳 4   🕐 85 mins

Ingredients:

4 tbsp. arrowroot
¼ tsp. salt
I tbsp. Apple cider vinegar
4 lemons, juiced
I cup cashews
3 cups baby spinach
I box lasagna noodles
2 zucchini
½ tsp. garlic powder
2 tsp. oregano
2 tsp. basil
2 tbsp. extra-virgin olive oil
½ cup nutritional yeast
16 oz. firm tofu
3 tbsp. tomato puree
I tbsp. onion powder
6 cloves of garlic
I white onion
2 cans crushed tomatoes
I cup red lentils, drained

Directions:

Put three cups of water in a saucepan with the lentils, then bring to a boil before reducing to a simmer for around twenty minutes. Drain the lentils and set aside.

In the same saucepan, add oil and the diced onion and let it cool down.

When the onion is soft, add finely diced garlic, generous pinches of salt and pepper, one tsp. of oregano and basil, the two cans of crushed tomatoes, and the tomato puree. Leave to simmer for 15 minutes, stirring every 5 minutes.

Add the lentils to this, then set aside. This is the marinara sauce.

Put one cup of cashews into a bowl with two cups of boiled water and set aside.

Wash and slice the zucchini into lengthwise strips that are long and relatively thin, then set aside.

Break up the tofu and add to the blender along with the juice from one lemon, one tsp each of basil and oregano, the nutritional yeast, garlic powder, and a little salt.

Keep pulsing until it is mostly smooth but still a little textured. Put into a bowl and set aside. This is your ricotta.

Drain the soaked cashews and put them into a clean blender with the apple cider vinegar, the juice from one lemon, tapioca starch, and a little salt. Pour in one and a half cups of water and blend until smooth.

Pour this into a saucepan on medium heat and stir until it becomes stretchy, then set aside. This is the cheese sauce.

In a baking dish, place a few spoonsful of the marinara sauce and spread it to cover the bottom and sides. Begin to layer the lasagna noodles, the ricotta, the zucchini, and the cheese sauce. Follow this with half of the spinach, more marinara, lasagna noodles, spinach, and the cheese sauce. Keep repeating until all ingredients have been used except for a small portion of the cheese sauce.

Put into a 350°F oven for 45 minutes on the highest shelf. Remove after 40 minutes and spoon the remainder of the cheese sauce over the top to resemble mozzarella blobs, then return to the oven for 5 to 10 more minutes. Let rest, then serve and enjoy!

NUTRITION FACTS: CALORIES 543KCAL FAT 14 G CARBOHYDRATE 76 G PROTEIN 34 G

VEGAN MAC AND CHEESE

 4   55 mins

Ingredients:

1 cup cashews
½ tsp. chili flakes
½ cup nutritional yeast
½ tsp. mustard powder
½ tsp. onion powder
½ tsp. garlic powder
3 cloves garlic
1 russet potato
1 white onion
2 tbsp. avocado oil
1 head broccoli
1 ½ tsp apple cider vinegar
2 cups buckwheat macaroni

Directions:

Peel and grate the potato. Finely dice the garlic. Heat a saucepan with oil over medium heat. Put onion and a little salt in the pot and cook until soft.

Add potato, chili flakes, garlic, mustard, onion, and garlic powders into the pot. Stir well until their flavors release, then add one cup of water and cashews. Keep stirring at a simmer until the potatoes are soft.

Pour the entire mixture into a blender with the apple cider vinegar and nutritional yeast, salt, and pepper. The consistency should be that of cheese sauce that is thick yet runny. If it is too thick, add more water. According to your taste, if it needs more salt or garlic powder, chili flakes, or vinegar, add them now.

Boil the pasta in salted water. In another pot, boil the broccoli in bite-sized florets until tender. When both are ready, transfer everything into one pot and cover with the cheese sauce. Combine well, serve, and enjoy!

NUTRITION FACTS: CALORIES 263KCAL FAT 14 G CARBOHYDRATE 36 G PROTEIN 4 G

VEGETABLE STEW

🍲 4　　🕐 32 mins

Ingredients:

3 potatoes
½ lb. pumpkin
1 zucchini
1 turnip
1 red onion, chopped
2 cloves garlic, crushed
2 stalks celery, chopped
½ Bird's Eye chili, chopped finely
1 red bell pepper, chopped
2 tbsp. extra-virgin olive oil
2 tbsp. mustard
3 tbsp. tamari
2 cups vegetable stock
2 tomatoes, chopped
1 tsp. basil
¼ tsp. thyme
1 bay leaf
1 handful parsley, chopped

Directions:

Scrub and trim the potatoes or peel and wash the yams, quarter lengthwise and cut in 1/2-inch cuts.

Cut the pumpkin, zucchini, and turnip the same thickness as the potatoes and steam them together.

Sauté the onion, garlic, celery, hot pepper, and sweet pepper in the extra-virgin olive oil until the onion is transparent.

Stir mustard, molasses, tamari, and stock.

Add the sauce/stock stir, steamed vegetables, sautéed vegetables, tomatoes, pimento grains, basil, thyme, bay leaf, and whole hot pepper in a saucepan.

Simmer for 10 minutes; season with salt and pepper. Top with parsley

Great when served with rice.

NUTRITION FACTS: CALORIES 199KCAL FAT 5 G CARBOHYDRATE 20 G PROTEIN 18 G

SIDE DISHES

BAKED EGGPLANT WITH TURMERIC AND GARLIC

 2 21 mins

Ingredients:
1 eggplant
2 tbsp. extra-virgin olive oil
2 whole dried red chilies
1 ½ tbsp. garlic, diced
1 tsp. green chili, chopped
¼ tsp. turmeric
¼ cup water
2 tbsp. white poppy seeds
½ tsp. salt
½ tsp. sugar

Directions:
Crush the poppy seeds with a drop of live oil to form a paste.

Preheat oven to 450°F. Cut eggplant lengthwise and place it on a baking sheet with the cut side down.

Bake for 30 to 34 minutes or until the eggplant wrinkles and feels soft to the touch when pressed. Cut. Set aside. Heat a skillet with oil over medium heat. Fry red chilies until they are soft.

Add garlic and green chili. Stir until garlic turns light brown. Add water and turmeric and bring to a boil. Lower the heat and stir in the eggplant cuts. Add poppy seed paste, salt, and sugar and mix well.

Simmer for 5 minutes. Trim with green onions and serve.

NUTRITION FACTS: CALORIES 160KCAL FAT 7 G CARBOHYDRATE 25 G PROTEIN 3 G

BEAN SALAD

 4   🕐 5 mins

Ingredients:
1 can black beans, drained
1 can corn, drained
½ cup parsley, chopped
¼ cup green onions, chopped
¼ red onions, chopped
⅓ cup lime juice
3 tbsp. extra-virgin olive oil
1 tbsp. cumin

Directions:
Stir together and let sit overnight.

NUTRITION FACTS: CALORIES 210KCAL FAT 3 G CARBOHYDRATE 26 G PROTEIN 3 G

BEETS WITH LEEK AND PARSLEY

 4   🕐 35 mins

Ingredients:
2 lbs. beets, chopped
1 lb. trimmed leeks, thickly chopped
1 tsp. ground cumin
1 tbsp. parsley, chopped
½ cups red wine

Directions:
Put the leeks with beets and spices in a pan. Add the wine, bring to a boil and simmer for 30 minutes until the beets are tender.

Season to taste with salt and pepper and serve, either hot or cold.

NUTRITION FACTS: CALORIES 178KCAL FAT 5 G CARBOHYDRATE 16 G PROTEIN 3 G

BUTTERNUT AND CHESTNUT HOLIDAY SAUTÉ

 4 50 mins

Ingredients:

1 cup dried lentils, soaked overnight
6 tbsp. olive oil
4 scallions, chopped
1 garlic clove, diced
1 butternut squash, chopped into cubes
1 lb. tomatoes, chopped and peeled
½ tsp. thyme
1 handful parsley, chopped
1 cup chestnuts, shelled

Directions:

Drain the lentils and wash them. Put them in a pan with fresh water. Bring to a boil and cook about 30 minutes, until the lentils are tender.

Heat a sauté pan with the oil and cook the garlic and scallions until tender.

Add the squash and cook for a few minutes. Add the tomatoes and thyme, and cook for 10 minutes. Add the lentils and cook for 10 more minutes or until all the vegetables are tender.

Add the chestnuts and warm through. Serve.

NUTRITION FACTS: CALORIES 206KCAL FAT 6 G CARBOHYDRATE 25 G PROTEIN 2 G

CARAMELIZED FENNEL

4 15 mins

Ingredients:

2 fennel bulbs
2 tbsp. extra-virgin olive oil
salt and pepper

Trim the fennel bulbs, removing the outer layers. Cut bulbs in half vertically and then into 1/8-inch-thick cuts.

Heat a sauté pan with olive oil over medium heat. Add fennel.

Cook, occasionally stirring, for 8 to 10 minutes until fennel is caramelized and tender. Season with salt and pepper.

Directions:

NUTRITION FACTS: CALORIES 104KCAL FAT 5 G CARBOHYDRATE 16 G PROTEIN 1 G

CHINESE-STYLE CHILI GREEN BEANS

 4   ⏱ 15 mins

Ingredients:

1 lb. green beans, trimmed
1 tbsp. olive oil
2 cloves garlic, crushed
½ tsp. dried red chili flakes
1 tsp. sesame oil
2 tbsp. soy sauce

Directions:

Heat a skillet with oil over high heat. Add the garlic, green beans, chili flakes, and soy sauce, and stir fry for 10 minutes until the beans are cooked.

Sprinkle with the sesame oil and serve.

These beans are also excellent when served at room temperature.

NUTRITION FACTS: CALORIES 145KCAL FAT 4 G CARBOHYDRATE 18 G PROTEIN 3 G

CURRY CHICKPEAS

4   ⏱ 25 mins

Ingredients:

15-oz. chickpeas, cooked
2 tbsp. red wine vinegar
2 tbsp. olive oil
2 tbsp. curry powder
½ tbsp. ground turmeric
¼ tbsp. ground cumin
⅛ tsp. ground cinnamon
¼ tbsp. salt
½ tbsp. pepper
1 handful parsley, chopped

Directions:

Gently crush chickpeas with hands in a medium bowl, removing skins.

Add oil and vinegar, and toss to coat. Add turmeric, curry powder, and cinnamon; mix gently to blend.

Put chickpeas in a single layer in the oven, and cook at 400°F until crisp, around 15 minutes, shaking them partway through cooking.

Move chickpeas to a bowl. Sprinkle with salt, pepper, and parsley, and toss to cover.

NUTRITION FACTS: CALORIES 173KCAL FAT 8 G CARBOHYDRATE 18 G PROTEIN 7 G

GARLIC-SALAD BRUSSELS SPROUTS

 4   30 mins

Ingredients:

3 tbsp. olive oil
2 garlic cloves
½ tbsp. salt
¼ tbsp. pepper
1 lbs. Brussels sprouts, chopped
½ cup buckwheat breadcrumbs
1 ½ tbsp. crisp rosemary

Directions:

Preheat Oven to 350°F. Stir fry the Brussels sprouts, halved, in a frypan with 1 tbsp. oil and garlic for 5 minutes.

Season with salt and pepper to taste. Move the sprouts to a ovenproof dish, sprinkle breacrumbs and rosemary, finely chopped.

Drizzle the remaining oil on top and cook in the oven for 15 minutes until golden brown.

NUTRITION FACTS: CALORIES 187KCAL FAT 7 G
CARBOHYDRATE 25 G PROTEIN 3 G

GINGER ZUCCHINI

 4   15 mins

Ingredients:

1 tbsp. olive oil
1 lb. zucchini chopped into 1/4-inch cuts
½ cup vegetarian broth
2 tsp. light soy sauce
1 tbsp. red wine
1 tsp. sesame oil

Directions:

Heat a skillet with oil and when it is hot, add the zucchini and ginger. Stir-fry for 1 minute, then add soy sauce, sherry, and broth.

Cook over high heat until the broth reduces and the zucchini is tender. Drizzle sesame oil and serve.

NUTRITION FACTS: CALORIES 160KCAL FAT 4 G CARBOHYDRATE 12 G PROTEIN 2 G

LEBANESE FRIED CUCUMBERS

 2   40 mins

Ingredients:

1 cucumber, peeled and chopped
½ cup flour
¼ tsp. garlic powder
½ cup green onions, finely chopped
3 tbsp. extra-virgin olive oil

Directions:

Sprinkle both sides of cucumber rounds with salt and allow to stand in a strainer for 30 minutes, draining excess water.

Mix pepper, garlic powder, and flour, then dip the cucumber slices in.

Heat frying pan on high. Add the oil and, when hot, fry cucumber slices until they turn evenly golden.

Place on a serving platter, then trim with green onions and serve.

NUTRITION FACTS: CALORIES 175KCAL   FAT 7 G   CARBOHYDRATE 12 G   PROTEIN 3 G

LEMON EGGPLANT

 2   40 mins

Ingredients:

1 eggplant, chopped
½ cup extra-virgin olive oil
2 cloves garlic, crushed
1 green pepper, very finely chopped
3 tbsp. lemon juice
6 tbsps. parsley, finely chopped

Directions:

Sprinkle eggplant cuts with salt, and drain water for 30 minutes, then pat dry using kitchen towels.

Heat a frying pan with oil and, when hot, fry the eggplant until golden brown. Set aside.

Prepare a sauce by mixing lemon juice, salt, and pepper to taste, and drizzle it over the eggplant.

Trim with parsley and serve.

NUTRITION FACTS: CALORIES 265KCAL   FAT 7 G   CARBOHYDRATE 18 G   PROTEIN 2 G

MASALA POTATOES

 4 25 mins

Ingredients:

3 tbsp. extra-virgin olive oil
1 tbsp. mustard seeds
1 bird's eye chili, chopped
2 red onions, chopped
1 red bell pepper, cored and diced
1 tsp. turmeric
½ tsp. masala powder
1 tsp. ground cayenne pepper
5 potatoes, chopped
juice of 1 lemon

Directions:

Warm the extra-virgin olive oil in a pan over medium heat. Add the mustard seeds and let them brown for 1 minute. Add the chili, onions, bell pepper, and sauté about 3 minutes, or until the onions are tender.

Add the turmeric, parsley, salt, ground cayenne, potatoes, ½ cup water, and lemon juice and stir well.

Reduce the heat to low and simmer, covered for 20 minutes.

NUTRITION FACTS: CALORIES 180KCAL FAT 5 G CARBOHYDRATE 25 G PROTEIN 2 G

PIQUANT COLESLAW

 6 25 mins

Ingredients:

2 lb. white cabbage
4 sticks celery
1 green pepper
1 red onion
12 green olives
3 tbsp. no-egg mayonnaise
5 drops of tabasco sauce

Directions:

Grate the cabbage. Cut the celery and green pepper. Cut the onion and olives finely.

Add all the veggies to a bowl and stir. Add the mayonnaise, tabasco, salt, and pepper to taste, toss to coat, and serve.

NUTRITION FACTS: CALORIES 160KCAL FAT 7 G CARBOHYDRATE 25 G PROTEIN 3 G

POTATO, MOREL, AND ONION FRICASSEE

 6 30 mins

Ingredients:

1 ½ lbs. potatoes, chopped
1 red onion, chopped
½ lbs. morels
3 tbsp. extra-virgin olive oil
¼ cup chopped parsley

Directions:

Boil the potatoes in salted water until soft, and the edges have started to break down. Drain and set aside. Cut the morels in half and wash them quickly in water. Sauté both morels in the extra-virgin olive oil over high heat. Let the juices evaporate in about 5 to 6 minutes. Fry the potatoes in a skillet

When the potatoes have started to turn golden brown, add the onions until potatoes are crispy and the onions start caramelizing. Add the morels, season with salt and pepper, and add parsley.

Toss and serve.

NUTRITION FACTS: CALORIES 350KCAL FAT 7 G CARBOHYDRATE 21 G PROTEIN 3 G

RAW ARTICHOKE SALAD

 2 5 mins

Ingredients:

2 Roman artichokes
1 lemon, juiced
1 tsp. extra-virgin olive oil
Salt and pepper

Directions:

Wash and peel the artichokes by removing the outer leaves. Cut them in two and gently remove the hair inside.

Cut them very finely (using a mandolin if you have one)

Put them in water and lemon so that they do not turn brown.

When ready to serve, drain the artichokes, mix them with olive oil, a few drops of lemon, salt, and pepper, and put them on a serving plate.

NUTRITION FACTS: CALORIES 100KCAL FAT 10.9 G CARBOHYDRATE 3.4 G PROTEIN 13.3 G

RED CAULIFLOWER

 4   28 mins

Ingredients:
1 cauliflower
2 tbsp. extra-virgin olive oil
1 garlic clove crushed
2 tbsp. chopped parsley
¼ cup. water
1 tbsp. tomato paste

Directions:
Divide the washed cauliflower into individual florets.

Heat the extra-virgin olive oil in a saucepan and fry the garlic for 1 minute. Add the cauliflower, stir and cook for 5 minutes, then add salt and pepper to taste, water, and tomato paste.

Cover the pan and cook over low heat until tender (about 15 to 20 minutes).

NUTRITION FACTS: CALORIES 190KCAL FAT 4 G CARBOHYDRATE 20 G PROTEIN 8 G

RICH ROASTED EGGPLANT

4   50 mins

Ingredients:
1 eggplant
2 tbsp. extra-virgin olive oil
1 green chili
1 cup red onion
1 garlic clove, crushed
1 tbsp. fresh ginger, peeled and diced
¼ tsp. turmeric
½ cup tomatoes, chopped
1 tbsp. parsley, chopped

NUTRITION FACTS: CALORIES 190KCAL FAT 7 G
CARBOHYDRATE 17 G PROTEIN 5 G

Directions:
Preheat oven to 450°F. Cut eggplant in half and place it on a baking sheet with the cut side down. Bake for 30 to 40 minutes until the eggplant skin has wrinkles and is soft to the touch. Let cool for 5 minutes, then remove the skin, finely cut the flesh, and roughly cut it with a knife.

Heat oil in a skillet over medium heat and fry chilies for 1 minute. Add onion and fry until transparent, 8 to 10 minutes. Add ginger, garlic, turmeric, green chili, salt, and tomatoes. Simmer until tomatoes have formed a sauce, about 20 minutes.

Add the eggplant and cook, covered, 10 minutes on low heat to combine flavors, occasionally stirring.

Remove from heat. Let stand covered for 15 minutes to combine the flavors. Add and serve.

SMOTHERED CABBAGE

 4   40 mins

Ingredients:

1 red onion, diced
2 tbsp. estra-virgin olive oil
1 cabbage, chopped
3 cloves garlic crushed
½ tsp. salt
¼ tsp. paprika
⅛ tsp. cayenne
½ cup water

Directions:

Heat a pan with the oil, and when hot, sauté onion, cabbage, and garlic for 10 minutes, stirring often.

Add the paprika, cayenne, water, salt, and pepper to taste and simmer for 15 to 20 minutes until tender.

NUTRITION FACTS: CALORIES 210KCAL FAT 6 G CARBOHYDRATE 25 G PROTEIN 3 G

SAUCES AND DRESSINGS

COCONUT AND PARSLEY CHUTNEY

 4 25 mins

Ingredients:
2 tbsp. lemon juice
1 cup shredded coconut
1/3 cup firm tofu, chopped
1 cup parsley
1-inch ginger, grated
1/2 green chili, chopped
1 tsp. ground cumin
1 tsp. extra-virgin olive oil

Directions:
Place ½ cup water, lemon juice, tofu, coconut, parsley, ginger, green chili, cumin, and salt in a blender.

Pulse until reduced to a thick puree; add a little more water if necessary.

Pour into a small bowl.

NUTRITION FACTS: CALORIES 199KCAL FAT 5 G CARBOHYDRATE 20 G PROTEIN 18 G

CREAMY CASHEW DRESSING

🍽 6   🕐 10 mins

Ingredients:
2 cups cashews, soaked 4 hours
1 cup walnuts, soaked 4 hours
1 cloves garlic
2 tbsp. lemon juice
½ cup green onions

Directions:
Blend cashews, walnuts, garlic, green onions, lemon juice, and salt until smooth.

Add water to thin the sauce to use it in salads. Leave it thick to season pasta dishes.

NUTRITION FACTS: CALORIES 199KCAL FAT 5 G CARBOHYDRATE 20 G PROTEIN 18 G

LOUISIANA MUSHROOM SAUCE

🍽 2   🕐 15 mins

Ingredients:
2 cups mushrooms, chopped
2 tbsp. extra-virgin olive oil
1 onion, diced
3 tbsp. almond butter
1 pinch cayenne
2 tbsp. tamari
½ cup walnuts, soaked

Directions:
Sauté the onion and mushrooms in oil for 10 minutes.

Add the almond butter, cayenne, tamari, and walnuts and blend until smooth.

Add a little water to make a thinner sauce.

NUTRITION FACTS: CALORIES 199KCAL FAT 5 G CARBOHYDRATE 20 G PROTEIN 18 G

PECAN DRESSING

 6   🕑 20 mins

Ingredients:
1 red onion diced
3 green onions diced
3 stalks celery diced
1 green pepper diced
1/3 cup oil
2 cups pecans, chopped
2 tsp. paprika
1 tsp. ground cumin
1/2 tsp. thyme
1/2 tsp. oregano
1 1/2 tsp. salt
1/8 tsp. cayenne

Directions:
Heat a saucepan with oil and sauté the green onions, celery, red onions, and bell pepper for 15 minutes.

Add paprika, cumin, thyme, oregano, salt, cayenne, and pecans and blend until completely smooth.

Perfect with steamed rice.

NUTRITION FACTS: CALORIES 199KCAL FAT 5 G CARBOHYDRATE 20 G PROTEIN 18 G

PISTACHIO DRESSING

🍽 2   🕑 15 mins

Ingredients:
2 tbsp. pistachio nuts, shelled
1 tbsp. red wine vinegar
2 soft dates, pitted
1 tbsp. soy sauce
3 tbsp. extra-virgin olive oil
1 garlic clove
1 scallion
2 tbsp. parsley
2 tbsp. basil

Directions:
Blend all ingredients and enjoy!

NUTRITION FACTS: CALORIES 199KCAL FAT 5 G CARBOHYDRATE 20 G PROTEIN 18 G

RED HOT RED PEPPER SALSA

 2   15 mins

Ingredients:

1 red onion, chopped
1 tbsp. extra-virgin olive oil
1 Bird's Eye chili
1 red bell pepper, diced

Directions:

Heat a pan with oil, and when hot, add the chili, onion, and bell pepper. Sauté for 4 minutes until the onion is transparent. Season with salt and pepper to taste, add ½ cup water and reduce the heat to low.

Cover and simmer for 10 minutes.

Puree in a food processor for 2 minutes until smooth. Serve warm.

NUTRITION FACTS: CALORIES 199KCAL FAT 5 G CARBOHYDRATE 20 G PROTEIN 18 G

SOUTHERN TOMATO SAUCE

 6   35 mins

Ingredients:

1 red onion, diced
2 bell peppers, thinly chopped
2 tsp. oil
3 stalks celery, diced
6 cloves garlic, crushed
12 tomatoes, diced
½ tsp. thyme
1 tsp. basil
1 tbsp. paprika
1 pinch cayenne

Directions:

Sauté the celery, onion, garlic, and bell peppers in the oil for 10 minutes.

Add the tomatoes, thyme, basil, paprika, and cayenne and cook on low heat for 20 minutes, stirring frequently.

Serve over rice or noodles.

NUTRITION FACTS: CALORIES 100KCAL FAT 5 G CARBOHYDRATE 15 G PROTEIN 3 G

TOMATO HUMMUS

🍲 4   🕐 40 mins

Ingredients:

1 cup chickpeas, soaked overnight
4 tbsp. extra-virgin olive oil
1 lb. green beans, trimmed
4 red onions, chopped
1 garlic clove, crushed
1 tbsp. tomato paste

Directions:

Heat oil in a saucepan and sauté garlic and onion for 5 minutes until golden. Add chickpeas and green beans and cook for 10 minutes.

Season with salt and pepper to taste, stir in the tomato paste, and blend until smooth.

NUTRITION FACTS: CALORIES 199KCAL FAT 5 G CARBOHYDRATE 20 G PROTEIN 18 G

SALADS

AVOCADO-POTATO SALAD

🍽 2　　🕐 35 mins

Ingredients:
1 ripe avocado, mashed
6 yukon gold or red potatoes
½ cup red onion, chopped
2 ribs of celery, chopped
½ cup sweet red bell pepper
1 handful parsley, chopped

Directions:
Steam and cook the potatoes until tender but not too soft. Stir thoroughly with all other ingredients. Keep refrigerated until ready to serve.

NUTRITION FACTS: CALORIES 213KCAL FAT 9 G CARBOHYDRATE 28 G PROTEIN 3 G

AVOCADO WITH RASPBERRY VINEGAR SALAD

 2   2h + 10 mins

Ingredients:

4 oz. raspberries

3 oz, red wine vinegar

1 tsp. extra-virgin olive oil

2 firm-ripe avocados

1 red endive

Directions:

Place half the raspberries in a bowl. Heat the vinegar in a saucepan until it starts to bubble, then pour it over the raspberries and leave too steep for 5 minutes.

Strain the raspberries, pressing the fruit gently to extract all the juices but not the pulp.

Whisk the strained raspberry vinegar together with the oils and seasonings. Set aside.

Carefully halve each avocado and twist out the stone.

Peel away the skin and cut the flesh straight into the dressing.

Stir gently until the avocados are entirely covered in the dressing.

Cover tightly and chill in the fridge for about 2 hours.

Meanwhile, separate the radicchio leaves, rinse and drain them, then dry them on kitchen paper. Store in the fridge in a polythene bag.

To serve, place a few radicchio leaves on individual plates.

Spoon on the avocado, stir and trim with the remaining raspberries.

NUTRITION FACTS: CALORIES 163KCAL FAT 4 G CARBOHYDRATE 15 G PROTEIN 14 G

BITTER GREENS, MUNG SPROUTS, AVOCADO, AND ORANGE SALAD

 4   🕐 19 mins

Ingredients:
1 cup baby spinach leaves
1 cup stir bitter greens (arugula, watercress, etc.)
1 cup Mung sprouts
1 orange, into wedges
½ cup diced avocado
¼ cup walnuts, soaked
2 tbsp. extra-virgin olive oil
1 tbsp. lemon juice
1 tsp. lemon zest
1 tbsp. tahini
½ tsp. fresh ginger, diced

Directions:
Heat 1 tbsp. of the oil in a skillet.

Toss in the spinach leaves and Mung sprouts, and stir briefly to wilt the spinach leaves. Remove to a bowl and cool.

Add the stir-fry, bitter greens, orange, and avocado to a bowl.

In another clean bowl, briskly whisk together the lemon juice, the rest of the olive oil, lemon zest, salt, pepper, ginger, and tahini.

Pour the dressing over the salad and toss to coat.

Trim with the cut walnuts and serve immediately.

NUTRITION FACTS: CALORIES 173KCAL FAT 4 G CARBOHYDRATE 15 G PROTEIN 9 G

CREAMY SEA SALAD

 4   10 mins

Ingredients:
1 head of lettuce
1 ripe avocado
3 Roma tomatoes
½ cucumber
A handful of dulse seaweed, soaked
2 tbsp. sesame seeds
1 tbsp. extra-virgin olive oil
Juice of ¼ lemon
A handful parsley, chopped

Directions:
Finely shred the lettuce into thin strips using a sharp knife or mandoline and place in a bowl.

Dice the avocado, tomatoes, and cucumber into medium-sized pieces and add to the bowl. Tear the dulse into small pieces and add to the bowl.

Make the dressing by stirring the above ingredients and pouring over the salad.

Stir everything together thoroughly and serve.

NUTRITION FACTS: CALORIES 220KCAL FAT 8 G CARBOHYDRATE 15 G PROTEIN 15 G

PEANUT TOPPED GREENS

 6   25 *mins*

Ingredients:

6 cups mixed greens: *kale, spinach, chard, collard, etc.*
2 tbsp. extra-virgin olive oil
I bay leaf
I whole dried red chili
I tsp. green chili, chopped
I tbsp. ginger, diced
¼ tsp. turmeric
⅛ tsp. black pepper
2 tsp. ground cumin
¼ tsp. salt
½ cup soy milk
¼ cup peanuts
¼ cup walnuts, chopped

Directions:

Steam the greens until tender and puree in a blender. Set aside. Heat oil in a skillet over medium-low heat. Fry bay leaf and red chili until the chili is soft.

Sprinkle in red chili. Stir in green chili, ginger, turmeric, black pepper, cumin, and salt. Add soymilk and cook until reduced to about half its volume, 3 to 5 minutes, stirring often.

Add the pureed greens.

Cover and place over low heat for 3 to 5 minutes to stir the flavors and heated through. Remove from heat.

Sprinkle peanuts on top.

NUTRITION FACTS: CALORIES 230KCAL FAT 8 G CARBOHYDRATE 26 G PROTEIN 14 G

ROMAINE HEARTS WITH TOFU AND CANDIED PECANS

 4   20 *mins*

Ingredients:

2 tsp. agave syrup
I tsp. extra-virgin olive oil
½ cup pecans
¾ tbsp. balsamic vinegar
I tsp. Dijon mustard
I tsp. parsley
I tsp. basil
3 tbsp. olive oil
2 romaine hearts, chopped
3½ oz. tofu

Directions:

Stir the agave syrup and melted soy butter with pecans and place in a preheated 300F oven.

Bake for 10 minutes or until lightly toasted and candied. Cool to room temperature.

Place the vinegar, mustard, salt, pepper, and parsley in a salad bowl and whisk. Slowly whisk in the olive oil.

Add the romaine and toss to coat. Top with the pecans and small pieces of tofu.

Serve immediately.

NUTRITION FACTS: CALORIES 210KCAL FAT 7 G CARBOHYDRATE 21 G PROTEIN 13 G

SIMPLE ARUGULA SALAD

 4   🕐 10 mins

Ingredients:
1 red onion, chopped
1 tbsp. red wine vinegar
2 cups arugula
¼ cup walnuts, chopped
2 tbsp. fparsley, chopped
2 garlic cloves, peeled and minced
2 tbsp. extra-virgin olive oil
1 tbsp. lemon juice

Directions:
In a bowl, mix the water and vinegar, add the onion, set aside for 5 minutes, and drain well. In a salad bowl, combine the arugula with the walnuts and onion, and stir.

Add the garlic, salt, pepper, lemon juice, parsley, and oil, toss well, and serve.

NUTRITION FACTS: CALORIES 200KCAL FAT 2 G CARBOHYDRATE 5 G PROTEIN 7 G

WHITE BEAN AND TOMATO SALAD

🍴 4   🕐 10 mins

Ingredients:
14 oz. cannellini beans, drained
1-pint grape tomatoes, halved
4 scallions, thinly chopped
2 tbsp. extra-virgin olive oil
1 handful parsley, finely chopped
1 tbsp. lemon juice

Directions:
Mix cannellini, tomatoes, scallions and parsley.

Season with oil, lemon juice, salt and pepper to taste and serve.

NUTRITION FACTS: CALORIES 199KCAL FAT 4 G CARBOHYDRATE 20 G PROTEIN 18 G

SOUP

ANASAZI BEAN SOUP

 4   2h

Ingredients:

1 cup Anasazi beans, dry —soaked overnight
1 red onion - chopped
2 garlic cloves - pressed or diced
¼ tsp. parsley
½ tsp. cumin
1 Bird's Eye chili, finely chopped
6 cups vegetable stock
1 handful parsley, chopped

Directions:

Add the stock into a pot with the beans, onion, garlic, cumin, and chili and bring to a boil. Simmer on low heat for 2 hours until beans are tender.

Season with salt and pepper to taste and serve hot topped with parsley.

NUTRITION FACTS: CALORIES 199KCAL FAT 5 G CARBOHYDRATE 20 G PROTEIN 18 G

ARMENIAN SOUP

🍴 44　🕐 45 mins

Ingredients:
2 oz. red lentils, washed
2 oz. dried apricots
1 potato
4 cups vegetable stock
juice of ½ lemon
1 tsp. ground cumin
3 tbsp. parsley, chopped

Directions:
Place lentils in a saucepan. Roughly cut the potato and add to the pan with the apricots and cumin. Bring to a boil, and simmer for 30 minutes.

Add lemon juice and blend until smooth.

Top with parsley and serve.

NUTRITION FACTS: CALORIES 219KCAL FAT 4 G CARBOHYDRATE 22 G PROTEIN 16 G

ASIAN MUSHROOM SOUP

🍴 4　🕐 35 mins

Ingredients:
½ oz. dried wakame seaweed
4 cups vegetable stock
8 oz. shiitake mushrooms, sliced
2 oz. miso paste
16 oz. firm tofu, diced
1 red onion
2 green onion, trimmed and diagonally chopped
1 Bird's Eye chili, finely chopped

Directions:
Soak the wakame in lukewarm water for 10 to 15 minutes before draining.

In a saucepan, add the vegetable stock and bring to a boil. Toss in the mushrooms and simmer for 2 to 3 minutes. Mix the miso paste with 3-4 spoons of vegetable stock from the saucepan until the miso is completely dissolved.

Pour the miso-stock back into the pan and add the tofu, wakame, green onions, and chili, then serve immediately.

NUTRITION FACTS: CALORIES 197KCAL FAT 4 G CARBOHYDRATE 19 G PROTEIN 18 G

BLACK BEAN SOUP

Ⓑ 4   🕑 40 mins

Ingredients:
1 chili, finely chopped
1 pinch cayenne pepper, chopped
1 cup boiling water
2 tbsp. extra-virgin olive oil
1 red onion diced
1 carrot diced
1 celery stalk diced
½ cup tomatoes
½ tsp. black pepper
¼ tsp. oregano
¼ tsp. ground cumin
1 (19 oz.) can black beans

Directions:
Heat the oil in a pot over medium heat. Add the onion, carrot, and celery and sauté for 2 to 3 minutes until the onion is transparent.

Blend the tomatoes for 1 minute, until smooth, and add it to the pot

Add the puree, beans, pepper, oregano, and cumin to the pot, bring to a boil, then reduce the heat to low.

Simmer for 30 minutes, then blend the soup in a blender until smooth.

Serve hot.

NUTRITION FACTS: CALORIES 199KCAL FAT 5 G CARBOHYDRATE 20 G PROTEIN 18 G

BLACK EYED PEAS SOUP

Ⓑ 4   🕑 40 mins

Ingredients:
3 tbsp. extra-virgin olive oil
2 red onions diced
1 pinch cayenne pepper
1 (15oz.) can black-eyed peas, rinsed
2 carrots chopped into ¼-inch cuts
1 tsp. parsley
2 cups water
⅛ tsp. ground cumin

Directions:
In a cast-iron skillet, melt 2 tbsps. of extra-virgin olive oil over medium heat. Add the onions and sauté 3 to 5 minutes until the onions are golden. Add cayenne pepper.

Place the black-eyed peas, carrots, parsley, salt, black pepper in a saucepan and cover with water. Bring to a boil. Add the sautéed onions and cayenne pepper, and simmer for 30 to 40 minutes.

Puree in a food processor with the remaining 1 tbsp. extra-virgin olive oil and the cumin. Serve.

NUTRITION FACTS: CALORIES 240KCAL FAT 5 G CARBOHYDRATE 28 G PROTEIN 18 G

CARROT APPLE AND WALNUT SOUP

 4   🕐 40 mins

Ingredients:

1 lb. carrots, chopped
1 white onion, chopped
1 potato, diced
1 apple, diced
2 tbsp. extra-virgin olive oil
2 pints vegetable stock
2 oz. walnuts, chopped

Directions:

Sauté the vegetables in a saucepan with oil for 5 minutes, stirring occasionally.

Add the stock, season with salt and pepper. Bring to a boil, and simmer for 30 minutes until the vegetables are soft.

Blend in a food processor until smooth and serve.

NUTRITION FACTS: CALORIES 195KCAL FAT 4 G CARBOHYDRATE 19 G PROTEIN 16 G

CARROT AND ASPARAGUS SOUP

🍲 2   🕐 45 mins

Ingredients:

1 cup asparagus, chopped
½ cups carrot, diced
2 tbsp. tahini
½ red onion

Directions:

Cook asparagus, red onion, and carrot in 2 cups salted water for 10 minutes.

Blend them with tahini until smooth. Season with salt and pepper to taste and serve.

NUTRITION FACTS: CALORIES 129KCAL FAT 2 G CARBOHYDRATE 20 G PROTEIN 18 G

CELERY SOUP

 2   35 mins

Ingredients:

½ cup red onion, chopped
4 cups celery, chopped
2 cloves garlic, diced
½ tbsp. extra-virgin olive oil
2 cups vegetable stock or water
¼ tsp. dill
1 cup soy milk

Directions:

Heat a pot with oil and, when hot, sauté the onion, celery, and garlic. Add the stock and simmer until soft.

Blend until creamy. Return to the soup pot, season with salt and pepper to taste. Add dill and soymilk, and serve hot.

NUTRITION FACTS: CALORIES 142KCAL FAT 3 G CARBOHYDRATE 10 G PROTEIN 8 G

CHIPOTLE SPLIT PEA SOUP

 4   45 mins

Ingredients:

2 cups dried split peas
3 cups boiling water
1 red onion chopped
2 cloves garlic diced
2 carrots chopped diagonally
2 stalks celery, chopped diagonally
½ cup chopped parsley
½ chipotle, finely chopped
1 tbsp. soy sauce

Directions:

Boil the split peas in the salted water for 40 minutes, until soft.

Add the onion, garlic, carrots, celery, chipotle, parsley, and soy sauce and continue cooking until the vegetables are tender.

Serve hot.

NUTRITION FACTS: CALORIES 206KCAL FAT 3 G CARBOHYDRATE 20 G PROTEIN 9 G

CHICKPEA SOUP

4   90 mins

Ingredients:

1 cup dried chickpeas, soaked overnight
2 tbsp. extra-virgin olive oil
2 red onions, chopped
4 cloves garlic, crushed
½ cup parsley
½ tsp. cayenne
½ tsp. turmeric
¼ tsp. mustard
3 cups vegetable broth

Directions:

Boil chickpeas in water for 65-70 minutes, and drain.

Heat the oil in a frying pan; stir fry onions and garlic until they begin to brown. Add parsley, cayenne, mustard, chickpeas, salt, and pepper to taste. Cook 5 minutes, then add 3 cups vegetable broth.

Cover and cook over medium heat for 15 minutes. Quickly blitz with a hand blender for a few pulses and keep cooking for 5 minutes to make it thick. Serve.

NUTRITION FACTS: CALORIES 205KCAL FAT 5 G CARBOHYDRATE 22 G PROTEIN 11 G

COCONUT SPINACH SOUP

4   15 mins

Ingredients:

1 cup coconut milk
3 cups spinach
1 tsp. curry paste
½ tsp. turmeric
½-inch fresh ginger, grated
1 tbsp. soy sauce

Directions:

Put spinach, coconut milk, curry, turmeric, ginger, and soy sauce in a pan and simmer until the spinach is cooked, around 15 minutes.

Blend until smooth and serve hot.

NUTRITION FACTS: CALORIES 234KCAL FAT 5 G CARBOHYDRATE 9 G PROTEIN 8 G

CORN VEGGIE CHOWDER

 4   🕐 40 mins

Ingredients:

4 cups corn
3 cups soy milk
1 red onion, diced
1 red bell pepper, diced
2 stalks celery, diced
2 tbsp. oil
2 potatoes, diced
1 cup water
1 tsp. paprika
¼ tsp. cayenne

Directions:

Blend 2 cups of the corn with the soymilk and set aside.

Sauté bell pepper, onion, and celery in oil for 10 minutes. Add the potatoes and cook for 15 minutes, stirring often. Add the corn mixture, the remaining 2 cups of corn, cayenne, and paprika, lower the heat, and simmer for 10 minutes.

NUTRITION FACTS: CALORIES 204KCAL FAT 3 G CARBOHYDRATE 25 G PROTEIN 3 G

CREAMY POTATO LEEK SOUP

 4   🕐 30 mins

Ingredients:

4 cups potatoes, diced
3½ cups water
2-3 leeks, diced
¼ lb. mushrooms, chopped
½ stalk celery, finely chopped
2 tbsp. extra-virgin olive oil
12oz. firm tofu

Directions:

Boil the potatoes in 3 cups of salted water until cooked, about 14 minutes. Don't drain.

Heat a pan and sauté the mushrooms and leeks in oil for 5 minutes, then add ¼ cup water until soft. Add them to the potatoes and blend until smooth and creamy.

Crumble the tofu into the pot, return it over medium heat for 3 minutes. Season with salt and pepper to taste.

NUTRITION FACTS: CALORIES 197KCAL FAT 5 G CARBOHYDRATE 20 G PROTEIN 18 G

CUCUMBER AVOCADO SOUP

 2   🕐 5 mins

Ingredients:
- 1 avocado
- 2 cucumber
- 1 cup vegetable broth
- 1 splash of lime juice
- ½ tsp. lime zest
- 1 tsp. extra-virgin olive oil

Directions:

Put the cucumber, avocado, water, and lime juice in a bowl and puree until creamy.

Season with salt and pepper to taste.

Put the soup in a deep plate, garnish with the lime peel and olive oil and serve.

NUTRITION FACTS: CALORIES 224KCAL FAT 4 G CARBOHYDRATE 9 G PROTEIN 8 G

FRENCH PEA SOUP

 4   🕐 40 mins

Ingredients:
- 1 red onion chopped
- 2 tbsp. oil
- 1 bay leaf
- 1 cup yellow split peas
- 2 cloves of garlic
- 1 tsp. of cumin

Directions:

In a soup pot, sauté onions, bay leaf, and garlic until soft.

Wash the peas and then add them to the pot with the garlic, salt/pepper to taste, 2 cups of water, and cumin.

Cook on medium-high for 35 minutes, stirring often and adjusting the water for the right consistency.

NUTRITION FACTS: CALORIES 203KCAL FAT 4 G CARBOHYDRATE 21 G PROTEIN 17 G

GOLDEN CHICKPEA SOUP

🍽 6   🕐 40 mins

Ingredients:

6 cloves fresh garlic, crushed
6 cups vegetable broth
1 lb. chickpeas, cooked
1 red onion, chopped
2 carrots, peeled and diced
2 tbsp. parsley
2 bay leaves
1 tbsp. extra-virgin olive oil
¼ tsp. ground black pepper
4 oz. buckwheat pasta

Directions:

Heat a pot with olive oil and, when hot, add the garlic and sauté for 2 minutes. Add chickpeas, red onion, carrots, bay leaf, and broth, bring to a boil, and simmer for 30 minutes. Remove the bay leaves from the soup.

Blend 2 cups of the soup until smooth, and put them back in the pot.

Add the pasta and simmer for 8 minutes. Serve hot.

NUTRITION FACTS: CALORIES 224KCAL FAT 5 G CARBOHYDRATE 25 G PROTEIN 8 G

GREENS SOUP

🍽 4   🕐 25 mins

Ingredients:

4 cups leafy greens, including kale, chopped
2 zucchini, chopped
2 bell peppers, chopped
1 onion, chopped
4 cups vegetable broth
1 tsp. turmeric
1 tsp. marjoram

Directions:

Put leafy greens, zucchini, bell peppers, onion, and broth in a pot and cook on medium heat until the vegetables are tender, about 25 minutes. Season with salt and pepper to taste.

Turn off the stove, let cool and blend until smooth.

NUTRITION FACTS: CALORIES 164KCAL FAT 3 G CARBOHYDRATE 12 G PROTEIN 8 G

HEARTY POTATO SOUP

🍲 4   🕐 40 mins

Ingredients:

6 potatoes, peeled and cubed
2 red onions, diced
2 carrots, chopped
2 stalks celery, chopped
3 cups vegetable broth
1 tsp. basil
¼ cup flour
1½ cups soy milk

Directions:

Add the potatoes, onions, carrots, celery, vegetable broth, basil, salt, and pepper in a pot.

Bring to a boil, cover, and cook over low heat until potatoes and carrots are cooked, about 35 minutes.

Whisk soy milk and flour until smooth and add them to the pot. Stir well and cook for 5 minutes until dense. Serve.

NUTRITION FACTS: CALORIES 378KCAL FAT 7 G CARBOHYDRATE 30 G PROTEIN 7 G

IRISH CABBAGE SOUP

 6   🕐 1h

Ingredients:

3 red onions
8 oz. raisins
½ cup brown rice, raw
15 oz. tomatoes, canned
1 can tomato paste
1 lb. cabbage, shredded
5 cups water
1 splash of vinegar

Directions:

Put cabbage, onions, raisins, and rice in a pot. Add water to cover generously.

Cook for 50 minutes until the cabbage is faded and the water is bright purple. Add tomatoes and vinegar. Season with salt and pepper to taste. Cook for another 10 minutes, then blend and serve.

NUTRITION FACTS: CALORIES 201KCAL FAT 4 G CARBOHYDRATE 20 G PROTEIN 6 G

ITALIAN BEAN SOUP

 4   ⏱ 60 mins

Ingredients:

2 celery stalks, chopped
2 carrots, chopped
1 red onion, chopped
1 zucchini, chopped
19oz white kidney beans, cooked
2 tbsp. extra-virgin olive oil
½ tsp. basil leaves
½ turmeric
16-oz. tomatoes, diced
2 cups vegetable broth
½ cup kale

Directions:

Place half white kidney beans in a bowl and mash them with a potato masher or fork.

Heat a saucepan over medium-high heat, add oil, carrots, onion, zucchini, basil, and pepper and cook until vegetables are tender and begin to brown, about 15 minutes.

Add tomatoes, vegetable broth, kale, mashed white beans, and 2 cups water. Bring to a boil, reduce heat to low, cover and simmer 15 minutes to blend flavors. Stir in remaining beans; heat through.

Serve.

NUTRITION FACTS: CALORIES 226KCAL FAT 3 G CARBOHYDRATE 28 G PROTEIN 18 G

KALE SOUP

4   ⏱ 50 mins

Ingredients:

1 red onion, chopped
5 cups vegetable broth
2 cups squash, diced
3 cups kale, stems removed and chopped
2 tsp. thyme
2 tsp. sage

Directions:

Heat 1 tbsp. of broth in a pot and sauté the onion over high heat for about 5 minutes.

Add the rest of the broth and bring to a boil. Reduce heat, add squash and let simmer for 25 minutes until tender.

Add the kale, thyme, and sage, and cook another 5 minutes. Serve hot.

NUTRITION FACTS: CALORIES 41KCAL FAT 10 G CARBOHYDRATE 7 G PROTEIN 3 G

JAMAICAN RED BEANS SOUP

🍲 4   🕐 2h + 20 mins

Ingredients:

8 oz. red kidney beans, soaked overnight
4 cups water
2 cups coconut milk
2 bay leaves
6 pimento grains
1 Bird's Eye chili
1 red onion, chopped
1 garlic clove
2 carrots, chopped
1 potato, cubed
½ lb. yellow yams, cubed
1 sweet potato, cubed
2 scallions, crushed
½ tsp. chili flakes
1 garlic clove, chopped
½ tsp. thyme

Directions:

Add beans, 4 cups of water, coconut milk, pimento, and bay leaves to a pot and bring to a boil.

Cook for 2 hours until the beans are almost tender. Add the onion, garlic, carrots, potato, yams, sweet potato, garlic, scallions, and chili flakes.

Cook another 20 minutes

Season with salt, pepper, and thyme. Puree half the soup to thicken, put it back in the pot with the other half, stir and serve hot.

NUTRITION FACTS: CALORIES 219KCAL FAT 5 G CARBOHYDRATE 20 G PROTEIN 15 G

LENTIL AND ONION SOUP

 2   ⏱ 40 mins

Ingredients:
1 red onion, chopped
2 tbsp. extra-virgin olive oil
1 bay leaf
1 cup red lentils
2 garlic cloves, chopped
1 ½ cups of water

Directions:
Sauté onions and garlic until soft. Add lentils, bay leaf, salt and pepper to taste, and water.
Cook for 30 minutes until the lentils are soft. Serve hot.

NUTRITION FACTS: CALORIES 149KCAL   FAT 5 G   CARBOHYDRATE 20 G   PROTEIN 7 G

LIMA BEAN SOUP

 6   ⏱ 50 mins

Ingredients:
1 red onion, diced
4 stalks celery, diced
1 bell pepper, diced
2 tsp. extra-virgin olive oil
8 cups water
1 lb. lima beans, cooked
1 garlic clove, diced
¼ tsp. cayenne
1 ½ tsp. salt
½ cup fresh parsley, diced

Directions:
Heat a pot with oil, add the onion, garlic, celery, bell pepper, and sautè for 5 minutes.
Add the beans, water, cayenne, salt, and pepper to taste, bring to a boil, and cook for about 40 minutes
Add the parsley on top and serve.

NUTRITION FACTS: CALORIES 179KCAL   FAT 4 G   CARBOHYDRATE 18 G   PROTEIN 8 G

MINESTRONE SOUP

 4   🕐 45 mins

Ingredients:

2 cups white beans, cooked
1 head cabbage chopped.
1 cup red onion
2 tbsp. extra-virgin olive oil
3 carrots, chopped
2 white turnips, chopped
1 lb. can of tomatoes
1 tomato, chopped
½ cup celery, chopped
2 tbsp. parsley, chopped
1 garlic clove, chopped
1 tbsp. basil
1 cup of buckwheat short pasta

Directions:

In a soup pot, fry the cabbage, garlic, and onion in the oil. Add the beans, carrots, turnips, tomatoes, celery, and 4 cups of water. Bring to a boil and cook for 30 minutes until vegetables are well done.

Then add the beans and the pasta and cook for 8 minutes until the pasta is done.

NUTRITION FACTS: CALORIES 147KCAL FAT 4 G CARBOHYDRATE 30 G PROTEIN 6 G

MUSHROOM AND BUCKWHEAT SOUP

 6   🕐 55 mins

Ingredients:

3 tbsp. extra-virgin olive oil
1 onion, chopped
1 leek, chopped
8 cups vegetable broth
1 lb. white potatoes, peeled and diced
1 carrot, chopped
2 cups buckwheat, cooked
3 bay leaves

Directions:

Separate mushroom stems from caps. Cut caps and set aside. Cut stems.

Heat extra-virgin olive oil in a saucepan over medium-high heat. Add mushroom stems, onion, and leek and sauté until tender, about 8 minutes. Stir in vegetable broth, potatoes, carrot, barley, and bay leaves.

Cover, stir and simmer 30 minutes.

Uncover soup, add mushroom caps, and continue simmering until vegetables are very tender, about 25 minutes. Season soup to taste with salt and pepper and serve.

NUTRITION FACTS: CALORIES 139KCAL FAT 3 G CARBOHYDRATE 18 G PROTEIN 16 G

PURE VEGETABLE SOUP

 6 50 mins

Ingredients:

1 cup yellow split peas, dried
½ cup parsnips, grated
½ cup carrots, grated
1 celery stalk
1 handful parsley
1 bay leaf
Salt and pepper to taste

Directions:

Cook the split peas in 4 cups water for 40 minutes. Halfway through cooking time, add parsnips, carrots, salt, and the bay leaf. Simmer with partially covered lid.

Remove bay leaf before serving. Blend until smooth and serve.

NUTRITION FACTS: CALORIES 89KCAL FAT 2 G CARBOHYDRATE 10 G PROTEIN 3 G

QUICK VEGGIE STROGANOFF

 4 25 mins

Ingredients:

1 red onion, thinly chopped
½ lb. white button mushrooms, chopped
2 cups Portobello mushrooms, sliced and grilled
2 tbsp. tomato paste
⅓ cup dry red wine
2 cups boiling water
1 tsp. dry mustard
1 tsp. extra-virgin olive oil

Directions:

Fry the onion and white mushrooms in a skillet with oil until the onion starts to soften.

Add the grilled mushroom and stir fry for 5 minutes. Add the tomato paste along with the wine. Stir in the boiling water, and add to the pan with wine and mustard.

Simmer over medium-low heat for 5 minutes.
Serve immediately.

NUTRITION FACTS: CALORIES 59KCAL FAT 1 G CARBOHYDRATE 10 G PROTEIN 5 G

RICE, VEGETABLE, AND TOFU SOUP

 4   🕐 25 mins

Ingredients:
1 stalk celery, diced
1 carrot, diced
4 mushrooms thinly chopped
1 ½ tbsp. extra-virgin olive oil
3 ¾ cups vegetable stock
1 ¼ cups cooked brown rice
1 tsp. grated ginger
1 ½ tbsp. soy sauce
1 cup tofu, chopped into small cubes

Directions:
Sauté celery, carrots, and mushrooms in a saucepan with oil for 5 minutes until tender.

Add the stock, rice, ginger, and soy sauce. Bring to the boil, stir in the vegetables and the tofu and cook for another 3 minutes.

Serve immediately.

NUTRITION FACTS: CALORIES 229KCAL FAT 6 G CARBOHYDRATE 22 G PROTEIN 17 G

ROASTED TOMATO SOUP

 6   1h + 15 mins

Ingredients:
2 lbs. tomatoes, halved
2 garlic cloves
4 leeks, chopped
3 red peppers, halved and seeded
6 tbsp. extra-virgin olive oil
6 cups water
1 cup red wine
2 cups tomato juice
3 sun-dried tomatoes, puréed
1 tbsp. paprika
1 cup parsley leaves
4 tbsp. soy milk

Directions:
Preheat oven to 450F° degrees. In a bowl, toss tomatoes, garlic, leeks, peppers, 3 tbsp. olive oil, and salt to taste. Spread them in one thin layer on a baking sheet and roast for 45 minutes, until vegetables are soft and charred.

Let cool. Add veggies, water, wine, tomato juice, sun-dried tomatoes, and paprika to a soup pot. Bring to a boil and then lower heat, and simmer for 30 minutes.

Add milk, then purée in a food processor until completely smooth. Salt and pepper to taste, trim with parsley.

NUTRITION FACTS: CALORIES 149KCAL FAT 5 G CARBOHYDRATE 16 G PROTEIN 6 G

SWEET POTATO SOUP WITH GINGER AND ORANGE

 6   40 mins

Ingredients:

6 cups sweet potato, diced
1 ½ cups red onions, chopped
1 tbsp. extra-virgin olive oil
2 cloves garlic, diced
5 cups vegetable broth
1 tbsp. orange zest
1 ½ tbsp. ginger, grated
1 tsp. ground cumin
½ tsp. salt
¼ tsp. pepper
Fresh parsley, chopped

Directions:

Oil a shallow baking pan. Add yams, onions, olive oil, and garlic.

Stir well. Roast, uncovered at 425F° for 25 minutes. Stir once, halfway through cooking time.

Transfer to a soup pot. Add broth, orange zest, ginger root, clove, cumin, salt, and pepper. Bring to a boil.

Reduce heat to medium-low and simmer, covered, for 10 minutes.

Working in batches, transfer soup into blender or food processor and purée until smooth.

Trim with fresh parsley and serve hot.

NUTRITION FACTS: CALORIES 168KCAL FAT 4 G CARBOHYDRATE 30 G PROTEIN 5 G

TOMATO BISQUE

 2   20 mins

Ingredients:

1 ½ cups tofu
1 cup water
14oz. tomatoes, diced
2 tbsp. tomato paste
½ red onion, chopped
1 cup vegetable broth
½ tsp. turmeric

Directions:

Blend the tofu and water until smooth. Add the tomatoes, tomato paste, red onion, turmeric, and broth and let simmer for 40 minutes.

Serve hot.

NUTRITION FACTS: CALORIES 190KCAL FAT 6 G CARBOHYDRATE 20 G PROTEIN 11 G

SQUASH AND PEPPERS SOUP

 6 39 mins

Ingredients:

½ cup buckwheat, cooked
½ lb. chickpeas, cooked
2 cups mushrooms, chopped
2 cups butternut squash, chopped
½ cup of chopped green peppers
½ cup of chopped red peppers
I red onion, chopped
2 Roma tomatoes, diced
½ gallon water
I tsp. dill
I tsp. red cayenne pepper
I tbsp. extra-virgin olive oil
I tsp. oregano
I tsp. basil

Directions:

Bring the water to a boil. Add mushrooms, peppers, onion, tomatoes, butternut squash, salt and pepper, and simmer for 30 minutes.

Add chickpeas, buckwheat, cayenne, oregano, and basil and heat through.

Add the olive oil on top and serve.

NUTRITION FACTS: CALORIES 44KCAL FAT 30 G CARBOHYDRATE 2 G PROTEIN 8 G

THAI TOMATO SOUP

 4   30 mins

Ingredients:
1 tbsp. ginger, grated
2 cups bok choy, chopped
1 cup kale
¼ cup basil leaves, chopped
2 cups stock
48 oz. tomato juice
3 tbsp. soy sauce
1 cup bean sprouts
½ cup coconut milk

Directions:
Cook the ginger, bok choy, and basil in a pot with boiling stock for 10 minutes.. Add the coconut milk, tomato juice, soy sauce, and bean sprouts and cook another 5 minutes.

Serve.

NUTRITION FACTS: CALORIES 136KCAL FAT 5 G CARBOHYDRATE 20 G PROTEIN 5 G

SNACKS

BUCKWHEAT GRANOLA

🍳 10   🕐 45 mins

Ingredients:
2 cups buckwheat, puffed
¾ cup pumpkin seeds
¾ cup walnuts, chopped
1 tsp. ground cinnamon
1 ripe banana, mashed
2 tbsp. agave syrup
2 tbsp. coconut oil

Directions:
Preheat your oven to 350°F. Place the buckwheat groats, pumpkin seeds, walnuts, cinnamon, and vanilla in a bowl and mix well. Add banana, honey, and coconut oil to the buckwheat mixture and mix until well combined.

Transfer the mixture onto a baking tray and spread it in an even layer. Bake for about 25–30 minutes, stirring once halfway through.

Remove the baking tray from the oven and set aside to cool.

NUTRITION FACTS: CALORIES 252KCAL FAT 14.3 G CARBOHYDRATE 27.6 G PROTEIN 7.6 G

CHOC NUT TRUFFLES

 8   3h + 15 mins

Ingredients:

5 oz. shredded coconut
2 oz. walnuts, chopped
1 oz. hazelnuts, chopped
4 Medjool dates
2 tbsp. cocoa powder
1 tbsp. coconut oil

Directions:

Place all of the ingredients into a blender and process until smooth and creamy. Using a teaspoon, scoop the mixture into bite-size pieces, then roll it into balls.

Place them in small paper cups, cover them and chill for 3 hours before serving.

NUTRITION FACTS: CALORIES 41KCAL FAT 3 G CARBOHYDRATE 4 G PROTEIN 1 G

CURRIED CASHEWS

 4   38 mins

Ingredients:

1 red onion
1 garlic clove
1 inch ginger
1 Bird's Eye chili
1 tsp. turmeric
1 cinnamon stick
2 cardamom pods
Zest of ½ lemon
¾ cup water
2 cups cashews
2 tbsp. coconut cream

Directions:

Cut the onion and chili finely, making certain the chili seeds have been discarded.

Crush the garlic and grate the ginger. Add these ingredients with all the spices and cover them with water in a saucepan. Simmer for a few minutes.

Add the cashews and coconut cream and simmer for a further 20 to 30 minutes.

Serve over rice.

NUTRITION FACTS: CALORIES 199KCAL FAT 7 G CARBOHYDRATE 10 G PROTEIN 18 G

ENERGY COCOA BALLS

 2   4h + 30 mins

Ingredients:
4 dates, pitted
1 tbsp. peanut butter
20 almonds
Cocoa powder for coating

Directions:
Blend all the ingredients, then put the mix in the refrigerator for 30 minutes. Form the balls and coat them with cocoa powder. Put them back in the refrigerator for 4 hours before eating.

NUTRITION FACTS: CALORIES 132KCAL FAT 5.3 G CARBOHYDRATE 22.8 G PROTEIN 4.6 G

KALE CHIPS

2   18 mins

Ingredients:
6 cups kale leaves, chopped
2 tbsp. extra-virgin olive oil
1 tbsp. soy sauce
1 tbsp. sesame seeds
½ tbsp. garlic
¼ tbsp. poppy seeds

Directions:
Wash and dry kale leaves. Cut them into 2-inch pieces and put them in a bowl. Mix olive oil and soy sauce massaging with clean hands to coat the kale. Add sesame seeds, garlic, poppy seeds, salt, and pepper to taste and mix again.

Cook the kale in batches at 375°F for 5 to 6 minutes until perfectly crisp.

NUTRITION FACTS: CALORIES 159KCAL FAT 8 G CARBOHYDRATE 10 G PROTEIN 7 G

DESSERTS

CHOCOLATE AGAVE WALNUTS

 15   45 mins

Ingredients:
½ cup pure agave syrup,
2 cups walnuts
½ cup dark chocolate, at least 85%
1 ½ tbsp. coconut oil, melted
1 tbsp. water
1 tsp. of vanilla extract

Directions:
Line a baking tray with parchment paper. In a skillet, combine the walnuts and ¼ cup of agave syrup and cook over medium heat, stirring continuously, until walnuts are entirely covered with syrup and golden in color, about 3 to 5 minutes.

Pour the walnuts onto the parchment paper and separate it into individual pieces with a fork. Allow cooling completely; at least 15 minutes.

In the meantime, melt the chocolate with the coconut oil, add the remaining agave syrup and stir until combined. When walnuts are cooled, transfer them to a glass bowl and pour the melted chocolate syrup over the top.

Use a silicone spatula to mix until walnuts are entirely covered gently.

Transfer back to the parchment paper-lined baking sheet and, once again, separate each of the nuts with a fork.

Place the nuts in the fridge for 10 minutes or the freezer for 3 to 5 minutes, until chocolate has completely set. Store in an airtight bag in your refrigerator.

NUTRITION FACTS: CALORIES 139KCAL FAT 10 G CARBOHYDRATE 19 G PROTEIN 24 G

CHOCOLATE MOUSSE

 1 5 mins

Ingredients:
½ avocado
1 tsp cocoa powder
1 tsp agave syrup

Directions:
Blend all ingredients and serve immediately.

NUTRITION FACTS: CALORIES 87KCAL FAT 1.1 G CARBOHYDRATE 11.8 G PROTEIN 1.6 G

COCONUT SCENTED RICE PUDDING

 4 30 mins

Ingredients:
¾ cup basmati rice
1 ½ cups water
2 tbsp. raisins
2 tbsp. walnuts, chopped
1 clove cardamom
3 dates, chopped
1 ¼ cups coconut milk
1 tbsp. cocoa powder

Directions:
Boil the rice in 1 ½ cups of water and cardamom until it is completely absorbed, around 20 minutes.

Add raisins, dates, milk, cocoa powder, and agave. Stir gently and cook until the mixture thickens, 5 to 10 minutes.

Remove from heat. Let cool slightly. Trim with walnuts and serve.

NUTRITION FACTS: CALORIES 180KCAL FAT 7 G CARBOHYDRATE 25 G PROTEIN 3 G

GOLDEN MILK ICE CREAM

 5   8h + 5 mins

Ingredients:

28 oz. full-fat coconut milk

2 tbsp. coconut oil

¼ cup agave syrup

2-inch fresh ginger, finely sliced

A pinch of sea salt

½ tsp. ground cinnamon

1 tsp. ground turmeric

⅛ tsp black pepper

⅛ tsp. cardamom

1 tsp. pure vanilla extract, unsweetened

Directions:

Place your ice cream churn and bowl in the freezer a night before to chill properly.

Add the agave syrup, turmeric, coconut milk, cardamom, fresh ginger, pepper, sea salt, and cinnamon into a pot and heat over medium heat.

Allow simmering, whisking continuously to mix the ingredients.

Then remove from heat and add the vanilla extract. Stir once more to combine.

If needed, adjust flavor, adding more agave syrup for sweetness, turmeric for intense flavor, salt to balance the flavors, or cinnamon for warmth.

Transfer the mixture plus the ginger slices into a mixing bowl and allow to cool to room temperature.

Cover the bowl and place in the refrigerator to chill overnight or for a minimum of 4 to 6 hours.

The next day, use a strainer or a spoon to remove the ginger slices.

Then add the coconut oil for more creaminess. Whisk to combine thoroughly.

Add the mixture to your ice cream maker and churn according to the manufacturers' instructions — this should take about 30 minutes.

In case you don't have an ice cream maker, skip this phase and go to the next one.

Move the ice cream to a freezer-safe container and smooth the top with your spoon.

Cover with a lid and place in the freezer for about 4 to 6 hours until firm. Bring out of the freezer ten minutes before serving to soften.

NUTRITION FACTS: CALORIES 140KCAL FAT 7 G CARBOHYDRATE 17 G PROTEIN 2 G

NO-BAKE STRAWBERRY FLAPJACKS

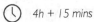 8   4h + 15 mins

Ingredients:

3 oz. porridge oats
4 oz. dates
2 oz. strawberries
2 oz. peanuts, unsalted
2 oz. walnuts
1 tbsp. coconut oil
2 tbsp. 100% cocoa powder

Directions:

Place all of the ingredients into a blender and process until they become a soft consistency. Spread the mixture onto a baking dish.

Press the mixture down and smooth it out. Put in the fridge for 4 hours, then cut it into 8 pieces and serve.

NUTRITION FACTS: CALORIES 191KCAL FAT 11 G CARBOHYDRATE 21 G PROTEIN 2 G

PISTACHIO FUDGE

 6   10 mins

Ingredients:

8 oz. Medjool dates, pitted
3½ oz. pistachio nuts, shelled
2 oz. shredded coconut
1 oz. oats
2 tbsp. water

Directions:

Place the dates, nuts, coconut, oats, and water into a food processor and process until the ingredients are well mixed.

Roll the mixture in a 1-inch thick roll a cut it into 6 pieces.

Refrigerate 2 hours and serve.

NUTRITION FACTS: CALORIES 280KCAL FAT 12 G CARBOHYDRATE 18 G PROTEIN 4 G

STRAWBERRY SORBET

 2   2h +15 mins

Ingredients:

3 cups fresh strawberries
juice of 2 lemons
⅓ cup cane sugar

Directions:

Blend the frozen strawberries in a blender. Add the lemon juice and the sugar and mix well.

Freeze for at least 4 hours and quickly blend again before serving.

NUTRITION FACTS: CALORIES 145KCAL   FAT 3 G   CARBOHYDRATE 18 G   PROTEIN 3 G

APPENDIX A – CONVERSION TABLES

MEASUREMENTS

CUPS	OUNCES	MILLILITRES	TABLESPOONS
8 CUP	64 OZ.	1895 ML	128 TBSP.
6 CUP	48 OZ.	1420 ML	96 TBSP.
5 CUP	40 OZ.	1180 ML	80 TBSP.
4 CUP	32 OZ.	960 ML	64 TBSP.
2 CUP	16 OZ.	480 ML	32 TBSP.
1 CUP	8 OZ.	240 ML	16 TBSP.
¾ CUP	6 OZ.	177 ML	12 TBSP.
⅔ CUP	5 OZ.	158 ML	11 TBSP.
½ CUPS	4 OZ.	118 ML	8 TBSP.
⅜ CUP	3 OZ.	90 ML	6 TBSP.
1/3 CUP	2.5 OZ.	79 ML	5.5 TBSP.
¼ CUP	2 OZ.	59 ML	4 TBSP.
⅛ CUP	1 OZ.	30 ML	3 TBSP.
1/16 CUP	½ OZ.	15 ML	1 TBSP.

WEIGHTS

OUNCES	GRAMS
½ OZ.	15 G
1 OZ.	29 G
2 OZ.	57 G
3 OZ.	85 G
4 OZ.	113 G
5 OZ.	141 G
6 OZ.	170 G
8 OZ.	227 G
10 OZ.	283 G
12 OZ.	340 G
13 OZ.	369 G
14 OZ.	397 G
15 OZ.	425 G
1 LB.	453 G

TEMPERATURES

FAHRENHEIT	CELSIUS
100 °F	37 °C
150 °F	65 °C
200 °F	93 °C
250 °F	121 °C
300 °F	150 °C
325 °F	160 °C
350 °F	180 °C
375 °F	190 °C
400 °F	200 °C
425 °F	220 °C
450 °F	230 °C
500 °F	230 °C
525 °F	264 °C
550 °F	288 °C

INDEX

CPSIA information can be obtained
at www.ICGtesting.com
Printed in the USA
LVHW062204221021
701183LV00005B/489